OXFORD MEDICAL PUBLICATIONS

Obstetric Anaesthesia

T0202384

Oxford Specialist Handbooks published and forthcoming

General Oxford Specialist Handbooks
Addiction Medicine
Applied Medicine and Surgery in Dentistry
Day Case Surgery
Infection in the Immunocompromised Host
Perioperative Medicine, 2e
Pharmaceutical Medicine
Postoperative Complications, 2e
Renal Transplantation
Retrieval Medicine

Oxford Specialist Handbooks in Anaesthesia
Anaesthesia for Emergency Care
Global Anaesthesia
Neuroanaesthesia
Obstetric Anaesthesia, 2e
Paediatric Anaesthesia, 2e
Regional Anaesthesia, Stimulation and Ultrasound Techniques
Thoracic Anaesthesia
Vascular Anaesthesia

Oxford Specialist Handbooks in Cardiology
Adult Congenital Heart Disease, 2e
Cardiac Catheterization and Coronary Intervention
Cardiovascular Computed Tomography, 2e
Cardiovascular Imaging
Cardiovascular Magnetic Resonance
Echocardiography, 2e
Fetal Cardiology, 2e
Heart Disease in Pregnancy
Heart Failure, 2e
Hypertension
Inherited Cardiac Disease
Nuclear Cardiology
Pacemakers and ICDs, 2e
Pulmonary Hypertension
Valvular Heart Disease

Oxford Specialist Handbooks in Critical Care
Advanced Respiratory Critical Care
Cardiothoracic Critical Care

Oxford Specialist Handbooks in End of Life Care
Dementia
Heart Failure
Kidney Disease
Respiratory Disease

Oxford Specialist Handbooks in Infectious Disease
Infectious Disease Epidemiology

Oxford Specialist Handbooks in Neurology
Parkinson's Disease and Other Movement Disorders, 2e
Stroke Medicine, 2e

Oxford Specialist Handbooks in Oncology
Practical Management of Complex Cancer Pain

Oxford Specialist Handbooks in Paediatrics
Community Paediatrics
Manual of Childhood Infections, 4e
Paediatric Dermatology 2e
Paediatric Endocrinology and Diabetes
Paediatric Gastroenterology, Hepatology, and Nutrition, 2e
Paediatric Intensive Care
Paediatric Nephrology, 3e
Paediatric Neurology, 3e
Paediatric Palliative Medicine, 2e
Paediatric Radiology
Paediatric Respiratory Medicine
Paediatric Rheumatology

Oxford Specialist Handbooks in Pain Medicine
Spinal Interventions in Pain Management

Oxford Specialist Handbooks in Psychiatry
Addiction Medicine, 2e
Forensic Psychiatry
Medical Psychotherapy

Oxford Specialist Handbooks in Radiology
Head and Neck Imaging
Interventional Radiology
Musculoskeletal Imaging
Thoracic Imaging

Oxford Specialist Handbooks in Surgery
Burns
Cardiothoracic Surgery, 2e
Colorectal Surgery
Current Surgical Guidelines
Gastric and Oesophageal Surgery
Hand Surgery, 2e
Oral and Maxillofacial Surgery, 2e
Otolaryngology and Head and Neck Surgery
Plastic and Reconstructive Surgery
Surgical Oncology
Urological Surgery
Vascular Surgery, 2e

Oxford Specialist Handbooks in Anaesthesia

Obstetric Anaesthesia

SECOND EDITION

EDITED BY

Rachel Collis
Consultant Anaesthetist,
University Hospital of Wales,
Cardiff, UK

Sarah Harries
Consultant Anaesthetist,
University Hospital of Wales,
Cardiff, UK

Abrie Theron
Consultant Anaesthetist,
University Hospital of Wales,
Cardiff, UK

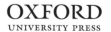

OXFORD
UNIVERSITY PRESS

OXFORD
UNIVERSITY PRESS

Great Clarendon Street, Oxford, OX2 6DP,
United Kingdom

Oxford University Press is a department of the University of Oxford.
It furthers the University's objective of excellence in research, scholarship,
and education by publishing worldwide. Oxford is a registered trade mark of
Oxford University Press in the UK and in certain other countries

© Oxford University Press 2020

The moral rights of the authors have been asserted

First Edition published in 2008
Second Edition published in 2020

Impression: 1

Published in the United States of America by Oxford University Press
198 Madison Avenue, New York, NY 10016, United States of America

British Library Cataloguing in Publication Data
Data available

Library of Congress Control Number: 2018966028

ISBN 978–0–19–968852–4

Printed and bound in China by
C&C Offset Printing Co., Ltd.

Dedication

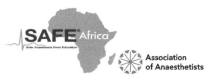

Reproduced with the kind permission of the Association of Anaesthetists.

Around the world people are suffering or dying unnecessarily from the lack of safe anaesthesia in surgery, something that is taken for granted in the UK.

The situation is critical in Africa, where millions lack access to safe anaesthesia.

This book is dedicated to patients globally who aspire to receive the safest possible anaesthesia care.

The authors will donate their royalties to **SAFE Africa**, which is the Association of Anaesthetist's fundraising campaign aiming to:

- Raise at least **£100,000**.
- Sale-up the delivery of three-day **SAFE Obstetrics and SAFE Paediatrics** training courses.
- Sustainably improve **anaesthesia education and care** in Africa long term.

Foreword

The delivery suite can be a very daunting place for the novice, or even experienced, anaesthetist. Obstetric anaesthesia is both rewarding and challenging. Helping a mother to give birth and witness all the joy that unfolds is
exhilarating. But childbirth is never without risk and difficulty and things can
go wrong at an alarming speed, threatening the wellbeing of both mother
and baby. Anticipation, early detection, and efficient management of complications are key to a successful outcome. What the obstetric anaesthetist
needs is a clear, practical, and easily accessible manual to assist them. This
Oxford Specialist Handbook is such a book.

I am proud to have been involved in the publication of the first edition
in 2008. Since then, however, obstetric anaesthesia practice has continued
to evolve and the publication of an updated second edition is long overdue
and I am sure, eagerly anticipated. Although some of the editors and authors have changed, it is reassuring to see that the book continues to be
authored by experienced obstetric anaesthetists who practice in busy units.
This ensures that the guidance given in this book is authoritative, practical,
and up to date.

As part of the updating of this edition there are four new chapters reflecting the importance of their subject: use of ultrasound, obesity in
pregnancy, the septic mother, and neonatal resuscitation. Ultrasound is becoming increasingly important to the anaesthetist and the chapter covers its
use to facilitate difficult neuroaxial block, its use in the increasingly popular
transversus abdominis plane block, and use in assisting central vascular access. The last couple of decades has seen a rise in the prevalence of obesity
in all populations and a chapter devoted to the management of the problems of the obese parturient is a welcome addition. Sepsis remains a major
cause of maternal mortality and morbidity and such an important topic now
warrants a chapter devoted to its prompt recognition and timely treatment,
essential to a successful outcome. Although neonatal resuscitation is usually
the responsibility of the neonatal team, it is important that the obstetric
anaesthetist has a good working knowledge of the subject and the skills to
support paediatric colleagues.

Finally, I'd like to personally thank the editors for donating all royalties
from the sale of this book to the Association of Anaesthetists' fundraising
campaign for SAFE AFRICA. SAFE (Safe Anaesthesia From Education) is
a ground-breaking project, supported by the Association of Anaesthetists
and the World Federation of Societies of Anaesthesiology, to roll out
educational anaesthesia courses in low- and middle-income countries,
empowering local educators to educate and train anaesthesia providers in
safe anaesthetic practice.

I also commend the editors for dedicating this book to all patients worldwide who aspire to receive safe anaesthetic care. This updated and improved second edition of *Obstetric Anaesthesia* makes a significant contribution to that laudable aspiration.

Paul Clyburn
Retired Obstetric Anaesthetist and Past President of the Association of
Anaesthetists of Great Britain and Ireland

Acknowledgements

This second edition of the *Oxford Specialist Handbook of Obstetric Anaesthesia* has been comprehensively revised with updated information and current evidence to support changes in practice, since publication of the first edition 10 years ago. We are very grateful to the authors that have contributed to this edition. However, this work would not have been possible without the contribution of the two past editors and all contributors to the first edition. We wish to sincerely thank and acknowledge the contribution of Dr Paul Clyburn and Dr Stuart Davies, as past editors, and the following first edition contributing authors; Drs Korede Adekanye, Rafal Baraz, Fiona Benjamin, Sue Catling, Monica Chawthe, Karthikeyan Chelliah, Doddamanegowda Chethan, Christine Conner, Libby Duff, Kath Eggers, Caroline Evans, Moira Evans, Claire Farley, Martin Garry, Shubhranshu Gupta, David Hill, Val Hilton, Felicity Howard, Jon Hughes, Saira Hussain, Aravindh Jayakumar, Eleanor Lewis, Anthony Murphy, Vinay Ratnalikar, Shilpa Rawat, Dan Redfern, Alun Rees, Leanne Rees, Hywel Roberts, Anette Scholz, Raman Sivasankar, Stephen Stamatakis, Gavin Sullivan, Daryl Thorp-Jones, Matt Turner, Ramesh Vasoya, Viju Varadarajan, Dave Watkins, Shreekar Yadthore.

Editors—Rachel Collis, Sarah Harries, Abrie Theron
March 2020

Acknowledgements

xi

Contents

Contributors

Korede Adekanye
Department of Anaesthetics,
University Hospital of Wales,
Cardiff, UK

Huda Al-Foudri
Department of Anaesthetics,
Al-Adan Hospital, Kuwait

James Bamber
Department of Anaesthetics,
Cambridge University Hospitals
NHS Foundation Trust,
Cambridge, UK

Rafal Baraz
Department of Anaesthetics,
University Hospital of Wales,
Cardiff, UK

Sarah Bell
Department of Anaesthetics,
University Hospital of Wales,
Cardiff, UK

Rachel Collis
Department of Anaesthetics,
University Hospital of Wales,
Cardiff, UK

Christine Conner
Department of Fetal Medicine,
Obstetrics & Gynaecology,
University Hospital of Wales,
Cardiff, UK

Stuart Davies
Department of Anaesthetics,
Singleton Hospital, Swansea, UK

Martin Garry
Department of Anaesthetics,
Singleton Hospital, Swansea, UK

Sarah Harries
Department of Anaesthetics,
University Hospital of Wales,
Cardiff, UK

Angela Hayward
Department of Neonatology,
University Hospital of Wales,
Cardiff, UK

David Hill
Department of Anaesthetics,
Ulster Hospital, Belfast, UK

Rhidian Jones
Department of Anaesthetics,
Princess of Wales Hospital,
Bridgend, UK

Gemma Keigthley
Department of Anaesthetics,
University Hospital of Wales,
Cardiff, UK

David Leslie
Department of Anaesthetics,
University Hospital of Wales,
Cardiff, UK

Eleanor Lewis
Department of Anaesthetics,
Singleton Hospital, Swansea, UK

Graeme Lilley
Department of Anaesthetics,
Nevill Hall Hospital,
Abergavenny, UK

Lucy De Lloyd
Department of Anaesthetics,
University Hospital of Wales,
Cardiff, UK

Nuala Lucas
Department of Anaesthetics,
Northwick Park Hospital,
Harrow, UK

Stephen Morris
Department of Anaesthetics,
University Hospital of Wales,
Cardiff, UK

Abrie Theron
Department of Anaesthetics,
University Hospital of Wales,
Cardiff, UK

Matthew Turner
Department of Anaesthetics,
Royal Gwent Hospital,
Newport, UK

Symbols and abbreviations

5-HT	5-hydroxytryptamine
A&E	Accident and Emergency
ABG	arterial blood gas
AC	abdominal circumference
ACE	angiotensin-converting enzyme
ACTH	adrenocorticotrophic hormone
ADP	accidental dural puncture
AF	atrial fibrillation
AFE	amniotic fluid embolus
AFI	amniotic fluid index
AFLP	acute fatty liver of pregnancy
AFV	amniotic fluid volume
AITP	autoimmune thrombocytopenia purpura
AKI	acute kidney injury
ALS	advanced life support
ALT	alanine aminotransferase
AoDP	aortic diastolic pressure
APTT	activated partial thromboplastin time
ARDS	adult respiratory distress syndrome
ARF	acute renal failure
ARM	artificial rupture of membranes
AS	aortic stenosis
ASD	atrial septal defect
AST	aspartate aminotransferase
AVA	aortic valve area
AVM	arteriovenous malformation
BD	twice a day
BMI	body mass index
BMR	basal metabolic rate
BP	blood pressure
bpm	beats per minute
CDP	computerized dynamic posturography
CEMACH	Confidential Enquiry into Maternal and Child Health
CEMD	Confidential Enquiry into Maternal Deaths
CHD	congenital heart defect
CKD	chronic kidney disease
cLMA	classic laryngeal mask airway
CNS	central nervous system
CO	cardiac output
COP	colloid oncotic pressure
CP	cerebral palsy
CPAP	continuous positive airway pressure
CPP	coronary perfusion pressure
CPR	cardiopulmonary resuscitation
CS	caesarean section
CSE	combined spinal–epidural
CSF	cerebrospinal fluid
CSM	Committee on the Safety of Medicines
CT	computed tomography
CTG	cardiotochograph
CTPA	CT pulmonary angiography
CVP	central venous pressure
DDAVP	1-desamino-8D-arginine vasopressin
DIC	disseminated intravascular coagulation
DVT	deep vein thrombosis
EBP	epidural blood patch
ECG	electrocardiograph
ECV	external cephalic version
EDF	end-diastolic flow
EEG	electroencephalograph
EF	ejection fraction
EFL	epidural for labour
EFM	electronic fetal monitoring
EFW	estimated fetal weight
ENT	ear, nose and throat
EXIT	ex utero intrapartum treatment
FBC	full blood count
FBS	fetal blood sample
FFP	fresh frozen plasma
FHR	fetal heart rate
FRC	functional residual capacity
FSE	fetal scalp electrode
FSH	follicle-stimulating hormone

GA	general anaesthesia		LMA	laryngeal mask airway
GAS	Group A Streptococcus		LMWH	low molecular weight heparin
GCS	Glasgow Coma Score		LSCS	lower segment caesarean section
GFR	glomerular filtration rate			
GIT	gastrointestinal tract		LV	left ventricle
GTN	glyceryl trinitrate		LVEDP	left ventricular end-diastolic pressure
GTP	gestational thrombocytopenia of pregnancy			
			LVF	left ventricular failure
Hb	haemoglobin		MAC	minimum alveolar concentration
HbF	fetal haemoglobin		MAP	mean arterial pressure
HC	head circumference		MAS	meconium aspiration syndrome
hCG	human chorionic gonadotrophin		MBRRACE-UK	Mothers and Babies: Reducing Risk through Audits and Confidential Enquiries across the UK
HDU	high dependency unit			
HELLP	haemolytic anaemia, elevated liver enzymes and low platelets			
			MCQ	multiple choice questions
HHT	hereditary haemorrhagic telangiectasia		MEOWS	Modified Early Obstetric Warning Score
HIT	heparin-induced thrombocytopenia		MMR	Maternal Mortality Ratio
			MPAP	mean pulmonary arterial pressure
HIV	human immunodeficiency virus			
HPV	human papillomavirus		MR	mitral regurgitation
HR	heart rate		MRI	magnetic resonance imaging
ICP	intracranial pressure		MSL	meconium-stained liquor
ICU	intensive care unit		MVP	mitral vein prolapse
IDDM	insulin-dependent diabetes mellitus		NeP	neuropathic pain
			NICE	National Institute for Health and Clinical Excellence
Ig	immunoglobulin			
IGP	intragastric pressure		NIDDM	Non-insulin dependent diabetes mellitus
IM	intramuscular			
INR	international normalized ratio		NIPP	non-invasive positive pressure ventilation
IPPV	intermittent positive pressure ventilation			
			NMDA	N-methyl-D-aspartate
ITP	idiopathic thrombocytopenia purpura		NNT	number needed to treat
			NOAD	National Obstetric Anaesthetic Database
ITU	intensive therapy unit			
IUGR	intrauterine growth restriction/retardation		NSAID	non-steroidal anti-inflammatory drug
IV	intravenous		NYHA	New York Heart Association
IVC	inferior vena cava		OAA	Obstetric Anaesthetists' Association
IVF	in vitro fertilization			
JVP	jugular venous pressure		ODP	operating department practitioner
kPa	kilopascal			
LA	local anaesthesia		OSA	obstructive sleep apnoea
LAP	left atrial pressure		Pa	pascal
LBP	low back pain		PCA	patient-controlled analgesia
LDF	leucocyte depletion filter		PCEA	patient-controlled epidural analgesia
LEHPZ	lower oesophageal high pressure zone			
			PCR	protein:creatinine ratio
LFT	liver function test		PCWP	pulmonary capillary wedge pressure
LH	luteinizing hormone			
			PDA	patent ductus arteriosus

PDPH	postdural puncture headache
PDSA	Plan Do Study Act
PE	pulmonary embolism
PEA	pulseless electrical activity
PEEP	positive end-expiratory pressure
PET	pre-eclampsia toxaemia
PFO	patent foramen ovale
PG	prostaglandin
PIH	pregnancy-induced hypertension
PMCS	peri-mortum caesarean section
PO	per os (orally)
PPH	postpartum haemorrhage
PR	per rectum
PT	prothrombin time
PTH	parathyroid hormone
PVR	pulmonary vascular resistance
QDS	four times a day
QI	Quality Improvement
RBBB	right bundle branch block
RBC	red blood cell
RCT	randomized controlled trial
RR	respiratory rate
RRT	renal replacement therapy
RV	right ventricle
RVF	right ventricular failure
SADS	sudden adult death syndrome or sudden arrhythmic death syndrome
SC	subcutaneous
SEP	somatosensory evoked potential
SFG	small for gestational age
SFH	symphyseal fundal height
SIRS	systemic inflammatory response syndrome
SLE	systemic lupus erythematosus
SNP	sodium nitroprusside
STAN	ST analysis of the fetal ECG

SV	stroke volume
SVD	spontaneous vaginal delivery
SVR	systemic vascular resistance
T3	tri-iodothyronine
T4	thyroxine
TB	tuberculosis
TBG	thyroxine-binding globulin
TDS	three times a day
TED	thromboembolism deterrent
TEG	thromboelastography
TENS	transcutaneous electrical nerve stimulation
THRIVE	transnasal humidified rapid-insufflation ventilatory exchange
TIBC	total iron binding capacity
TORCH	toxoplasmosis, rubella, cytomegalovirus and herpes simplex
TSH	thyroid-stimulating hormone
TTP	thrombotic thrombocytopenia purpura
TV	tidal volume
U&E	urea and electrolytes
UA	umbilical artery
UFH	unfractionated heparin
UO	urine output
URTI	upper respiratory tract infection
UTI	urinary tract infection
V/Q	ventilation/perfusion
VAE	vascular air embolism
VBAC	vaginal delivery after caesarean section
VHA	viscoelastometric haemostatic assay
VR	venous return
VSD	ventricular septal defect
VTE	venous thrombo-embolism
vWF	von Willebrand factor
WCC	white cell count
WHO	World Health Organization

Thinking about obstetric anaesthesia

Rachel Collis

Surviving the labour ward A–Z

The labour ward can be a stressful and demanding experience for all anaesthetists, junior and senior alike. Start off by seeing yourself as part of a team comprising anaesthetists, midwives, and obstetricians. Your level of seniority will often determine how you are viewed within that team, but the principles of team-working are always the same.

Obstetricians and midwives may need an anaesthetist to aid in the safe delivery of mother and baby, as well the multidisciplinary management of a whole host of complications associated with childbirth such as postpartum haemorrhage and sepsis. The anaesthetist, however, cannot work effectively, dealing with the multitude of problems on the delivery suite, without the skills of both midwives and obstetricians. No one is better or more important than anyone else; only experience should change how you function within the team.

When the anaesthetist starts working on the delivery suite for the first time, it can feel like one of the most frightening and out of control places in the hospital. The anaesthetist can feel they are working to their maximum capability, at flat out pace with heightened emotion in nearly every setting. By the end of a shift it can be natural to feel exhausted, and perhaps grateful that no major mistakes have been made and both mothers and babies are safe.

Before you start, think how you can function optimally. The best way to start is to think ahead. This means not only familiarizing yourself with local protocols and the layout of the maternity unit before your first shift but also constantly thinking ahead as each situation arises. You need to minimize the tendency to react to a situation and start to learn to anticipate potential problems. You will feel more in control, and that control will enable you to work in a calmer and more effective manner.

> The A–Z layout sets out ways that can help you cope without emphasizing one point above others. No single suggestion is more important than another and no single action will help without taking into account many of the others.

A–Z of survival

A

- *Advice*: ask for advice if you are not sure. Never be afraid to ask. It may be a very simple question but, if you don't know the answer, it can lead to problems later on.
- *Anaesthetic alert*: has the patient been to an anaesthetic antenatal clinic? If so, what are the likely anaesthetic problems and what is the plan? Familiarize yourself with the local mechanism of alert; there may be clinic letters, special anaesthetic alert pages in the maternity notes, or a separate folder kept on the labour ward.
- *Anticipate*: almost all problems on the labour ward can be anticipated. The 'crash section' is rarely so—it's that you only just found out about it and now everything has to be done immediately in a hurry.

- *Assessment*: before you perform any general or regional anaesthetic, always assess the patient. It is routine practice in all other fields of anaesthesia but can be overlooked on the labour ward. Learn to do it the same on every occasion so nothing is missed, even if time is of the essence. Many units have assessment proformas—use them.

B

- *Bleeps*: give your bleep number to the midwife who is coordinating the labour ward. Make sure that the bleep numbers of consultants, operating department practitioners (ODPs), and senior cover are known to you and clearly displayed on a contact information board. Most units have one. If you have duties away from the labour ward, inform the senior midwife how best to get hold of you.
- *Blood*: blood loss can be rapid. Find out local blood policy: how to get hold of it in a hurry, who to ask, and what forms need to be filled out. Most hospitals will provide O negative blood, group-specific blood, and full cross-match depending on the urgency. Give a clear account to the blood bank of how urgent the situation is and find out how long the blood will take to reach the labour ward. If the situation changes and becomes more or less urgent, inform the blood bank.
- *Board*: all labour wards have a board with details of patients, current obstetric progress, and management. Abbreviations are nearly always used and there could be over 30 different ones. Some are universal such as P for parity or a number for centimetres of cervical dilatation. Some others can be unique to an individual unit. Make sure you know what everyone means, otherwise you could be missing an essential piece of information. If you don't know, ask. The information on the board can change rapidly. Review it regularly.
- *Breaks*: it is important to sit down and have a drink and something to eat as often as you can, even if it is only for a few minutes. When the delivery suite is busy, it can be difficult to get to the hospital canteen, so bring some snacks to work. Don't spend long periods of time away from a busy unit during a break as you can be caught unawares regarding pending problems.
- *Busy*: if the labour ward is very busy, let another anaesthetist in the hospital know if possible, so help can be quickly summoned if required.

C

- *Calm*: if you stay outwardly calm, even if inwardly you feel the opposite, the people around you will trust you and stay calmer themselves, thus making a difficult situation easier to handle.
- *Caesarean section (CS)*: find out the urgency for surgery. This can be categorized into:
    1. Threat to life of mother or baby that requires immediate delivery.
    2. Compromise to mother or baby that requires early delivery.
    3. Early delivery where neither the baby nor mother is compromised.
    4. Elective CS.

This classification does not dictate the type of anaesthetic you should give, but provides an approximate time frame for you to give a safe anaesthetic in the situation.

- *Check your epidurals*: see all the women with an epidural at the beginning of your shift. Examine and document the block. See them again even if not called by the midwife when you have time.
- *Communicate*: clear and concise communication with the ODP, midwife, and other members of the labour ward team is crucial. Take adequate time to communicate with the mother and her birthing partner. Taking a little time early on can save time later. Inadequate communication is the basis for many complaints and legal claims.
- *Confrontation*: this can quickly arise, especially in a stressful situation. It never helps, so take a deep breath and don't get involved. If there is a point you feel strongly about, be polite or get someone more senior to deal with it. Sort out ongoing confrontation later and away from the clinical setting when there is plenty of time for a long discussion.
- *Consultant:* know who the consultant anaesthetist is and how to call them in an emergency.
- *CTG*: the cardiotochograph is a printed or electronic record of the fetal heart rate (FHR) with a pressure gauge reading of the mother's contractions which is below the FH reading. Knowing the basic patterns associated with fetal well-being and impending fetal compromise will allow you to think ahead as you provide epidural analgesia or anaesthesia for CS.
- *Consent*: this should be obtained before all anaesthetic procedures, either written or verbal informed consent. There is much debate regarding the capacity of a labouring woman to give informed consent; therefore it is good practice to ensure that consent is witnessed by her birthing partner, if present, and the attending midwife.

D

- *Debrief*: things do go wrong. Sometimes you may feel responsible and sometimes you are an onlooker. In all situations, talk to someone senior about it.
- *Drugs*: draw up all drugs that may be required in an emergency. Label each syringe with content, concentration, and the time and date that the drug was drawn up; remember that a different anaesthetist may have to use them. Store them in a drug fridge.

Find out where non-anaesthetic emergency drugs are kept, particularly those used for eclampsia.

Familiarize yourself with the entire content of the drug cupboard. Know what is routinely kept on delivery suite and how they are stored, e.g. alphabetically or groups of drugs by function.

E

- *Emotions*: happiness, sadness, fear, aggression, and helplessness are all normal and commonly encountered emotions on the labour ward. You will feel them in yourself and see them in others. Work out how you can cope with them before they happen, and stay focused. If you become distracted, you can miss something important.
- *Epidural*: almost every labour ward will have an epidural policy. Follow it, even if you have used something different elsewhere. All the other staff will be used to it and it is dangerous to do your own thing. If you want to make changes, talk to the policy makers.

- *Equipment*: always check all anaesthetic equipment at the beginning of the shift. This must include the anaesthetic machine, monitoring, and airway equipment. You may need to use them in a hurry later.
- *Experience*: appreciate the limitations of your expertise. When you reach your limit, ask for help.

F

- *Fear*: this is a normal reaction to a situation that you don't understand, is happening too quickly, or is outside your control or competence. Recognize the signs early and ask for help before it gets the better of you.
- *Flag issues*: if you are concerned about a particular problem, flag it up early with a senior midwife, obstetrician, or a senior anaesthetist.
- *Fluids*: know where they are kept, what to give, and when. Fluid requirements can be difficult to estimate in a labouring mother.
- *Forceps delivery*: find out the local policy on where they should be carried out—delivery room or operating theatre. Always get involved, even if the mother does not want or already has an epidural. You can at least make an assessment of the situation so you are not completely caught out when a forceps delivery turns into a 'crash section'. If the mother has an epidural, assess the adequacy of her analgesia, give an appropriate top-up, and stay with her to monitor her and the situation until the baby is delivered, and the risk of haemorrhage has passed.

G

- *Guidelines*: most delivery suites have them. Find out where they are kept, read them before you start, and refer back to them regularly.

H

- *Handovers*: usually happen at the beginning of the morning shift, at and at the start of the night shift. They should involve midwives, obstetricians, and anaesthetists, and will provide useful information about women who have not required anaesthetic intervention at that time. You may also find out about potential problems that are on the ante- or postnatal wards, medical wards, or A&E.

Within your shift pattern there should be adequate time for anaesthetic handover. Make full use of it. A useful mnemonic is **SAFE** handover: **S**-mothers who are Sick; **A**-Anticipated problems; **F**-who needs Follow-up; **E**-who has an epidural and is it working well.

- *Help*: where is it? Who is it? How long will it take to get to you?
- *Helpful*: if what you have been asked to do is within your competence, be helpful when you have time, even if you think it is not your direct responsibility. A common example is being asked to site IV access. If you genuinely don't have time to help, be polite.

I

- *Information*: labour is a dynamic process. Situations progress and change rapidly. Stay well informed about all mothers in labour, not just the ones with an epidural.
- *Intravenous access*: make sure you use a 14G or 16G drip in all mothers who have an epidural or need an obstetric anaesthetic.

J

• *Jehovah's Witness*: there are Association of Anaesthetists of Great Britain and Ireland (AAGBI) and local guidelines for the management of a Jehovah's Witness. You should be informed when a Jehovah's Witness is admitted, and have a management plan. Most Jehovah's Witnesses will have signed an advanced directive in the antenatal clinic with a list of blood products and procedures they will accept.

K

• *Knowledge*: keep up to date and discuss controversial issues surrounding patient management.

L

• *Labels*: label all syringes and infusions with the drug name and concentration.
• *Labour*: understand the normal and abnormal patterns of labour. Abnormally prolonged labour very frequently requires anaesthetic intervention at some time.

M

• *Meetings*: attend the multidisciplinary labour ward meeting or organize one if you don't happen. It is a forum to raise concerns and issues.
• *"My name is....."* There is no more important place to do this—even if the mother is distressed.
• *Multidisciplinary team*: you are a member of a team. Don't work in isolation. Understand what you are expected to do during a major obstetric emergency.

N

• *Notes*: legible notes are very important. Discuss and document plans, procedures, and advice received. *'If you have not written it down, you have not done it'*. Every entry should be timed and dated with a legible signature. If notes are written in retrospect, make that clear.

Read the patients notes, especially if there is additional medical information and a high risk obstetric plan.

O

• *Obstetric emergencies*: there are a number of obstetric emergencies including antenatal and postpartum haemorrhage, shoulder dystocia, and eclampsia which you may see and will be expected to be involved with. Find out what you need to do in each and ask about teaching or 'obstetric fire drills' when it is quiet.
• *Organize*: Organize your workload for the shift by prioritizing and delegating to others if appropriate. If a mother is thinking about an epidural, it is usually possible to tell her and her midwife whether you anticipate other more pressing anaesthetic procedures. Remember you can only be in one place at a time.
• *Oxytocics and prostaglandins*: give these drugs slowly. Find out how the different drugs should be given and diluted. Be aware as you step up the therapeutic ladder from oxytocin bolus to oxytocin infusion to prostaglandin that blood loss can be considerable and difficult to estimate. An obstetric patient will appear to be cardiovascularly stable until she has lost 25–30% of her blood volume, and blood loss can be insidious.

P

- *Passwords*: in many hospitals, blood results and X-rays can only be accessed electronically. Familiarize yourself with the computerized system and have an up-to-date access code and password.
- *Position*: make sure the mother is in the ideal position for your regional technique. Taking your time and being patient, especially if she is in a lot of pain, will save time later. When sitting or lying a mother down, take great care to avoid aorto-caval compression. Explain to the mother why this is important.
- *Problem epidural*: work out what you are going to do if an epidural for labour is not working well. Replace it early if you have got time, or recognize that you may need to do a spinal anaesthetic should the mother need a CS.

Q

- *Questions*: there must be time for patients to raise concerns. Always ask mothers if they have any questions.

R

- *Rapport*: build a rapport with the midwives. They can help you a lot.
- *Resuscitaire*: this is where a baby that requires resuscitation is placed. They can be complex to use, but find out how to operate the basic functions. Babies are frequently born unexpectedly requiring help, and with good airway skills the anaesthetist is ideally placed to give initial resuscitation until a paediatrician can attend. Find out about the basic principles of neonatal resuscitation and how they differ from other life support algorithms.
- *Risk management*: this is a part of clinical governance and is important for patient safety. Raise any concerns and report them to the appropriate person, who is frequently one of the senior midwives.

S

- *Smile*: it may seem a small thing but to appear relaxed and friendly will go a long way on a labour ward.
- *STAN*: Stands for ST analysis and is a sophisticated form of fetal scalp monitoring. If your labour ward uses this form of monitoring in high risk labours, find out about it, as interpretation is different to usual CTG analysis.
- *Stress*: the labour ward can be a very stressful place to work and fear can be a normal response. Accept it and have a way of coping with it.

T

- *Teach*: teaching and training—get involved and show initiative. Valuable informal teaching should take place with midwives looking after a mother with an epidural and with midwifery and medical students. A midwife who understands more about an epidural will call you to troubleshoot less often.
- *Time*: there is a tendency for the obstetrician to demand a general anaesthetic when time is short. The question in reply should be 'how quickly does the baby need to be delivered?'

U

- *Use*: use quiet time to practice difficult scenarios or learn about equipment you are less familiar with.
- *Utilize*: utilize all your resources. The haematologist, general physicians, and surgeons can all be invaluable in an emergency or when there are complex management issues with a sick mother.

V

- *Value*: value the opinion of midwives and others in the team. Many will be more experienced than you and can offer an opinion that, although different from yours, can be equally valid and helpful in the long run.
- *Vulnerable*: the patient can feel vulnerable, which can come across as rude and aggressive behaviour. Put yourself in her place.

W

- *Ward rounds*: all mothers who have had an obstetric anaesthetic should be followed-up. Feedback is important and you will learn a lot from listening to her.

X

- *(E)Xpectations*: it is easy to underestimate the mother's expectations in a stressful environment like the labour ward. She may not be able to differentiate one doctor from the other. Introduce yourself, be courteous and be clear. For the doctors, one situation can merge into the next. For the mother, she will remember her personal experiences for many years.

Y

- *Y*: why are you doing what you are doing? Watch and learn from others to improve your own practice.

Z

- *Plan Z*: always have one before things go wrong.

Asking the right questions OR where do you look for the answers?

There are different questions that should be directed to the patient, obstetrician, and midwife. The questions you ask will depend upon the time you have, but most of the information below will need to be obtained, even if time is very short. Directing your questions to the right person can save time.

The midwife

Has the pregnancy and labour been normal? The midwife will have carefully reviewed the mother's notes and will be aware of problems that may alter your anaesthetic management:
- History of blood pressure (BP) problems or pre-eclampsia, which could cause clotting or platelet abnormalities.
- History of low platelets (ITP).
- History of thrombosis. Is the mother on heparin?

The midwife will also be able to tell you if the pattern of labour up to that point has been normal or abnormal and if the CTG has been reassuring or suggestive of fetal compromise.

- *Is this a first or subsequent labour?* A mother who has laboured before is more likely to deliver quickly, and this may alter your anaesthetic management.
- *Is this a spontaneous or induced labour?* An induced labour is more likely to be slow and complicated.
- *How many centimetres of cervical dilatation has the labour progressed to?* An early request for an epidural may already indicate a slow labour with excessive pain from an occipito-posterior presentation of the fetal head. An epidural will need to be effective for many hours. You may consider late requests for an epidural to be inappropriate as delivery is possibly imminent. However, it may reflect major obstetric difficulties in the latter stages of labour, when epidural analgesia can be difficult to achieve and operative delivery is likely.
- *Has the mother had a previous CS?* If so, she is more likely to have another one.
- *Is this labour slow and is augmentation with oxytocin likely?* If so, an epidural may be required for many hours and needs to be effective.
- *Is the CTG normal or abnormal?* If it is abnormal, is fetal scalp blood sampling or early operative delivery anticipated?

The obstetrician

There will be overlap between the questions you can direct towards the midwife and obstetrician, especially about the obstetric history, but a clearer overview of the labour and likelihood of operative delivery can usually be obtained from the obstetrician.
- *How long do I have to do this anaesthetic?* Is the anaesthetic urgent for fetal blood sampling or operative delivery, or can I take more time?

- *When do you anticipate obstetric intervention?* This may be in the next few minutes or in several hours if there has been inadequate progress in labour.
- *Is it likely the baby will be delivered by forceps or need a caesarean delivery?* If an operative vaginal delivery is likely, is there a high risk of proceeding to CS? In which case the anaesthetic needs to be effective for both procedures before the obstetrician starts.

The mother

The mother will be able to tell you if she has any past medical complications. There is usually a tick box questionnaire in her notes that will have been filled out in early pregnancy, but there may be a need for clarification. The mother should also tell you what she understands about the procedure you have been asked to carry out.

- *What do you know about epidurals?* There are issues about consent in labour, but it is important that the mother understands the major issues. If she tells you that she has read the information from a well-recognized source and discussed it with a midwife or anaesthetist in the antenatal period, the information you need to give her is brief. If she says she knows nothing, you must spend some time in giving her a good explanation.
- *What are your expectations?* The mother may have very high or unrealistic expectations. Listen carefully and give good information back. If she has low expectations, be reassuring.

A systematic review of questions

Many obstetric units have a dedicated obstetric anaesthetic chart because the information that needs to be documented is different from other theatre work. It is helpful if the chart is subdivided into systems and has some tick boxes so a history and examination can be carried out quickly without overlooking important factors.

Past medical history
- *Medical problems*: systems review.
- Previous surgery: what?
- *Anaesthesia*: any previous problems with regional or general anaesthetic?

Drug
- *Current medication*: diabetic, hypertensive or epileptic?
- Heparin or gastric acid prophylaxis given recently?
- *Allergies* especially latex and antibiotics.

Obstetric history
- *Gravidity (G)*: the number of pregnancies.
- *Parity (P)*: the number of births. P0 long labour, high expectation compared with P3 short labour, higher risk of uterine atony/postpartum haemorrhage (PPH).
- *Mode of delivery*: spontaneous vaginal delivery (SVD), elective caesarean section (lower segment caesarean section (LSCS)), emergency LSCS, and why?
- *Mode of anaesthesia*: nil, epidural for labour (EFL) ± top-up/spinal/combined spinal–epidural (CSE).

Current pregnancy

Problems—mother, placenta, or fetus.

- *Mother*: raised BP, proteinuria, diabetes.
- *Placenta*: insufficiency, praevia; minor or major, anterior or posterior.
- *Fetus*: congenital anomaly requiring early delivery or transfer to another unit, multiple pregnancy, poly/oligohydramnios, large/small baby, prematurity.

Planned delivery

- SVD, LSCS, and why?

Examination

Examination of the patient can provide a lot of answers. Particular attention should be given to:

Airway

Higher incidence of failed intubation, 1:250.

Assessment includes Mallampati score and mouth opening, dentition, thyro-mental distance, occlusion of the teeth, and neck movement. In pregnancy, a high body mass index, oedema, and large breasts can also present greater difficulties.

Body mass index (BMI)

BMI is becoming an increasing problem in obstetrics and may predict a difficult regional and general anaesthetic.

Systems examination

- *CNS, HR, BP, heart sounds*: be aware of the cardiovascular changes in normal pregnancy and how maternal disease will influence your findings (see Chapter 3).
- *Respiratory*: breath sounds. Physiological changes that underline the importance of pre-oxygenation.
- *GIT*: reflux. Note the delayed gastric emptying in labour. Look at your labour ward starvation policy. Prescribe omeprazole and don't forget to give sodium citrate prior to emergency anaesthesia.
- *Spine*: increased lumbar lordosis and higher BMI, deformed anatomy, previous spinal surgery. Look and feel for lumbar spaces.

Investigations

The majority of mothers requesting a routine epidural for labour do not need current investigations. Women have a large number of investigations in pregnancy, which screen for complications such as a low haemoglobin or platelet count. The likelihood of picking up further pathology during labour if the pregnancy has proceeded without other complications is minimal and will only delay analgesia and anaesthesia when required.

- The midwife should know the results from the mother's most recent tests, which could be 8 weeks old.
- If the mother has signs or symptoms of pre-eclampsia, a platelet count within the last 4h should be known before an epidural or spinal is inserted. U&Es, LFTs and a clotting screen can also be useful.
- If a mother has a history of a low platelet count, other than from pre-eclampsia, then a platelet count within the last 12h should be known before an epidural or spinal is inserted.
- An emergency anaesthetic may need to be given before recent investigations are known. Unless major abnormalities are suspected, then the lack of blood results should not delay you.
- In cases of emergency anaesthesia, make sure that a full blood count and at least a blood 'group and save' is on its way to the laboratories.

Dealing with difficult behaviour

The labour ward is a stressful environment. Problems can progress rapidly and this can lead to patients, partners and colleagues behaving in a difficult and inappropriate manner. It helps to try and understand why they may be behaving in this way. Think, however, how your behaviour may appear to others, to prevent yourself becoming the problem.

The midwife

- Senior midwives and those in charge of the labour ward often have direct and assertive personalities. Don't take things too personally; they do a difficult job.
- Midwives can be thought of by some as difficult people. The reality is that they are highly qualified professionals, working in the best interests of the mother and baby, and therefore may have a forceful but valid opinion.
- High workload is a big factor affecting behaviour; midwives may be looking after more than one patient and juggling other tasks.
- It is highly stressful to look after a difficult or demanding patient for many hours.
- The difficult behaviour of a patient may be taken out on you. Take a deep breath.
- Lack of breaks. Many labour wards suffer from midwifery shortages. This can lead to inadequate or absent breaks, not even time for a drink. Try to be sympathetic.

How you can help

- Try and help out; be calm and polite.
- If a particular midwife is always a problem, speak to your seniors and ask if they can help.

The obstetrician

- High work intensity can lead to behavioural changes.
- You may recognize that the obstetrician is inexperienced, out of their depth, or has lost time perspective.

How you can help

- You can help by being non-confrontational and offering support. Remember there may be occasions where you need their help.
- They may see calling for help as a failure on their part; constructively suggest senior or additional assistance if inexperience is leading to difficult behaviour as the situation will only become worse.

The mother

- A mother may spend the majority of her pregnancy worrying about how she will cope with labour and the responsibility of a new baby. This can spill out into apparently difficult behaviour.
- Most difficult behaviour during labour is caused by pain.
- Fear for her unborn baby can also be a major concern.
- A mother may have had very little preparation for her experience. This is most common during a first labour, but can also happen unexpectedly when a labour is very different from one already experienced.
- Individual preconceived ideas, media, and social and cultural background can contribute to the mother's attitude.
- There can be a real sense of disappointment that labour and analgesia choices have not gone to plan.

How you can help

- The pain of labour is made worse by anxiety. If a mother observes competency and efficiency in the staff dealing with her, confidence can be more easily gained.
- Give full but concise information.
- Never shout back.
- Sometimes the simple act of sitting down, coming properly into the mother's view, and taking time to allay anxiety will transform the situation.
- Stay calm.
- If the mother is finding it very difficult to listen, then only one person must talk to her. It may be better to leave the room and let a confident midwife regain control.
- A lot of communication by an anaesthetist is from behind a face mask and from behind the mother. If she is finding it difficult to understand and co-operate, walk round in front of her, remove your mask, and talk face to face.

The partner

A birthing partner is a person who has been designated by the mother to accompany them in labour. It is well recognized that a calm and supportive birthing partner can reduce anxiety, which in turn can lead to a better outcome in labour. Unfortunately, many birthing partners are ill prepared for the experience, and their anxiety can easily become difficult behaviour.

- The hospital environment can be frightening and alien.
- Sometimes medical and nursing staff as patients can be the most difficult. It is somehow expected that they should know about labour and hospitals, but they may not have been on a labour ward for many years. The environment may seem as alien to them as to someone who has never been to hospital before.
- Confusion may arise from the large number of individuals involved in the mother's care.
- The partner may feel fearful for the unborn child and the labouring mother.
- They want to be protective but can't be.

- A partner may have a job where they control a work situation or a workforce. They can find themselves unable to control the pain their loved one is experiencing, or control the midwifery and medical staff who are in attendance. This can rapidly appear as aggressive behaviour. Stay calm.
- The birthing experience of a mother accompanying her daughter may be helpful, but can also result in overprotective behaviour.
- There can also be real disappointment that the labour and anticipated analgesia have not gone to plan.

How you can help
- It is important that difficult and overanxious behaviour from a partner is rapidly defused to prevent the labouring woman also becoming anxious and difficult herself.
- Introduce yourself clearly by name, and explain the role you have in attending the mother.
- Bring the partner into the conversation.
- Bring the partner into the decision making.
- Explain clearly what you are doing and why.
- Never shout.
- Occasionally, it is better to have a conversation with the partner away from the labouring woman, especially if there are raised voices.
- Very occasionally, the partner may be aggressive or confrontational whatever you do. Tell them calmly that you feel their behaviour is unacceptable and that measures will be taken to remove them from the ward. Don't get into personal arguments over this; senior midwifery staff will help. They frequently have a great deal of experience in dealing with these problems.

Dealing with malformation and death

Fetal malformations are common and always cause great anxiety to the mother and birthing partner. The degree of malformation may not reflect the degree of anxiety, and minor abnormalities can cause significant emotional problems. Most severe congenital anomalies will be picked up on antenatal ultrasound scanning, but many minor problems will not. Some mothers will choose not to have antenatal scans and, occasionally, babies will be born with unexpected significant major problems.

Some large maternity centres will look after many mothers who are known to carry babies with major abnormalities because of regional fetal medicine and neonatal surgical services. The anaesthetist working on such units will meet these mothers on an almost daily basis and needs to understand rapidly the specific needs of the baby's parents.

Maternity units that deal with these problems will frequently have staff who are specifically trained to counsel the parents. The anaesthetist should be guided by the experts and listen carefully to any advice offered.

Expected malformation

The mother and partner have been told about the malformation, but they may or may not have come to terms with it.

Mid-trimester termination of pregnancy

In the UK, a mother has a right to choose to end her pregnancy up to the 24th week gestation for social reasons. A mother can undergo a termination of her pregnancy for significant fetal anomalies at any gestation, although it is uncommon after 24 weeks gestation as most problems are picked up on a 20-week anomaly scan. If the pregnancy is beyond 21 weeks plus 6 days when a decision is made to terminate the pregnancy, a specially trained obstetrician undertakes a feticide, where potassium is injected through the mother's abdominal wall into the fetal heart so that the baby is delivered dead. The mother will then be given prostaglandins to induce labour.

- Formal anaesthesia or major sedation is not usually required for feticide procedures so the anaesthetist will not have to be directly involved. See Chapter 14 for further details on feticide management.
- It is recognized that some anaesthetists, because of strongly held moral or religious views, do not give anaesthesia or sedation for these procedures. If as a professional you feel unable to be involved, your views must be made known to the service providers so alternative arrangements can be made. You have a moral obligation as a professional to ensure the mother receives the best care there is, which could require you personally to find an alternative anaesthetist.
- Some anaesthetists will not directly involve themselves in the termination or feticide, but will provide necessary analgesia or anaesthesia for complications such as a retained placenta. Make sure your colleagues and the midwife in charge knows what you are prepared to do.

- It is never right to impose your views on the situation, as the mother and partner will already have had time to reflect, be counselled, and have made their choice.
- Many mothers will have significant pain during the labour of a mid-trimester termination. They have a right, like any labouring mother, to have a choice of analgesia.
- Many women find regular opioid-based analgesia enough, whilst occasionally others may request an epidural.
- An epidural can safely be given, but the usual safety aspects of providing it must be rigorously upheld. Because there is no reason for the midwife to monitor the fetus they often do not stay in the room the whole time. Make sure that the mother is adequately monitored depending on her analgesia choice.
- When providing analgesia in these situations, there is frequently a very difficult atmosphere in the delivery room. There is often a real sense of guilt and grief. The usual rules about the number of birthing partners are frequently flouted, and you can find yourself addressing a large number of people.

- Be sensitive to the situation.
- Never voice personal views.
- Don't be judgmental.
- Talk primarily to the patient but make sure everyone else understands what you are doing.
- It can be useful to find out who are friends and family members. The midwife looking after the patient usually knows.
- If you find the situation difficult or upsetting, talk to someone about your feelings.

Term deliveries of a baby with known congenital malformation

The anaesthetist may be involved in providing regional analgesia during labour but is also frequently involved when anaesthesia for CS is required. During a CS, it is usual for the anaesthetist to take on the role of primary carer of the mother from the midwife. This is considerably more demanding when the baby has congenital abnormalities. The anaesthetist will then meet the mother again during a postnatal ward round. The mother is frequently distressed, but it is important to ascertain that there has been good recovery from the anaesthetic and that analgesia is effective. The mother must have the opportunity to talk over problems or concerns she may have about her anaesthetic, just as every mother should.

- Before you get involved in the care of the mother, find out from the obstetrician and midwife the nature and degree of abnormality.
- Is the baby expected to live or die?
- Is the baby expected to need neonatal resuscitation and transfer to a special care neonatal unit?
- Talk to the mother very carefully about what type of anaesthetic (general or regional) she wants for her CS.

- It is normal for any patient to be anxious about being awake for a CS. This normal anxiety is heightened when the baby is known to have an anomaly.
- Most mothers, however, do want to be awake when their baby is born; it may be very important so that the mother and partner can more quickly come to terms with the problem.
- This is especially so if the baby is likely to die or need immediate transfer to the neonatal unit.
- A general anaesthetic may seem the easier option, but it is only moving the emotional problems out of the operating theatre and from the anaesthetist's view.
- Some parents want to see the defect immediately and others want the baby carefully wrapped, therefore hiding the problem. Listen very carefully to their wishes.
- Partners need to be made welcome and feel included.
- Acknowledge the malformation if appropriate.
- Some mothers become very remote after the baby is born, while others want to talk. Facilitate the emotion she wants to show at that time.
- Dealing emotionally with this situation can be very difficult for a doctor who has not had to deal with this situation before. Talk to someone about it afterwards.

Unexpected malformation

Babies are quite frequently born with obvious abnormalities that have not been picked up on routine antenatal ultrasound screening. The abnormalities that are picked up at birth are usually highly visible and therefore distressing, but may also become apparent over the first few minutes of life when a baby that is expected to be healthy fails to breath or to become pink because of an underlying respiratory or cardiac problem.

- Always acknowledge to the mother and partner that there is a problem. They will have already noticed that the baby is causing concern to the staff and will immediately know if they are lied to.
- The parents are likely to be extremely shocked and may behave in a difficult or overtly emotional way.
- The midwife will always be involved but it is possible that she will have only just met the parents. Work together.
- A paediatrician will usually be involved but they may also be inexperienced in dealing with the situation.
- Be informative about the abnormality if it is within your knowledge, but don't be reassuring if you are not certain.
- If the partner wants to see the baby and the baby is stable, invite him/her to the resuscitaire.
- It may be difficult for the mother to see the abnormality even if she wants to. A simple explanation is appropriate at this stage.

- Sometimes the partner wants to stay with the mother and support her; sometimes the partner may become emotionally detached and even leaves the operating theatre or delivery room. In the latter situation, the mother will need additional support from the medical and midwifery staff. Never be critical of the partner.
- Dealing emotionally with this situation can be very difficult for a doctor who has not had to deal with this situation before. Talk to someone about it afterwards.

The death of a baby

The admission of a mother whose baby is found to have died *in utero* is sadly common. The death of a baby at any gestation can be devastating for the mother and partner. A common euphemism for death is 'loss' or 'lost'. Be very careful when using these words because they may also imply a degree of carelessness. The mother may already have a huge feeling of guilt associated with her baby's death, and the use of these words may aggravate this.

The anaesthetist frequently becomes involved with these mothers because labour has to be induced and may be prolonged and painful. She is also less likely to cope with labour pain.

The anaesthetist may encounter the death of a baby whilst administering an anaesthetic for fetal distress if the paediatricians are unable to resuscitate the baby. Advice on dealing with stillbirth is available on the Stillbirth and Neonatal Death (SANDS) charity website, http://www.uk-sands.org. Antenatal Results and Choice (ARC) http://www.arc.org.uk is a UK national charity, who provide non-directive support and information to parents throughout antenatal testing, and where there has been a diagnosis of fetal anomaly. They will also support healthcare professionals.

General anaesthesia

- If the mother needs a general anaesthetic, don't become distracted. Stay focused on the anaesthetic and keep the mother safe.
- She will have gone to sleep knowing that there was a problem; she is likely to ask about it as soon as she awakes. Be truthful.

Regional anaesthesia

- The mother may have had a regional technique and her partner may be with her. They will be immediately aware that there is a significant problem.
- The mother and partner must not be allowed to interfere with the resuscitation, but it is acceptable that they are allowed to look on from a distance. If the parents can see that the medical staff are working effectively and calmly to save their baby's life, it can help them to come to terms with the baby's death later.
- The anaesthetist and midwife must form a link between the resuscitation and the couple.

Aftermath
- It is natural to feel extremely sad. Expressing how you feel in a controlled fashion can help the couple, as they will appreciate your empathy.
- You must carry on communicating with them as they are in an alien hospital environment and will need emotional support.
- Some parents want to see the baby straight away and some may not wish to see the baby until they are quietly together after the delivery is over. Help facilitate whatever the parents want.
- It is common to want to criticize your anaesthetic technique and feel a personal sense of guilt. Did you do everything possible to save the baby's life? Don't express these feelings to the parents at this time.
- Never start blaming other medical personnel in front of the parents, even if you feel that their actions may have contributed to the baby's death. These types of concerns need to be discussed at length with senior medical and midwifery staff later.
- As soon as possible afterwards, write down the sequence of events with times from the start of your involvement in the death. There will almost certainly be an internal enquiry and occasionally there may be a formal complaint or court case.
- Dealing emotionally with this situation can be very difficult for a doctor who has not had to deal with this situation before. Talk to someone about it afterwards. There may be a Bereavement Midwife or Specialist Nurse in your unit who may be able to support you.
- Remember that your anaesthetic assistant may not have faced death before; they may need to talk afterwards too.

The death of a mother

Thankfully, the unexpected death of a mother in the peripartum period is uncommon in the UK (1:10,000). However, any maternal death is always catastrophic and unexpected. The death of a baby is relatively common and many midwives will have plenty of experience dealing with bereaved parents and will help you. However, it is very unlikely that there is anybody immediately available who has much experience of dealing with a maternal death.

- Stay focused calm and professional.
- Ask for help from a senior colleague.
- You will feel deeply upset, and it is usual to experience guilt if you have been either a passive onlooker or deeply involved in the mother's care.
- Recriminations and blame are common. Don't get emotionally involved; there will be plenty of time afterwards for proper reflection.

The relatives
- Senior staff must present a unifying front to the relatives and provide accurate information.
- It is important that the relatives do not feel that there is a cover-up from the hospital staff.

The aftermath

- A proper debriefing is essential for all staff involved. This is best carried out the following day. If you feel very distressed, talk to someone sooner.
- As soon as possible afterwards, write down the sequence of events with times from the start of your involvement in the death. There will be an internal enquiry and coroner's inquest.
- It is a personal decision as to whether you feel able to carry on to the end of your shift. However, if you have been closely involved, arrangements should be made for you to hand over duties and go home.

The mother who does not speak English

The mother who does not speak English on a labour ward can be either a visitor, or a legal or an illegal resident. She is likely to come from an ethnic group with a different social and cultural background, with varying views on childbirth and pain relief. These views can sometimes lead to many problems, as well as not having the same language in common.

She may find all aspects of her care difficult to understand, and the problems of pain and anxiety seen in many labouring mothers will make communication more difficult.

Translators

- It is common for the mother's birthing partner to speak more English than she does.
- The birthing partner can be a husband or female relative. A female partner may be from the husband's family and can sometimes forcefully express the husband's viewpoint.
- Sometimes the partner's views can be strongly felt and divergent from those of the medical staff.
- In this situation, it is important that an independent translator is used if at all possible. The mother must be told in accurate terms what she is to expect, otherwise her care could be compromised.
- Most hospitals provide some type of independent translation service, although this can be language dependent.
- It is common and acceptable to use hospital staff in these situations. Some hospitals organize training and a register of staff that are willing to help. This is particularly helpful in the emergency situation.
- Registered translators are routinely used in many antenatal clinics, but it is unusual to have these translators available on a 24h basis. Some hospitals subscribe to a 24h telephone or video translation service. It can be difficult to talk via a third unseen party on the telephone but can be useful and should be used if available.
- The Obstetric Anaesthetists' Association (OAA) has a large number of translated patient information leaflets relating to obstetric analgesia and anaesthesia on their website www.oaa-anaes.ac.uk. There are detailed information booklets as well as simple sheets with common words and useful diagrams. The latter are more useful in an emergency. All are free to download.
- In a real emergency, translation services can be difficult to use and an English-speaking member of the family may have to be used.

General advice

- Remember that the mother's expectations of childbirth may be as high as those of many English-speaking mothers. It is your duty as a professional to facilitate the care that she needs.
- Assess the level of English she can speak and understand. Women may understand much more English than they are willing to speak. Sometimes plenty of signs and the use of simple words are all that is required.
- Use non-verbal communication to establish a rapport; a simple handshake or smile can help.
- It is especially difficult to inform in the usual detail about regional techniques for labour analgesia and CS. This should not mean that the mother should not have an epidural or that she must have a general anaesthetic for an operative delivery. There are risks associated with deviating from your usual practice simply because it cannot be explained easily to the patient. Use a translation service if at all possible.
- Inability to understand the language, pain and fear can make behaviour appear difficult. The tone of your voice and a sympathetic manner in which you approach the mother can help her cope in this situation.
- Keep the relatives informed, but always address the mother even if the relatives seem to be doing all the talking.
- Do provide time for any questions from the mother or the relatives. All mothers experience the same feelings and emotions through labour, wherever they are from. It is easy to underestimate this.

Audit and quality improvement in obstetric anaesthesia

Audit and quality improvement is an integral and important part of medical practice, acting as a means of improving service delivery, as an aid to research, as a means of accountability and quality control, and to facilitate efficient management.

Definition and principles of use

The different principles of research, audit and quality improvement are set out in Table 1.1.

Table 1.1 Comparison of research and audit/QI principles

Research	Clinical audit/QI
Asks what we should be doing	Asks whether we are doing what we should
Creates new knowledge (evidence)	Assesses whether best practice (often informed by research evidence) is being used
Often experimental	Never experimental
Hypothesis generated	Measures against predetermined standards
May involve new or untried treatment	Treatment always previously evaluated
Often involves randomization of patients to treatment and use of placebos	No randomization (patient choice). No placebo
Uses statistical tests and power analysis	Descriptive statistical analysis only

Audit in obstetric anaesthetic practice

A high standard of care within obstetric anaesthesia is essential to achieve acceptable levels of maternal satisfaction and a low incidence of complications, and to maintain a high degree of safety within the service. New service initiatives and developments should be introduced with monitoring by audit.

Quality improvement (QI)

Aims to improve the patient experience and is usually focused on more holistic issues. QI can be done using the plan, do, study, act (PDSA) framework. PDSA cycles are iterative and have short time spans allowing improvement to be incorporated quickly.

Guide to audit and QI

The focus is generally on quality issues and compliance with national guidelines.

- Adequacy of staffing.
- Timely anaesthetic involvement in the care of high risk mothers.
- Information about obstetric anaesthesia and analgesia.
- Pain management in labour.
- Consent given by women during labour.
- Response times for the provision of intrapartum analgesia and anaesthesia.
- Monitoring levels for regional analgesia.
- Technique of anaesthesia for CS.
- Pain relief after CS.
- Monitoring of obstetric patients in recovery and the High Dependency Unit (HDU).
- Airway and intubation problems during general anaesthesia for CS.
- Anaesthetic complications and side-effects such as postdural puncture headache (PDPH) rate and regional to general anaesthesia conversion rates.
- The use of antacid prophylaxis in labour and for CS.

These topics and themes can then be incorporated into QI projects with PDSA cycles to demonstrate implementation and sustainability of change.

Regional audits
- Regional audits allow analysis of a much larger data set.
- Larger numbers can increase inaccuracies within the data collected—especially quantitative numbers—but are very good at looking at relatively rare problems and complications within obstetric anaesthesia.
- They are probably a more satisfactory way of looking at trends.
- The setting up of a regional database will also improve communications between neighbouring maternity units, and will facilitate service development as it can more easily justify a need when a problem is relatively rare.

National audits
National audits usually have a broad framework and have looked in general terms at setting up good maternity services and analysing the risks associated with very rare complications.

National postal questionnaires
- A useful network of key personnel that provide obstetric anaesthetic services in the UK has been set up through the OAA.
- Are helpful adjuncts to local audit.
- Provide a snapshot of current practice across a large number of units and allow current local practice to be evaluated against national trends.

UK Obstetric Surveillance System (UKOSS)
- To develop a UK-wide Obstetric Surveillance System to describe the epidemiology of a variety of uncommon disorders of pregnancy.

- To use the knowledge gained to make practical improvements in prevention and treatment and allow for more effective service planning.
- To provide a system capable of responding rapidly to emerging conditions of major public health importance.

MBRRACE-UK: Mothers and Babies: Reducing Risk through Audits and Confidential Enquiries across the UK

- Is the longest running audit project in the world.
- Known as CEMD (Confidential Enquiry into Maternal Death), which started in 1952.
- Reports are now produced on a rolling yearly basis and highlight main factors responsible for maternal mortality.
- The confidential enquiries have had one of the greatest influences in reducing mortality relating to general anaesthesia in obstetrics.
- This UK-based audit has had far-reaching influence across the world relating to maternity care, and many countries have used it to set their own standards.
- Recommendations on the broader involvement of anaesthetic services within maternity services have reduced maternal mortality relating to a number of obstetric emergencies, including the management of PPH and severe sepsis.

Further reading

Smith RL et al. Analgesia for medically induced second trimester termination of pregnancy: A randomized trial. *Journal of Obstetrics and Gynaecology: Canada*. 2016; 38: 147–153.
Obstetric Anaesthetist Association translations: http://www.labourpains.com/home
UK Obstetric Surveillance System UKOSS: www.npeu.ox.ac.uk/ukoss/publications-ukoss
MBRRACE confidential enquires: www.npeu.ox.ac.uk/mbrrace-uk/reports
The termination of pregnancy for fetal abnormalities: www.rcog.org.uk/globalassets/documents/guidelines/terminationpregnancyreport18may2010.pdf
UK based bereavement organizations:
Stillbirth and Neonatal Deaths, www.sands.org.uk
Antenatal Results and Choice, www.arc.org.uk

Confidential Enquiries into Maternal Deaths

Nuala Lucas and James Bamber

Introduction

- A reduction in maternal mortality is one of the United Nations Sustainable Development Goals, with the aim to reduce Global Maternal Mortality Ratio (MMR) to fewer than 70 per 100,000 live births. In 2015, the Global MMR was estimated to be 196 per 100,000 births.
- To deliver improvement in the quality of maternal health and reduce the MMR, it is important to understand the structures and processes that leads to a maternal death—described by the WHO as going 'beyond the numbers'.
- Different methodologies, depending on the healthcare setting and resources available, can be utilized to identify areas for quality improvement and reduce maternal mortality.
- The Confidential Enquiry into Maternal Deaths (CEMD) is one methodology. It is the UK's longest running audit of practice, and represents an international gold standard for detailed investigation and improvement in maternity care.
- From the first triennial report reviewing deaths in 1952–54 to the triennial report for 2012–14, the CEMD has reviewed the deaths of 10,301 women; 6685 deaths from Direct causes and 3616 deaths from Indirect causes.
- Many of the lessons highlighted in its reports are applicable in other healthcare settings, including developing nations.

History

- The CEMD was started in England and Wales in 1952. Since then the CEMD has expanded to include the rest of the UK from 1985, as well as the Republic of Ireland since 2012.
- In 1952, the MMR for England and Wales was 54.6 per 100 000 live births. It was 4.65 per 100,000 live births for the 2012–2014 triennium in the UK. The UK Government has set a target to halve the number of maternal deaths for England by 2030.
- The rate estimate from routine sources of data is much lower, i.e. about half, than the actual rates as identified through the UK CEMD, which uses multiple sources of death identification.
- From its introduction until 2011, the CEMD published triennial reports on the causes of maternal deaths.
- Following a Government review of the value of the CEMD in 2011, the report moved to annual publication, in order to facilitate a more rapid response to emerging patterns of disease, preventing a time-lag in dissemination and learning from cases.
- To ensure anonymity and confidentiality of the deaths reported, the CEMD reports the number of deaths as a rolling triennial number by cause of death. The chapter reviews of specific causes of death, presented previously, are now divided between annual reports spread over a three-year cycle.
- The Healthcare Quality Improvement Partnership (HQIP) currently commissions the CEMD as part of the Maternal, Newborn and Infant Clinical Outcomes Review Programme (MNI-CORP), which also includes the Perinatal Confidential Enquiry.

- The current reporting system is now managed by the National Perinatal Epidemiology Unit at the University of Oxford as MBRRACE-UK (Mothers and Babies—Reducing Risk through Audits and Confidential Enquiries across the UK).

The aims of the CEMD have remained consistent since its inception

- To reduce maternal mortality and morbidity by identifying not just the causes of and trends in maternal deaths, but also identifying avoidable or substandard factors that should be changed to improve care.
- To promulgate these findings and subsequent recommendations to all healthcare professionals involved in caring for pregnant women, and to ensure that their uptake is audited and monitored.
- To make recommendations concerning improvement of clinical care and service provision, including local audit, to commissioners of obstetric services and to suggest directions for future areas for research and audit.

The CEMD methodology

Case ascertainment
- Maternal deaths are notified to MBRRACE-UK by healthcare staff through a reporting system or by other sources (e.g. coroners, media reports).
- A unique feature of the CEMD is the meticulous case ascertainment.
- To ensure completeness of data, notified deaths are cross-checked with national records e.g. registered deaths.
- Full medical records are obtained for all women who died, which are then anonymized before undergoing a confidential review process by assessors.

Cause of death
- A pathologist determines the cause of each death from review of the anonymized records, with an obstetrician or physician as required.
- The definitions of maternal deaths are summarized in Table 2.1.

Case review and report publication
- The care of each woman is assessed using the anonymized medical records by 10–15 expert reviewers, who include obstetricians, midwives, pathologists, anaesthetists, and other specialist assessors as required, e.g. psychiatrists, general practitioners, physicians, emergency medicine specialists, and intensive care experts.

Table 2.1 Classification of maternal deaths

Maternal death	Death of a woman while pregnant or within 42 days of the end of pregnancy*, from any cause related to or aggravated by the pregnancy or its management, but not from accidental or incidental causes
Direct	Deaths resulting from obstetric complications of the pregnant state (pregnancy, labour, and puerperium) from interventions, omissions, incorrect treatment, or from a chain of events from any of the above
Indirect	Deaths resulting from previous existing disease, or disease that developed during pregnancy and which was not the result of direct obstetric causes, but which was aggravated by the physiological effects of pregnancy
Late	Deaths occurring between 42 days and 1 year after the end of pregnancy that are the result of Direct or Indirect maternal causes
Coincidental**	Deaths from unrelated causes which happen to occur in pregnancy or the puerperium

*Includes giving birth, ectopic pregnancy, miscarriage or termination of pregnancy.

**Termed 'Fortuitous' in the International Classification of Diseases (ICD).

Adapted from Maternal mortality ratio (per 100 000 live births). World Health Organization.

Classification of care

Care is classified as:
• Good care.
• Improvement to care* which would have made no difference to outcome.
• Improvement to care* which may have made a difference to outcome.

*Improvements in care are interpreted to include adherence to guidelines where these exist and have not been followed, as well as other improvements which would normally be considered part of good care, where no formal guidelines exist.

• The expert reviews are collated and examined by a multidisciplinary writing group, which is responsible for identifying the main learning themes and recommendations for future improvements in care.
• These are published in the annual reports, with rolling three years of UK statistical surveillance data.

Statistical analysis

• The CEMD calculates maternal mortality rates, with 95% confidence intervals using the number of maternities, i.e. women giving birth at or beyond 24 weeks' gestation, derived from national statistics as the denominator.
• The number of pregnancies is not used as the denominator as it is impossible to know the number of pregnancies, as not all pregnancies result in a registrable birth, i.e. live or stillbirth.
• In contrast, international MMRs use live births as the denominator, as not all nations have accurate records of stillbirths in their national statistics.
• National data is used to obtain denominator data for the calculation of mortality rates for age, country of birth, ethnicity, and socio-economic groups. The CEMD also publishes MMR data to allow for international comparisons.
• Mortality data may also be presented as deaths from obstetric causes per million women aged between 15–44 years, as this allows comparison with other causes of women's deaths. However this lacks the precision of confining the rate calculated to women who were actually pregnant.

CEMD Report structure

• Each annual Report is subdivided into sections on surveillance and epidemiological data, e.g. causes and trends, clinical reviews of deaths by particular cause with recommendations for care improvement, with an executive summary of report recommendations for action by policy makers, healthcare organizations, and healthcare professionals.
• The statistics are presented as maternal mortality rates per 100,000 maternities as a rolling three-year average, with recent historical data presented for comparison and describing trends.
• Deaths are analysed by cause and grouped as either direct or indirect causes.

Classification of maternal deaths used in CEMD

Direct causes
- Pregnancy related infections—Sepsis*.
- Pre-eclampsia and eclampsia.
- Thrombosis and thromboembolism.
- Amniotic fluid embolism.
- Early pregnancy deaths.
- Haemorrhage.
- Anaesthesia.
- Psychiatric causes—Suicides.

Indirect causes
- Cardiac disease.
- Indirect sepsis—Influenza.
- Indirect sepsis–Pneumonia/others.
- Indirect neurological conditions.
- Psychiatric causes–drugs/alcohol/others.
- Indirect malignancies.
- Other Indirect causes.
- Coincidental.
- Homicide.
- Other.
- Late deaths.

Unascertained
*Genital/ urinary tract sepsis deaths, including early pregnancy deaths as a result of genital/ urinary tract sepsis. Other deaths from infectious causes are classified under indirect causes.

- The report contains an analysis of the women's socio-demographic characteristics, e.g. age, ethnicity, socio-economic status, and summary information of the classification of the quality of care received by the women.
- The causes of death are considered in topic-specific chapters, which are divided over a three-year cycle. Each annual report has a different group of topic-specific chapters until the cycle repeats.
- To compliment the lessons learned from maternal deaths, MBRRACE-UK has also introduced topic-specific Confidential Enquiries into Maternal Morbidity (CEMM), which reports alongside the annual CEMD Report. This is in recognition of the significantly larger number of women who survive their complications of pregnancy with severe morbidity, i.e. up to 100 times more survive than die. Investigation into the care of these women also provides important lessons for improving care.
- There is an annual application process for organizations and individuals to submit topics to be chosen by an MBRRACE-UK advisory group.
- Over the last 30 years, the classification and review of maternal deaths has continued to evolve.
- A separate chapter with a focus on deaths from mental illness was first published in the 1994–96 triennial report. Prior to this, maternal deaths

from mental illness had been included within chapters that reviewed deaths from miscellaneous causes.

- Early reports included a specific chapter for deaths following uterine rupture. In later reports, this complication is present with deaths from genital tract trauma. As the number of these deaths declined, they are now included in the Haemorrhage chapter.
- Other changes include the inclusion of all deaths from sepsis within a Sepsis specific chapter since the 2006–08 report, whereas previously sepsis deaths had been included in those deaths reviewed in the chapter on early pregnancy deaths.
- The chapter on deaths associated with caesarean section (CS), which was a feature of early reports, was removed in the 1994–96 report.

CEMD trends

- Between 1847 and 1935, the maternal mortality rate had been ~400 per 100,000 deliveries, with nearly 50% of deaths due to sepsis.
- The maternal mortality rate in England and Wales began to fall from 1935, when antibiotics to treat puerperal sepsis became more available.
- There was a continued decrease in maternal mortality rate during the Second World War, leading up to the introduction of the first CEMD instigated in 1952.
- Since introduction of the CEMD process, the maternal mortality rate has continued to decrease, but the rate has plateaued over the past 30 years, see Fig 2.1.
- During this plateau, the number of maternal deaths attributed to direct causes has been overtaken by deaths attributed to indirect causes. The number of deaths due to indirect causes exceeded the number of deaths from direct causes in the 1997–1999 triennium and this pattern has persisted since.
- As traditional causes of maternal death have declined, newer causes or themes are being identified.
- Maternal death from sudden adult death syndrome (SADS): 'sudden arrhythmic cardiac death in an adult with a morphological normal heart' was categorized for the first time in the 2000–2002 report.
- In a review of cardiac deaths for the triennium 2009–2014, deaths from SADS represented over a third of the cardiac deaths and constitute the largest category of cardiac death.

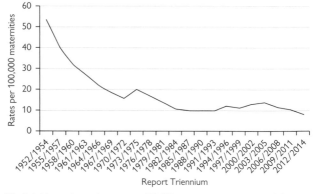

Fig. 2.1 Maternal mortality rates per 100,000 maternities since the start of the CEMD. Note: Data prior to 1985/1987 Triennium is England and Wales only and data since 1985/1987 is for UK.

Source data from: CEMD Reports (1970–1972; 1988–1990; 2000–2002; 2013–2015)

- As the CEMD reports have evolved to reflect the changes in the number and causes of maternal deaths, there has also been change within the maternity population.
- The maternity population is becoming older and more obese; both are independent risk factors for maternal death.
- Socioeconomic status and ethnicity are additional risk factors for maternal death.
- An increase in risk factors within the maternal population may be one reason why the maternal mortality rates have plateaued.

Standards of care

- Since the first report, the CEMD has evaluated the standard of care received by the women who died.
- The classifications of standards of care have changed over the past 60 years.
- The term 'avoidable deaths' was used in the early reports to describe cases assessed by the reviewers to have an avoidable factor that should have been recognized, anticipated, or managed differently to avoid a fatal outcome.
- In later reports the terms 'minor' and 'major' substandard care were used.
- 'Major substandard care' was defined as failures of care that contributed significantly to the death of the mother and in many, but not all cases, where different treatment may have altered outcome.
- The most recent reports use categories by which the care is judged to have been 'good', 'improvements to care which would have made no difference to outcome', or 'improvements to care which may have made a difference to outcome'.
- Sub-optimal standards of care have been identified as a contributory factor in 40–50% of maternal deaths from direct causes since the first CEMD report.

Lessons for care

The key purpose of the CEMD has always been to review maternal deaths, so that lessons can be learnt to improve care and reduce the future number of deaths. This purpose has been emphasized in reports produced by MBRRACE-UK, with chapter titles including the wording 'Lessons', 'Learning', 'Messages', and 'Prevention'.

Key lessons: Direct causes in Reports since 1988

Haemorrhage

- There has been an increase in the number of deaths from haemorrhage, particularly related to abnormally invasive placentation.
- A variety of lessons have been identified from evaluation of deaths of haemorrhage.

These include:

- The importance of early recognition of the severity of haemorrhage, as the failure to recognize and treat postpartum haemorrhage (PPH) has consistently been highlighted as a factor associated with a poor outcome.
- Young fit women with robust cardiovascular systems can compensate effectively in the face of significant blood loss, and maintain a relatively normal heart rate and blood pressure.
- PPH is not always clinically obvious and may be concealed. Clinicians must have a low index of suspicion when assessing a woman with potential haemorrhage, and use other indicators of end organ perfusion, e.g. urine output.
- Clinicians may be falsely reassured by a result from a single point of care haemoglobin testing device, which is likely to be erroneous if adequate resuscitation has not taken place.
- The impact of a woman's weight on blood volume and their ability to tolerate PPH. In smaller women, i.e. <55kg, modest PPH will represent a greater percentage of total blood volume.
- The importance of resuscitation and proactive management: the anaesthetist is often the main point of contact responsible for communicating with the surgeons and blood bank to ensure that timely and appropriate resuscitation is occurring.
- Immediate access to blood and blood products is crucial. O-negative blood may be required for initial immediate resuscitation in severe cases.
- There has been repeated emphasis on the potential for massive obstetric haemorrhage in women with placenta praevia associated with previous uterine scar.
- Other recurring important messages include; the presence of a unit specific massive obstetric haemorrhage protocol, regular drills to practice the protocol, early senior involvement in the management of women with anticipated massive obstetric haemorrhage or uncontrolled bleeding, the availability and timely administration of blood products, early recourse to hysterectomy if bleeding is uncontrolled.

Hypertension

- There has been a dramatic decline in deaths from hypertensive disorders of pregnancy. In the 1985–87 triennium, hypertensive disorders accounted for 19% of the direct causes of death, whereas in 2012–14 triennium hypertensive disorders accounted for 3% of the direct deaths.
- The low rate of maternal deaths from pre-eclampsia in the UK contrasts dramatically with the international perspective, where an estimated 40,000 women die each year from pre-eclampsia.
- Reports from the 1980s demonstrated that deaths in women with pre-eclampsia primarily occurred as a result of pulmonary oedema and intracerebral haemorrhagic events.
- The widespread use of fluid-restricting protocols led to the disappearance of pulmonary oedema as a cause of death in these women in the UK following the 2000–02 report.
- Guidance from the UK National Institute for Health and Care Excellence (NICE) on the use of anti-hypertensive medication to control BP to lower targets, i.e. less than 150/100 mmHg has been associated with a reduction in deaths from intracerebral haemorrhage
- The use of low-dose aspirin as prophylaxis for hypertension has been a NICE recommendation from 2010, which is likely to have had further impact.
- The use of magnesium for anticonvulsant treatment and prophylaxis against further fits is recommended, as the results from randomized controlled trials informed the reports' recommendations.
- Other lessons emphasized in successive reports indicate the importance of screening for hypertensive disorders, with regular blood pressure checks throughout pregnancy and the early puerperium.

Thrombosis and thromboembolism

- Thrombo-embolic disease is currently the leading cause of direct deaths in the UK. Deaths from thrombosis and thromboembolism accounted for 30% of the direct deaths in 2012–14 triennium.
- However, there has been a significant decline in the numbers of deaths from thromboembolic disease since the early 2000s.
- This was largely attributed to the publication of the first national guidelines by the Royal College of Obstetricians and Gynaecologists, recommending better identification of at-risk women and the more widespread use of thrombo-prophylaxis.
- The maternal mortality rate due to thrombo-embolism has been relatively static in the last four Reports.

Recent Reports continue to highlights strategies to reduce deaths from thromboembolism

- Avoidance of medication gaps and inadequate dosing in high BMI women. Delivery for high risk women who have been prescribed prophylactic or therapeutic low molecular heparin requires careful planning to minimize prolonged gaps in thrombo-prophylaxis medication, particularly when medication has been stopped to enable neuraxial anaesthesia or minimize blood loss at delivery.

- Maternal weight in obese women should be remeasured in the third trimester to enable the calculation of correct doses of thromboprophylaxis.
- Pulmonary embolus (PE) can be difficult to diagnose. New onset tachycardia with shortness of breath mandates further investigation for PE; dizziness and collapse may also be symptoms.
- A woman who presents with symptoms that may be due to a venous thrombosis or thromboembolism should be anticoagulated pending the results of imaging to confirm or exclude the diagnosis.

Sepsis
- During the evolution of CEMD reports, the sepsis chapter has expanded to include all maternal deaths from sepsis, i.e. sepsis from direct causes (genital tract sepsis) and indirect causes (including influenza, pneumonia).
- The importance of using prophylactic antibiotics for CS was recommended in the 1988–90 Report.
- Sepsis emerged as the leading cause of direct deaths in the 2006–2008 CEMD report, which lead to a renewed drive to improve the management of peripartum sepsis.

The aspects of care identified that required improvement
- The recognition of and response to sepsis in an obstetric patient.
- The timeliness of antibiotic administration.
- The importance of fluid management in a septic obstetric patient.
- The removal of the septic focus.

- These messages have coincided with a major public health initiative to improve outcomes from sepsis in all patients.
- The 2009–12 report message was to 'Think Sepsis' when presented with an unwell woman.
- The 2013–15 report recommended that whenever sepsis is suspected or presents, a sepsis protocol should be activated, analogous to the activation of a major obstetric haemorrhage protocol.
- The application of a defined sepsis care bundle including; arterial blood gas with lactate measurement, blood cultures, commencement of intravenous antibiotics within 1 hour, fluid resuscitation, and urine output measurement is essential. This should be associated with continued appropriate monitoring and management.
- The importance of screening for sepsis by recording observations of HR, BP, SpO_2 (oxygen saturation), respiratory rate, and temperature on an early warning score chart has been highlighted, particularly in the community setting.
- The number of deaths from an influenza epidemic has led recent reports to emphasize the importance of influenza vaccination for all pregnant women.

Anaesthesia
- There were 19 maternal deaths directly attributed to anaesthesia in England and Wales in the 1982–84 triennium. By the next triennium report in 1985–87, there were 6 deaths. In the 2012–14 report, there were 2 deaths.
- This is in the context of a rise in the CS rate from 10% of deliveries in 1982–84 triennium, to 26% in the 2012–14 triennium.
- Nearly all the direct anaesthetic deaths throughout all the reports have been associated with general anaesthesia, and particularly the associated complications of aspiration, failed intubation, and hypoxia.
- The reduction of deaths from anaesthesia are likely to be a combination of increased use of neuraxial anaesthesia, better availability and use of monitoring (especially pulse oximetry and capnography), and better training and supervision of trainee anaesthetists.
- Report recommendations over the past 30 years have highlighted the importance of women receiving the same standard of perioperative care, including postoperative recovery, as other hospital patients.
- Dedicated obstetric anaesthetic services in consultant obstetric units, early referral, and assessment of high risk women by a consultant obstetric anaesthetist and the involvement of an obstetric anaesthetist in multidisciplinary planning of care have also been repeatedly highlighted.
- The importance of skills training for the management of potential anaesthetic catastrophes and the prompt early involvement of consultant anaesthetists in the peripartum management of women at high risk (cardiac disease, obesity, major haemorrhage) has been emphasized.

Key lessons: Indirect causes in Reports since 1988

Cardiac disease
- Reports have repeatedly highlighted the importance of multidisciplinary planning of care in women with known cardiac disease.
- The need for pre-pregnancy counselling of women with cardiac disease and early recognition of the symptoms and signs of cardiac disease, which require prompt assessment, investigation, and specialist review are key.
- The diagnosis of sudden arrhythmic cardiac death (SADS) has become an important recognized cause of cardiac death in recent reports.
- A post mortem diagnosis of death due to SADS has important implications for a woman's family, as they may also be at increased risk.
- The risk of maternal cardiac death is important as the maternity population becomes older and more obese.

Mental illness
- A report chapter on deaths from psychiatric causes first appeared in the 1994–1996 triennial report.
- Recurrent themes related to mental illness have been included the importance of identifying women at risk of mental illness, and ensuring service protocols and guidelines are in place to manage those women at risk.

- Specialist perinatal mental health services should be available to assess, support, and treat women at risk of perinatal mental illness, particularly in the postpartum period.
- Specific recommendations include the necessity to take a mental health history of all women at the antenatal booking visit. At risk women should be referred to specialist perinatal mental health services, with an assessment by a psychiatrist for those women with a prior history of serious mental illness.
- The important need for specialist mother and baby mental health units to be made available for the admission of women with mental illness.
- Other recommendations include the need for health professionals and maternity services to recognize that women who have been referred to child protection services are at high risk of medical or mental health problems, and may actively avoid engagement with maternity services.
- A recent recommendation to be cautious when diagnosing mental illness in women whose only symptoms are physical or show distress and agitation, particularly if the woman has no prior history of mental illness, does not speak English, or comes from an ethnic minority, to avoid inaccurate labelling of mental illness

Other important messages

Critical care
- The first chapter dedicated to critical care issues in maternal deaths appeared in the 1991–93 report.
- Women who died in intensive care generally received excellent care; however, they died from an overwhelming disease process despite best treatment.
- Pregnancy can make the differential diagnoses of critical illness more complex. The physiological changes of pregnancy can overlap with the pathophysiological changes of diseases process such as sepsis. It is important for clinicians to consider diagnoses beyond common pathologies of pregnancy.
- Early recognition of critical illness and prompt involvement of senior clinical staff, coupled with multidisciplinary team working, remain the key factors in providing high quality care to sick pregnant and postpartum women.
- Critical care support can be initiated in a variety of settings. Critical care clinicians must work in partnership with the labour ward team to provide care before transfer to the critical care unit.
- Inter-hospital referral of a sick pregnant or postpartum woman should be directed by the principle 'one transfer to definitive care'. It is unlikely to be appropriate to move a sick antenatal woman to a facility without an on-site obstetric facility.
- Obstetricians and obstetric anaesthetists must remain closely involved in the clinical management of women with obstetric specific conditions, such as pre-eclampsia. These conditions are rarely seen on the general critical care unit but are common problems on the labour ward.

Further reading

United Nations. Transforming our world: the 2030 Agenda for Sustainable Development. Sustainable Development Knowledge Platform.

https://sustainabledevelopment.un.org/post2015/transformingourworld (accessed 13/04/2018)

Kassebaum NJ et al. Global, regional, and national levels of maternal mortality, 1990–2015: a systematic analysis for the Global Burden of Disease Study 2015. *Lancet* 2016; 388: 1775–1812.

World Health Organization. Beyond the numbers: reviewing maternal deaths and severe morbidity to make pregnancy safer. Geneva: WHO, 2004. http://www.who.int/maternal_child_adolescent/documents/9241591838/en/ (accessed 13/04/2018).

Knight M et al. on behalf of MBRRACE-UK. Saving Lives, Improving Mothers' Care—Lessons Learned to Inform Future Maternity Care from the UK and Ireland Confidential Enquiries into Maternal Deaths and Morbidity 2009–12. Oxford: National Perinatal Epidemiology Unit, University of Oxford, 2014.

Knight M et al. on behalf of MBRRACE-UK. Saving Lives, Improving Mothers' Care—lessons learned to inform maternity care from the UK and Ireland Confidential Enquiries into Maternal Deaths and Morbidity 2013–2015. Oxford: National Perinatal Epidemiology Unit, University of Oxford 2017: 24–36.

Maternal physiology

Korede Adekanye and Abrie Theron

Cardiovascular system

There are a number of physiological adaptations to pregnancy in the cardio-vascular system. It is important to be aware of what is considered 'normal' for pregnancy, in order to promptly recognize and manage common medical conditions, e.g. hypertension.

Blood volume

See Fig. 3.1.

- The most striking maternal physiological alteration during pregnancy is the increase in blood volume. The magnitude of this increase depends on the size of the mother, parity, and the number of fetuses.
- The increase in blood volume continues until term, with an average increase of 45–50%, which is needed for extra blood flow to the uterus, the metabolic needs of the fetus, and increased perfusion of organs, especially the kidneys.
- The extra volume also compensates for maternal loss during delivery. The average blood loss with a vaginal delivery is 500–600mL, and 700–1000mL during a caesarean section (CS).

Red blood cells

See Fig. 3.1.

- Red blood cell (RBC) mass increases by approximately 33%. In early pregnancy, plasma volume increases faster than RBC volume and this creates a 'physiological' anaemia.
- The haematocrit falls until the end of the second trimester, when the increase in RBCs starts to equal that of the plasma volume. The haematocrit then stabilizes or may increase slightly nearer term.

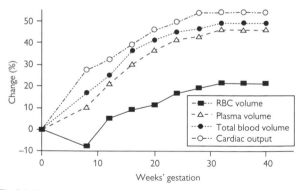

Fig. 3.1 Blood volume and cardiac output changes in pregnancy.

This figure was published in *BJA CEPD Reviews*, 3, Heidmann BH and McClure JH, Changes in maternal physiology during pregnancy, pp. 65–68. Copyright The British Journal of Anaesthesia Ltd. 2003, with permission from Elsevier.

Haemodynamic changes in pregnancy

- There is a progressive fall in systemic vascular resistance (SVR) of up to 40%: this causes a decrease in mean arterial pressure (MAP), which is most significant at the end of the first trimester.
- The average SVR in pregnancy is two-thirds that of non-pregnant woman.
- There is an initial 5–15mmHg decrease in diastolic BP, before it starts to rise to non-pregnant levels at term. The systolic BP remains unchanged throughout pregnancy.
- Heart rate increases from ~72 to 85 beats/min (bpm) and stroke volume (SV) increases by up to 30%. This combined with the reduction in SVR increases cardiac output (CO).
- By 24 weeks gestation CO reaches a maximum of 50% above non-pregnant levels (see Table 3.1). This is sustained until term, except in the supine position during the third trimester when it falls as a consequence of the gravid uterus compressing the inferior vena cava (IVC), reducing venous return (VR).
- CO increases further during labour, even with effective epidural analgesia. It peaks immediately after delivery as a result of uteroplacental transfusion into the maternal intravascular volume. It is during this period, when the preload and afterload of the heart are changing rapidly, that women with impaired cardiac function are at greatest risk.
- Left ventricular wall thickness and mass increase progressively throughout pregnancy by up to 30% and 50%, respectively.
- CO returns to almost pre-pregnancy levels 2 weeks after delivery.

Aorto-caval compression

Illustrated in Fig. 3.2.

- Uteroplacental blood flow is not auto-regulated and is dependent upon uterine BP.
- Aorto-caval occlusion occurs when the gravid uterus rests on the aorta and IVC. The reduction in VR is partially compensated for by an increase in distal venous pressure forcing blood through the compressed IVC and collateral veins. This is in part regulated by the autonomic nervous system.
- Even in the absence of maternal hypotension, placental blood supply may be compromised in the supine position. From 20 weeks gestation, a left lateral tilt should always be maintained.
- The severity of this effect depends upon:
  - Patient position: in the supine position 5–8% of pregnant women experience a substantial drop in BP (supine hypotension syndrome).
  - Gestation: IVC compression develops as early as 13 weeks gestation and is maximal at 36–38 weeks.
  - Uterine size: aorto-caval compression is increased in multiple pregnancies and polyhydramnios.
  - Systemic BP.
  - Presence of a sympathetic block.

- In the unanaesthetized state, most women are able to compensate for the decrease in SV by increasing SVR and heart rate. There are also alternative venous pathways; the paravertebral and azygos systems, that will continue to fill the heart.
- During anaesthesia, these compensatory mechanisms are reduced or abolished and significant hypotension may rapidly develop.

Haemodynamic changes during labour
- In labour, between uterine contractions, CO increases from pre-labour values by ~10% during the early first stage, 25% during late first stage, and 40% during the second stage.
- These changes result from increased SV with minimal change in heart rate. Systolic and diastolic BPs also rise.
- A progressive rise in sympathetic nervous system activity, which peaks at the time of delivery, accounts for these changes by increasing myocardial contractility, SVR, and VR. Central venous pressure (CVP) also rises.
- CO and SVR increase by a further 15–25% during contractions, with lesser increases of 10–15% with effective analgesia.

Haemodynamic changes during the puerperium
- There is a state of relative hypervolaemia and an increase in VR following a vaginal delivery.
- This results from the relief of caval compression, a reduction of maternal vascular capacitance, and uteroplacental transfusion.
- CVP rises, and SV and CO increase by as much as 75% above pre-delivery values.
- Mothers with significant cardiac disease are at increased risk during this period.

Distribution of the increased cardiac output
- There is an increased blood flow to the uterus, kidneys, and skin.
- Uterine blood flow is ~10–12% of CO. Mammary artery blood flow increases early in pregnancy causing breast tenderness and swelling.
- Flow to the liver and brain remains unchanged.

Fluid balance during pregnancy
- Arterial dilatation creates a relatively 'under-filled' state, which stimulates the renin–angiotensin–aldosterone system, resulting in sodium and water retention throughout pregnancy. This leads to a 6–8L rise in total extracellular fluid volume.
- An increase in plasma volume is apparent by 6 weeks gestation and continues until week 32, when it is 40% (~1.2L) above non-pregnant levels.

- Furthermore, shortly after conception, the osmotic threshold for thirst falls and plasma osmolality drops by 10mosmol/kg. A concomitant fall in the threshold for secretion of antidiuretic hormone (arginine vasopressin) prevents a water diuresis and sustains low plasma osmolality until term.
- During the second half of pregnancy, placental production of vasopressinase increases maternal antidiuretic hormone degradation, but plasma antidiuretic hormone levels remain stable as pituitary secretion of antidiuretic hormone increases 4-fold.
- Plasma atrial natriuretic peptide levels are normal until the second trimester, when they rise by ~40%.

Cardiac size/position/ECG
- The heart changes both in size and position which can lead to electrocardiograph (ECG) changes.
- The heart is enlarged due to both chamber dilation and hypertrophy. Dilation across the tricuspid valve can initiate mild regurgitation, resulting in a normal grade I or II systolic murmur.
- Upward displacement of the diaphragm by the enlarged uterus causes the heart to shift to the left and anteriorly, so that the apex beat is moved outward and upward.
- These changes lead to common ECG findings of left axis deviation, sagging of ST segments, and frequent T wave inversion or flattening in lead III.

Clinical implications of cardiovascular changes
- Despite the increased workload of the heart during pregnancy and labour, healthy women have no impairment.
- In contrast, in pregnant women with heart disease and low cardiac reserve, the increase in the work of the heart may cause ventricular failure and pulmonary oedema.
- In these women further increases in cardiac workload during labour must be prevented by effective pain relief (including sympathetic nervous system blockade), provided by an epidural, low dose spinal analgesia, or a combination of both, i.e. low dose CSE.
- Since CO is highest in the immediate postpartum period, sympathetic blockade should be maintained for several hours after delivery and weaned off slowly.
- Aorto-caval compression can be very detrimental during pregnancy, especially when the parturient lies supine; left uterine displacement must always be maintained.
- Downregulation of α and β receptors is an additional important factor, which may necessitate an increased dose of vasopressors.

(a)   (b)

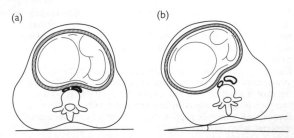

Fig. 3.2 Aorto-caval compression. (a) In the supine position, blood flow through the vena cava and aorta is significantly reduced, causing maternal and fetal compromise. The efficacy of left lateral displacement was demonstrated in 1972. The full left or right lateral position completely relieves aorto-caval compression. (b) Elevating the mother's hip 10–15cm completely relieves aorto-caval compression in 58% of term parturients.

Table 3.1 Summary of cardiovascular changes in pregnancy

Measurement	Change	% Change
Heart rate	Increase	20–30%
Systolic blood pressure	Decrease	10–15% mid-trimester
Stroke volume	Increase	20–50%
Cardiac output	Increase	30–50%
Central venous pressure	No change	—
Systemic vascular resistance	Decrease	20%
Pulmonary artery pressure	Decrease	30%
Pulmonary capillary wedge pressure	No change	—

Respiratory system

Major physiological and anatomical changes occur in the respiratory system during pregnancy due to a combination of hormonal and mechanical factors. Dyspnoea is a common complaint in pregnancy, affecting over half of women at some stage.

Ventilatory changes during pregnancy

See Fig. 3.3.

- The increased metabolic demands of pregnancy lead to a progressive increase in oxygen consumption, reaching almost 20–30% by term. Carbon dioxide production follows similar changes to that of oxygen consumption.
- During labour, oxygen consumption is further increased (up to and over 60%) as a result of the exaggerated cardiac and respiratory workload.
- To compensate pregnant women breathe more deeply, with tidal volume (TV) increasing from ~500 to 700mL, while the respiratory rate remains unchanged.
- Effective alveolar ventilation (increased by ~50%) actually surpasses the body's demand for oxygen and carbon dioxide production (increased by ~30–40%), creating a respiratory alkalosis with a decrease in $PaCO_2$ from 5.0 to 4.0kPa.
- Over breathing is a direct effect of progesterone on the respiratory centre, particularly increasing the sensitivity to CO_2.
- During labour, ventilation may be further accentuated, either voluntarily (Lamaze method of pain control and relaxation) or involuntarily in response to pain and anxiety.

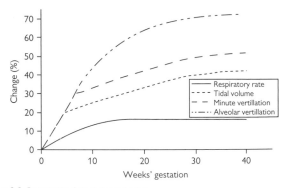

Fig. 3.3 Respiratory changes in pregnancy.

This figure was published in *BJA CEPD Reviews*, 3, Heidmann BH and McClure JH, Changes in maternal physiology during pregnancy, pp. 65–68. Copyright The British Journal of Anaesthesia Ltd. 2003, with permission from Elsevier.

Anatomical changes

- Hormonal changes to the mucosal vasculature of the respiratory tract lead to capillary engorgement and swelling of the lining in the nose, oropharynx, larynx, and trachea.
- Upward displacement by the gravid uterus causes a 4-cm elevation of the diaphragm, but total lung capacity decreases only slightly because of a compensatory increase in the transverse and antero-posterior diameters of the chest. These changes are brought about by hormonal effects that loosen ligaments and flaring of the ribs.
- Abdominal muscles have less tone and are less active during pregnancy, causing respiration to be more diaphragmatic. Despite upward displacement, the diaphragm moves with greater excursions during breathing. In fact, breathing is more diaphragmatic than thoracic during pregnancy, an advantage in the supine position and following high regional blockade.
- Lung compliance is relatively unaffected, but chest wall compliance is reduced, especially in the lithotomy position.

Lung volume changes

- A progressive increase in minute ventilation starts soon after conception and peaks at 50% above normal around the second trimester.
- TV increases by 45%.
- Functional residual capacity (FRC) decreases by 20–30% due to a reduction in the expiratory reserve volume of 25% and a 15% reduction in residual volume.
- Closing capacity can encroach on FRC, increasing ventilation/perfusion (V/Q) mismatch with the occurrence of hypoxia.
- Inspiratory capacity increases by 15%.
- Since dead space remains unchanged, alveolar ventilation is ~70% higher at the end of gestation.

Acid–base status
- The $PaCO_2$ declines to almost 4kPa by 12-week gestation and remains so throughout the rest of pregnancy.
- A gradient exists between the end-tidal CO_2 and $PaCO_2$ in non-pregnant individuals, but in pregnancy the two are equal.
- PaO_2 rises due to the decrease in $PaCO_2$. An average PaO_2 of 13.7kPa persists throughout pregnancy.
- The arteriovenous O_2 difference increases due to increased peripheral oxygen consumption.
- Metabolic compensation for the respiratory alkalosis of pregnancy reduces the serum bicarbonate concentration to ~20mmol/L. Only CO_2 levels <3.7kPa will lead to a respiratory alkalosis.
- Hyperventilation during labour results in marked hypocarbia and severe respiratory alkalosis, which can lead to cerebral and uteroplacental vasoconstriction and a left shift of the oxygen dissociation curve. This causes reduced release of oxygen from haemoglobin with consequent decreased maternal tissue oxygenation.
- The changes are detailed in Table 3.2.

Table 3.2 Ventilation and acid–base in pregnancy and labour

	Pregnancy	Labour	Non-pregnant
Respiratory rate (min^{-1})	15	22–70	12
Tidal volume (mL)	480–680	650–2000	450
$PaCO_2$ (kPa)	4.1	2–2.7	5.3
PaO_2 (kPa)	14	13.5–14.4	13.3

This figure was published in *BJA CEPD Reviews*, 3, Heidmann BH and McClure JH, Changes in maternal physiology during pregnancy, pp. 65–68. Copyright The British Journal of Anaesthesia Ltd. 2003, with permission from Elsevier.

Clinical implications of respiratory changes

- Symptoms of nasal congestion, change in voice, and upper respiratory tract infection may be present throughout gestation.
- The changes in respiratory function have significant clinical relevance for the anaesthetist. Most importantly, increased oxygen consumption and a decreased reserve, due to the reduced FRC, may result in rapid falls in arterial oxygen tension, despite careful maternal positioning and pre-oxygenation.
- Even with short periods of apnoea, airway obstruction, or inhalation of a hypoxic mixture of gas, the gravida has little reserve to protect her against the development of hypoxia.
- The increased minute ventilation combined with decreased FRC hastens inhalation induction or changes in depth of anaesthesia when breathing spontaneously.
- Airway management is more challenging. Laryngoscopy may be hindered by weight gain and breast engorgement. Avoid intranasal manipulation as the swollen mucosa is prone to bleeding.
- In cases with fluid overload or oedema associated with pregnancy-induced hypertension (PIH) or pre-eclampsia, manipulation of the airway can result in profuse bleeding from the nose or oropharynx and tracheal intubation can be difficult.
- Reduced compliance necessitates higher airway pressures to maintain adequate ventilation. Maintain lower 'normal' levels of $PaCO_2$ (4.0kPa) during mechanical ventilation.
- See Table 3.3 for a summary of the respiratory changes in pregnancy.

Table 3.3 Summary of respiratory changes in pregnancy

Measurement	Change	% Change
Rate	No change	—
Tidal volume	Increase	40%
Minute volume	Increase	40%
Alveolar ventilation	Increase	40%
Vital capacity	Increase	100–200mL
Functional residual capacity	Decrease	20%
Total lung capacity	Decrease	5%
Residual volume	Decrease	15%

Renal function

The renal system undergoes marked changes in function during pregnancy due to hormonal effects, the increased metabolic load, and due to outflow obstruction of the ureters by the enlarging uterus. See Table 3.4.

Renal changes during pregnancy

- There is an 80% increase in renal blood flow and a 55% increase in glomerular filtration rate (GFR) by 16-week gestation.
- The rise in renal blood flow causes the kidneys to swell so that they appear ~1cm longer on ultrasonography.
- The renal pelvis and ureters dilate, sometimes appearing obstructed to those unaware of these changes.
- Serum levels of creatinine and urea fall, so that levels considered normal outside pregnancy suggest renal impairment in pregnancy.
- Proteinuria increases slightly during pregnancy, but levels >260mg/24h should be considered abnormal. Aminoaciduria due to reduced absorption is normal in pregnancy and tubular reabsorption of sodium is increased.
- Gestational glycosuria reflects reduced tubular glucose reabsorption and does not necessarily indicate abnormal carbohydrate metabolism.
- Reduced tubular absorption of bicarbonate creates a metabolic acidosis that compensates for the respiratory alkalosis, maintaining maternal pH at 7.4.
- The production of all three renal hormones—erythropoietin, vitamin D, and renin—increases during healthy pregnancy, but their effects are masked by other physiological changes.
- In early pregnancy, peripheral vasodilatation exceeds the renin-aldosterone mediated plasma volume expansion, with BP falling by 12-week gestation.
- The 40% expansion of plasma volume exceeds the effect of a 2–4 fold increase in maternal serum erythropoietin levels, which stimulates only a 25% rise in red cell mass.
- This creates a 'physiological anaemia', but should not in normal circumstances cause haemoglobin concentration to fall to <95g/L.
- Similarly, active vitamin D circulates at twice non-gravid levels, but concomitant halving of parathyroid hormone (PTH) levels as well as hypercalcuria and increased fetal requirements, keep plasma ionized calcium levels unchanged.

Table 3.4 Changes in the renal system

Plasma concentration	Non-pregnant	Pregnant
Urea (mmol/L)	2.5–6.7	2.3–4.3
Creatinine (mmol/L)	70–150	50–73
Urate (mmol/L)	0.2–0.35	0.15–0.35
Bicarbonate (mmol/L)	22–26	18–26

Clinical implications of renal changes

- Normal parturients' urea and creatinine values are 40% less than non-pregnant women. The normal range for urea and creatinine should be adjusted for the pregnant state, as values within the normal range for the non-pregnant state may indicate significant impaired renal function.
- Physiological diuresis during the postpartum period occurs between 2 and 5 days with the glomerular filtration rate and urea concentration slowly returning to non-pregnant values by the 6th week postpartum.

Haematological changes

- The plasma volume increases by up to 50% at term.
- Red cell volume also increases due to increased erythropoietin production, but not by enough to prevent the dilutional anaemia of pregnancy, which causes a 15% drop in the measured haemoglobin.
- Blood viscosity is also slightly reduced, causing a small decrease in cardiac work.
- Normal pregnancy is associated with a demand of 1000mg of additional iron—500mg to increase maternal RBC volume, 300mg gets transported to the fetus, and 200mg to compensate for normal iron loss. Serum iron is decreased and there is an increase in total iron binding capacity (TIBC) and transferrin.
- Platelet turnover increases during pregnancy, and the measured platelet count decreases due to a dilutional effect.
- There is an increase in white blood cell count, peaking in labour.
- There is a decreased concentration in plasma protein due to the increase in plasma volume. This results in a drop in colloid oncotic pressure leading to the oedema seen in pregnancy. There is a ~15% fall in total protein and albumin, with a 25% drop in plasma cholinesterase levels.
- Table 3.5 summarizes all expected haematological changes.

Coagulation

- In anticipation of haemorrhage at childbirth, normal pregnancy is characterized by low grade, chronic intravascular hypercoagulation in both the maternal and uteroplacental circulation.
- There are increased levels of clotting factors (V, VIII, and X), decreased levels of the endogenous anticoagulant protein S and decreased fibrinolytic activity. These changes lead to an acquired protein C resistance in up to 38% of pregnant women.
- Therefore, pregnancy is a relatively hypercoagulable state, but neither clotting nor bleeding times are abnormal.

However, postpartum contraction of the uterus by oxytocin is probably more effective at preventing haemorrhage than any changes to the co-agulation system.

Table 3.5 Summary of haematological changes in pregnancy

Measurement	Change	% Change
Haemoglobin	Decrease	20%
Platelets	Decrease	10–20%
Clotting factors (except XI)	Increase	50–250%
Factor XI	Decrease	

Clinical implications of haematological changes

- Pharmacokinetics of protein-bound drugs are affected due to reduced protein binding.
- There is a slightly prolonged action of suxamethonium due to reduced levels of plasma cholinesterase.
- Due to the hypercoagulable state of pregnancy, there is an increased incidence of thromboembolic disease; thrombosis and thromboembolism remain a leading cause of direct maternal mortality in developed countries.

Gastrointestinal system

Anatomical changes

- The stomach is displaced upwards to the left side of the diaphragm and its axis rotated 45° to the right of its normal vertical position.
- This displaces the intra-abdominal segment of the oesophagus into the thorax in most pregnant women.
- As a result the lower oesophageal high pressure zone (LEHPZ), which normally prevents reflux, is reduced in size.
- The intragastric pressure (IGP) is elevated, especially in the last trimester. Therefore, the barrier pressure (LEHPZ – IGP) is reduced.

Physiology of the GIT

- Nausea and vomiting affect ~60% of women during the first trimester.
- Relaxation of intestinal smooth muscle by progesterone creates many of the gastrointestinal changes in pregnancy.
- Gastric motility and small bowel transit times are slowed, especially during labour.
- The gallbladder enlarges and empties more slowly in response to meals.
- A decrease in lower oesophageal pressure makes gastro-oesophageal reflux more common and there is an increased risk of aspiration. Pulmonary aspiration of gastric contents can follow either vomiting (active) or regurgitation (passive).
- The pH of gastric contents is lower (more acidic) in pregnancy.

Liver metabolism during pregnancy

- The size of the liver and its blood flow appear not to change during healthy pregnancy; hence liver blood flow accounts for proportionately less of the CO as pregnancy progresses.
- There are, however, changes to hepatic synthetic function and metabolism. Circulating concentrations of fibrinogen, ceruloplasmin, transferrin, and binding proteins, such as thyroid-binding globulin increase, while serum albumin levels fall by ~20%.
- Serum cholesterol increases by 50% and triglycerides by up to 300%. The normal ranges for aspartate transaminase, alanine transaminase, gamma glutamyl transferase, and bilirubin decrease by at least 20% from the first trimester until term.
- After the 5th month, placental production of alkaline phosphatase increases maternal plasma levels by up to 4-fold.
- Telangiectasia and palmar erythema are common signs of healthy pregnancy and resolve postpartum.

Clinical implications of the gastro-intestinal changes

- Pregnant woman should be considered to have a 'full stomach', with increased risk of aspiration from the start of the second trimester, or earlier if symptomatic.
- During general anaesthesia (GA), airway protection by means of a cuffed tracheal tube is mandatory.
- Precautions should be taken, even when induction to intubation time is expected to be brief, to prevent regurgitation.
- Preoxygenation prior to induction and no positive pressure ventilation prior to insertion of the tracheal tube is recommended to prevent distension of the stomach with gas (i.e. rapid sequence induction).
- Cricoid pressure (Sellick's manoeuvre) during induction should be maintained until correct tracheal tube placement has been confirmed. This manoeuvre occludes the oesophagus and obstructs the path for regurgitation.
- Aspiration of solid material causes atelectasis, obstructive pneumonitis, and lung abscesses, while aspiration of acidic gastric contents results in chemical pneumonitis (Mendelson's syndrome).

Endocrine system

The principle hormone of pregnancy is progesterone. Soon after fertilization the developing placenta produces human chorionic gonadotrophin (hCG). This sustains the corpus luteum until 6–8 weeks of pregnancy, enabling it to produce progesterone. Thereafter the placenta becomes the main source of progesterone. The placenta also produces human placental lactogen.

Pituitary function

- Once ovulation has occurred and the uterus is prepared for implantation, the maternal pituitary makes only a small contribution to a successful pregnancy.
- The only pituitary hormone to increase significantly during pregnancy (by ~10-fold) is prolactin, which is responsible for breast development and subsequent milk production.
- Pituitary secretion of growth hormone is mildly suppressed during the second half of pregnancy by placental production of a growth hormone variant.
- Placental production of adrenocorticotrophic hormone (ACTH) leads to an increase in maternal ACTH levels, but not beyond the normal range of non-pregnant subjects.
- Free cortisol levels double and in the second half of pregnancy may contribute to insulin resistance and the appearance of striae gravidarum.
- High oestrogen levels during pregnancy stimulate lactotroph hyperplasia, resulting in pituitary enlargement. These high levels, together with those of progesterone, suppress luteinizing hormone (LH) and follicle-stimulating hormone (FSH).
- Plasma FSH levels recover within 2 weeks of delivery, but pulsatile LH release is only resumed in women who do not breastfeed. In these mothers, prolactin inhibits gonadotrophin-releasing hormone and hence LH.

Thyroid function

- Pregnant women should remain euthyroid. There is an increase in total thyroxine (T_4) and tri-iodothyronine (T_3), but high oestrogen levels induce hepatic synthesis of thyroxine-binding globulin (TBG). Free T_4 and T_3 therefore remain unchanged.
- Increased renal clearance of iodine and loss to the fetus create a state of relative iodine deficiency. In geographical areas where dietary iodine intake is low, pregnancy stimulates growth of thyroid goitres.
- Placental hCG shares structural similarities with thyroid-stimulating hormone (TSH) and has weak TSH-like activity. Although hCG rarely stimulates free T_4 levels into the thyrotoxic range, trophoblastic disease, and hyperemesis gravidarum are associated with high hCG levels and can lead to hyperthyroxinaemia. In these circumstances, the mother remains clinically euthyroid.
- The basal metabolic rate (BMR) increases to 15–20% above normal.
- There is lowered T_3 uptake during pregnancy.
- TSH does not cross the placenta.

Calcium metabolism

- Pregnancy and lactation are associated with an increased in calcium demand, and there is an increased loss of urinary calcium. These factors necessitate a 2-fold increase in vitamin D-mediated gut absorption of calcium.
- PTH is reduced in pregnancy, but PTH-related peptide is produced by the placenta and has a compensatory role in maintaining calcium balance.

Carbohydrate metabolism

- The islets of Langerhans and β-cells increase in number during pregnancy as does the number of receptor sites for insulin.
- During the first trimester women are more sensitive to insulin than when non-pregnant.
- From 20-week gestation, insulin resistance develops and women in the second half of pregnancy respond to a glucose load by producing more insulin with less effect.
- Obese women who are already insulin resistant are more likely to develop gestational diabetes.
- Hormones that might mediate this insulin resistance include cortisol, progesterone, oestrogen, and human placental lactogen (a growth hormone-like protein).
- Placental production of human placental lactogen coincides temporarily with insulin resistance.

Central nervous system

The central and peripheral nervous system undergo significant changes during pregnancy.

- There are substantial pressure and volume changes in the epidural and subarachnoid spaces, which have important effects on the spread of local anaesthesic (LA) solutions.
- This is in part due to the engorgement of the epidural veins due to aorto-caval compression, and also Valsalva manoeuvre, when pushing in labour.
- This leads to a reduction in the volume available for the spread of LA in the vertebral canal. Less LA volume is required to produce the same effect in pregnancy compared with the non-pregnant state.
- In addition, the nerve tissue is more sensitive to a specific concentration of LA, an effect mediated via increased levels of oestrogen and progesterone.
- Cannulation of an epidural vein when performing epidural catheter insertion (bloody tap) is more common.
- The constituents of cerebral spinal fluid (CSF) do not change during pregnancy but its pressures are high due to reduced capacitance.
- Between contractions, the CSF pressure is ~28mmHg, but during contractions this may rise to as much as 70mmHg. It is therefore advised not to advance an epidural needle or insert an epidural catheter during a contraction, for risk of puncturing the dura and subsequent expulsion of CSF at a high pressure.
- The increased concentrations of progesterone and endogenous opioids (β-endorphin especially) are the most likely explanation for the observed reduction in minimum alveolar concentration (MAC) for volatile anaesthetic agents.
- There is a similar increase in sensitivity to opioids, sedatives, and other GA drugs.
- Emotional changes during pregnancy are common. Reduced cognitive ability and memory loss have been demonstrated. Depression, both antenatally and in the postnatal period, is well recognized.

Summary of physiological changes relating to anaesthesia

The hormonal changes that occur from very early on in pregnancy cause a complex series of physiological and anatomical changes that affect every system of the body. To illustrate how all these changes may alter or affect anaesthetic management, it is useful to classify them in terms of GA and regional anaesthesia.

General anaesthesia
- Careful attention to the assessment of the airway and any necessary preparation to deal with a potentially difficult airway in the preoperative period.
- Tracheal intubation—increased risk of failed intubation, a smaller tracheal tube required, increased risk of trauma with nasotracheal intubation and increased risk of pulmonary aspiration of gastric contents.
- Maternal oxygenation—increased physiological shunt when supine, increased rate of decline of PaO_2 during apnoea.
- Preoxygenation is essential and should be with a tight-fitting mask for at least 3 minutes.
- When positioning the patient on the operating table, remember to practice left uterine displacement, using either left tilt of between 15 and 30° on the table or a wedge under the right buttock to minimize aorto-caval compression.
- Rapid sequence induction with the application of cricoid pressure is mandatory.
- Intubation may be difficult and so adjuncts for difficult intubation should be available.
- The trained anaesthetic assistant should be careful when applying cricoid pressure if there is a left tilt on the operating table. The temptation to exert cricoid pressure vertically downwards can distort the view at laryngoscopy.
- Once the airway is secured, ventilation should be aimed at keeping the $PaCO_2$ in the normal range for pregnancy.
- There is an increased sensitivity to opioids, sedatives, and other GA drugs. The MAC of volatile anaesthetic is slightly reduced.
- Volatile agents cause relaxation of the uterus (uterine atony) and this may result in significant haemorrhage after delivery of the foetus.
- There is decreased sensitivity to endogenous and exogenous catecholamines. Therefore, if vasopressors are required to maintain adequate BP, the necessary dose may be increased.
- Extubation should be done with the patient fully awake in the lateral position, to reduce the risk of aspiration of gastric contents.

Regional anaesthesia

- There is an increased lumbar lordosis and thoracic kyphosis.
- There is a tendency towards a head-down tilt in the lateral position because of greater hip than shoulder dimensions.
- These factors lead to increased rostral subarachnoid spread of LA solution when injected in the lateral position.
- The subarachnoid dose requirement is reduced (~25%).
- There is increased sensitivity to LA agents.

Further reading

Gaiser R. Physiologic changes of pregnancy. In: Chestnut DH, ed. *Obstetric Anaesthesia: Principles and Practice*, 5th edn. Mosby, 2014, 15–38.

Wilkey AD, Millns JP. Pregnancy and fetal physiology. In: Hutton P, ed. *Fundamentals Principles and Practice of Anaesthesia*. Martin Dunitz, 2002, 563–565.

Maternal pathophysiology

Korede Adekanye and Abrie Theron

Principles of managing cardiac disease

Overview of cardiac disease

Cardiac disease is the most common cause of indirect maternal death and a leading cause of maternal death in the UK. Women with cardiac disease during pregnancy require specialist assessment and management during pregnancy, childbirth, and in the postpartum period.

Cardiac disease affecting pregnancy falls into three categories:
- Known pre-existing cardiac disease before pregnancy.
- Known pre-existing risk factors for developing cardiac disease during pregnancy, e.g. heavy smoker, strong family history of ischaemic heart disease.
- A condition arises during pregnancy when there were no known risk factors, e.g. peripartum cardiomyopathy.

There are two distinct management challenges:

Women with previously diagnosed cardiac disease
- All women should be risk assessed and receive pre-pregnancy counselling from an experienced cardiologist or obstetrician.
- All should be seen early in pregnancy and regularly thereafter by an appropriate multidisciplinary team (cardiologist, obstetrician, and anaesthetist), who can formulate a management plan for pregnancy and delivery.

Women who develop cardiac disease during pregnancy
- Surveillance should be in place to identify those women with risk factors for developing cardiac disease.
- Surveillance should also identify early symptoms and signs of the disease progression in women who develop a cardiac condition, in order to promptly institute treatment.
- When acquired cardiac disease presents, a multidisciplinary management approach is essential.

Antenatal assessment
See Chapter 5, pp. 138–141.
- Careful functional assessment and adherence to the correct New York Heart Association (NYHA) classification will help identify women at risk.
- High risk women must have early multidisciplinary care.

Principles of analgesia and anaesthesia
- There remains controversy over the preferred mode of delivery for patients with high risk cardiac conditions:
  - Elective CS allows delivery on a planned date, and avoids an unplanned, emergency CS, with higher risk.
  - In general, labour is haemodynamically more stable than operative delivery, particularly if a low dose epidural is in place.
  - Decisions for mode of delivery should be influenced more by obstetric considerations than by the cardiac disease.
  - Regular assessment by an experienced multidisciplinary team is essential. If there is evidence of significant disease progression during pregnancy, either symptomatically or on echocardiogram findings, delivery should be expedited.

- If regional anaesthesia is chosen for operative delivery:
  - A rapid onset sympathetic block with haemodynamic instability following a single-shot spinal technique is undesirable.
  - Incremental epidural anaesthesia provides greatest haemodynamic stability.
  - An alternative is a CSE technique, with a low initial spinal dose (5–7.5mg 0.5% heavy bupivacaine + opioid), followed by gradual incremental epidural extension, titrated against block height and invasive BP.
- Invasive monitoring should follow a careful risk/benefit analysis:
  - Intra-arterial cannulation has a low complication rate and is useful for accurately monitoring changes in BP.
  - Although central venous catheters (and pulmonary artery catheters) may provide useful information in some conditions regarding cardiac filling pressures and allow for infusion of cardio-active drugs, they are difficult to insert in a pregnant woman with cardiac disease, as they may not tolerate a head-down position. The information provided may be difficult to interpret in complex congenital heart conditions and will confer an increased risk of infection and air embolism.
  - Insertion of an IV long line in the antecubital fossa is an alternative method for measuring central venous pressure (CVP). It is usually better tolerated and is likely to be inserted easily because of the associated vasodilatation in pregnancy.
- Meticulous care should be taken to avoid aorto-caval compression.
- Care should be taken with the use of oxytocin as it causes vasodilatation, particularly when given as a rapid bolus.
- If the patient is on heparin, the timing of regional anaesthesia in relation to the administration of the heparin is very important.
- Patients may be prone to develop complex cardiac dysrhythmias. Cardiology advice on management should be sought in advance.

Myocardial disease

Recent reports of the Confidential Enquiry into Maternal Morbidity and Mortality demonstrated an increase in deaths resulting from acquired cardiac disease, in particular ischaemic heart disease (IHD) and sudden arrhythmic death syndrome. This has been attributed to an increased maternal age, maternal obesity, other known risk factors, and improved recognition of cardiac pathology during autopsy. The number of deaths related to IHD is set to increase further.

Ventricular failure

- Understanding ventricular failure is easier when considering the dynamic relationships between pressure and volume. See Fig. 4.1a–e.
- In a normal heart the end-systolic pressure–volume relationship is relatively steep, while for a failing heart it is flatter.
- The end-diastolic pressure–volume relationship is flatter for a normal heart compared with a failing heart.
- A failing heart responds to changes in vascular resistance by smaller changes in systolic pressure, larger increases in diastolic pressure, and decreases in SV and CO, compared to a normal heart.
- Drugs which impair the inotropic state of the myocardium have more effect in a failing heart than a normal heart.
- The failing heart also has a greater potential for self-perpetuating myocardial depression in the presence of poor coronary perfusion.

Right ventricular failure (RVF)

The right ventricle (RV) fails when there is pressure or volume overload, or myocardial disease. RVF is associated with enlargement of the liver, peripheral oedema, and pleural effusion.

Aetiology
- Pulmonary hypertension.
- Pulmonary valve stenosis.
- RV and tricuspid valve pathology.
- Right ventricular infarction.
- Right ventricular cardiomyopathy.
- Diseases of the pericardium.

Pathophysiology
- Acute RVF may be precipitated by hypoxia and/or hypercapnia. Short episodes of hypoxia associated with difficult intubation or inadequate ventilation during recovery from anaesthesia, can precipitate acute pulmonary arteriolar constriction.
- As the pericardium is relatively non-compliant, acute right ventricular dilatation caused by pulmonary hypertension may precipitate leftward shift of the interventricular septum, so that failure of left ventricular filling complicates right ventricular ejection.
- In patients with severe pulmonary hypertension and right ventricular hypertrophy (cor pulmonale), RV function may be acutely deranged if systemic arterial pressure decreases, causing reduced coronary perfusion pressure (CPP) to the RV with ischaemia.

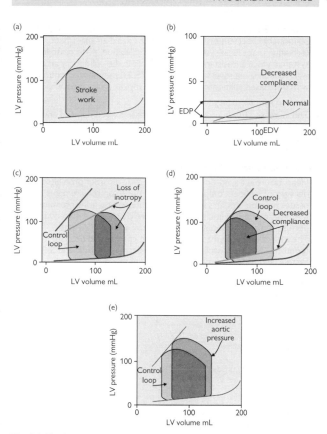

Fig. 4.1 The dynamic pressure and volume relationships in normal and dysfunctional ventricles. (a) SW ≈ SV × MAP. The normal end-diastolic pressure volume relationship (EDPVR) lower curve and end-systolic pressure volume relationship (ESPVR) upper curve. (b) The position of the end-diastolic pressure (EDP) on the EDPVR as compliance decreases, i.e. an upward / leftward shift in the EDPV curve. (c) A downward shift towards the right of the ESPV curve, i.e. the negative effect of poor contractility on the ESPVR (ventricular systolic dysfunction). (d) Diastolic dysfunction. Pathological conditions such as ischaemic heart disease and ventricular hypertrophy shift the EDPVR up to the left. (e) The effect of increasing afterload on the ventricular EDPVR and ESPVR.

- When RVF is associated with a ventricular septal defect (VSD) and pulmonary hypertension, it is important to avoid an anaesthetic technique that causes systemic arteriolar dilatation. A decrease in systemic vascular resistance relative to that in the pulmonary arteries will result in shunt reversal through the VSD (Eisenmenger syndrome), with decreased pulmonary blood flow, hypoxia, and acute RVF.

Interaction with pregnancy
- The increased CO in pregnancy will increase oxygen demand and increase the risk of ischaemia and failure.
- A fall in SVR may increase a right to left shunt, increasing hypoxia and worsening right ventricular failure.

Left ventricular failure (LVF)
- Heart failure is a syndrome in which a cardiac disorder prohibits the delivery of sufficient output to meet the perfusion requirements of tissues metabolism. This may occur despite normal filling pressure.
- It is characterized by multisystem adaptive changes and inadequacy in perfusion may be associated with both low and high CO states.
- The reduction in CO that underlies these changes can be systolic (contractility) and diastolic (compliance, decreased filling, and SV). Systolic and diastolic dysfunction are commonly related.
- Diastolic dysfunction is associated with severe pre-eclampsia.
- Heart failure associated with an elevated CO is most commonly seen in hypermetabolic states, which are typically associated with a low SVR. Examples include pregnancy, anaemia, and thyrotoxicosis.

Aetiology
- IHD/coronary artery disease (CAD).
- Cardiomyopathy:
  - Peripartum.
  - Non-peripartum (idiopathic, alcohol, myocarditis, familial).
- Hypertension.
- Severe anaemia.
- Sepsis.
- Hypo- or hyperthyroidism.
- Drugs (β-blockers, Ca^{2+} channel blockers, antiarrhythmic drugs, and chemotherapy).

Pathophysiology
- In compensated heart failure, arteriovenous oxygen difference is normal at rest, but rapidly widens during stress or exercise.
- Mechanisms of compensation include increasing preload and sympathetic tone, activation of the renin–angiotensin–aldosterone system, releasing arginine vasopressin and ventricular hypertrophy. See Fig. 4.2.
- An increased preload serves to maximize SV by improving cardiac function (moving up on the Starling curve). An increase in ventricular end-diastolic volume can maintain a normal SV, even when the ejection fraction is reduced.
- Worsening venous congestion and excessive ventricular dilatation cause a fall in CO (downward slope on the Starling curve).

- LVF results in pulmonary vascular congestion and progressive transudation of fluids into the pulmonary interstitium and alveoli (pulmonary oedema).
- Increased sympathetic tone can initially maintain CO by increasing heart rate and contractility, but the increased afterload due to vasoconstriction reduces CO and exacerbates ventricular failure.
- The renin–angiotensin–aldosterone system causes a further increase in peripheral vascular resistance and left ventricular afterload as well as sodium and water retention. See Fig. 4.3.
- Volume overload can maintain a normal resting SV, but cause progressive diastolic dysfunction.

Interaction with pregnancy
- Pregnancy is associated with increased CO and oxygen consumption, increasing the risk of decompensated LVF. The physiological reduction in afterload will counteract this to a degree.
- Acute LVF caused by peripartum cardiomyopathy rapidly leads to decompensation with pulmonary oedema.

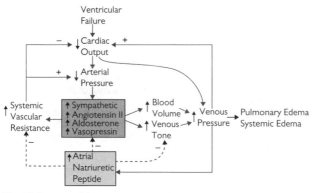

Fig. 4.2 Summary of the compensatory mechanisms.
Reproduced with permission from Klabunde RE, *Cardiovascular Physiology Concepts*, Copyright Lippincott Williams & Wilkins, 2005.

Hypertrophic obstructive cardiomyopathy

Characteristics
- Genetically transmitted cardiac disease with left ventricular hypertrophy and poor left ventricle (LV) compliance.
- Pregnancy can be well tolerated depending on the prenatal NYHA functional status. Pre-pregnancy counselling should be considered for women with NYHA function III as a grossly thickened left ventricle with poor compliance greatly increases the risk of decompensation.
- Reduction in preload and afterload results in poor LV filling (fixed CO state).

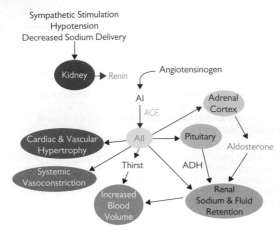

Fig. 4.3 The renin–angiotensin system.
Reproduced with permission from Klabunde RE, *Cardiovascular Physiology Concepts*, Copyright Lippincott Williams & Wilkins, 2005.

Key points
- Regular cardiology assessment with echocardiography.
- β-blockers are frequently prescribed as tachycardia of pregnancy increases functional obstruction.
- Caution with regional anaesthesia due to effect on afterload, although low dose techniques successfully used during labour and CS.
- Can develop LV fluid overload and pulmonary oedema. Give IV fluids with caution and consider diuretics early.
- Invasive monitoring is required.
- Phenylephrine is the vasopressor of choice, avoiding large swings in afterload.

Peripartum cardiomyopathy

Characteristics
- Rare disorder: 1 in 1500–4000 live births with a high mortality.
- Aetiology unknown with poorly understood pathology.
- Defined as onset of cardiac failure with no identifiable cause within the last month of pregnancy or within 5 months after delivery, in the absence of heart disease before the last month of pregnancy.
- Associated with older maternal age, greater parity, Afro-Caribbean race, and multiple gestation.
- Symptoms are fatigue, dyspnoea, pedal oedema, paroxysmal nocturnal dyspnoea, nocturnal cough, new regurgitant murmur, raised jugular venous pressure, hepatomegaly, and pulmonary crackles.

Key points
- A high degree of suspicion is important.
- Low threshold for echocardiogram. ECG may be normal, sinus tachycardia, left ventricular hypertrophy, inverted T waves, or non-specific ST changes. Echo will show new LV systolic dysfunction.
- Chest x-ray shows cardiomegaly.
- Treatment involves salt restriction, diuretics, and vasodilators.
- If the ejection fraction is <35%, low molecular weight heparin (LMWH) therapy is indicated.
- The fetus should be delivered once mature enough.
- Need close input from the cardiologists.
- Epidural good for labour but beware if anticoagulated.
- Regional or GA suitable for CS, dependent on maternal status and anticoagulation.
- If GA, should be a cardiovascular stable anaesthetic with invasive monitoring. Avoid tachycardia and swings in BP. Use phenylepherine as vasopressor if tachycardic. Obtund pressor response to intubation.
- Early critical care referral is essential.
- ACE inhibitors are beneficial in the postpartum period.

Ischaemic heart disease

Aetiology
- Atherosclerosis.
- Severe hypotension.
- Severe hypertension.
- Tachycardia (in association with left ventricular hypertrophy).
- Hypoxaemia.
- Anaemia.
- Coronary artery vasospasm, aneurysm, dissection, haematoma.
- Cocaine abuse.

Pathophysiology
- Myocardial ischaemia is caused by a metabolic oxygen demand that exceeds oxygen supply. The myocardium cannot increase oxygen extraction to compensate for a decrease in coronary blood flow.
- The average resting coronary blood flow is 250mL/min. Coronary blood flow changes in parallel with myocardial oxygen demand.
- The myocardium autoregulates blood flow between perfusion pressures of 50–120mmHg, beyond this range it is pressure dependent.
- Normal CPP is given by the equation: CPP = AoDP - LVEDP.
- An increase in left ventricular end-diastolic pressure (LVEDP) or a decrease in aortic diastolic pressure (AoDP) can reduce CPP.
- A significant tachycardia also decreases coronary perfusion due to a reduction in the duration of the diastolic phase of the cardiac cycle, the period when coronary perfusion occurs.
- The endocardium is most vulnerable to ischaemia as a result of a decrease in CPP.
- See Table 4.1 for balance between myocardial oxygen supply and demand.

Interaction with pregnancy
- Pregnancy increases heart rate, myocardial wall tension, contractility, basal metabolic rate, and oxygen consumption.
- Labour causes a further increase in oxygen consumption.
- Pain increases maternal concentrations of catecholamines, which increase myocardial oxygen demand.
- Each uterine contraction results in an autotransfusion of 300–500mL of blood into the central circulation, which increases preload and may further stress the balance between oxygen supply and demand.
- Oxygen consumption peaks at delivery. Maternal efforts at delivery may result in a 150% increase in oxygen consumption.
- Even an elective CS can increase the CO by up to 50% and oxygen consumption can be 25% higher in the postpartum period.

Table 4.1 Balance between myocardial oxygen supply and demand during pregnancy.

Parameter	Effect of pregnancy
Supply	
Diastolic time	Decreased
CPP	Decreased
Arterial oxygen content	
Arterial oxygen tension	Increased
Haemoglobin concentration	Decreased
Coronary vessel diameter	Unchanged
Demand	
Basal oxygen requirement	Increased
Heart rate	Increased
Wall tension	
Preload (ventricular radius)	Increased
Afterload	Decreased
Contractility	Increased

Acute coronary syndrome
- Coronary artery dissection is the most common cause of death, with 78% of mothers having no risk factors for CAD.
- Consider early angiography if acute coronary syndrome suspected.
- Coronary stenting or bypass grafting is treatment of choice immediately postpartum.
- Tissue plasminogen activator does not cross placenta, also suitable for thrombolysing after early post-partum period although may increase risk of PPH.

Key points
- Consider differential diagnoses: aortic dissection, pulmonary embolism, pre-eclampsia, haemorrhage, sickle crisis, sepsis.
- Use of anticoagulant or antiplatelet drugs will affect the choice of anaesthetic for labour or surgical delivery.
- Cautious use of ergometrine in mothers at risk of ischaemic heart disease.

Anaesthetic management
Labour
- Epidural anaesthesia is beneficial in that it reduces oxygen requirements and afterload.
- A CSE with intrathecal opioids can establish analgesia rapidly without haemodynamic compromise.
- Adequate preload is important—avoid aorto-caval compression and treat haemorrhage early.
- Fluid balance must be meticulously maintained to prevent fluid overload.
- Breathlessness and low oxygen saturation may be an early sign of pulmonary oedema and must be adequately monitored.

Caesarean section
- Single dose spinal anaesthesia should be avoided because of the possibility of rapid haemodynamic changes.
- Use a CSE with a small initial intrathecal dose to establish a sacral block followed by careful topping up via the epidural.
- GA, if required, should be supplemented with a short-acting opioid (e.g. fentanyl or alfentanil) during induction to obtund the pressor response to laryngoscopy and intubation.
- Aim to maintain normal heart rate and BP during delivery.

Post-delivery
- Major fluid shifts and uterine autotransfusion increase the risk of ischaemia and fluid overload.
- The reduction in sympathetic block as regional anaesthesia regresses can worsen this effect.
- The mother must be monitored for at least 24h in a high dependency area with BP, heart rate, urine output, oxygen saturation, and respiratory rate (RR).

Cardiac shunts

Cardiac shunts may be described as left to right, right to left, or bidirectional and as systemic to pulmonary or pulmonary to systemic. The direction is controlled by the left and/or right heart pressures, by a biological or artificial valve, or both. The presence of a shunt can affect left and/or right heart pressure either beneficially or detrimentally.

- They can also be classified into two groups:
  - Congenital
  - Acquired (biological/mechanical).
- The most common congenital heart defects (CHDs), which cause shunting are; atrial septal defect (ASD), VSD, patent ductus arteriosus (PDA), and patent foramen ovale (PFO).
- In isolation, these defects may be asymptomatic or produce symptoms which can be mild to severe.
- Shunts are often present in combination with other defects, which can also be asymptomatic, or mild to severe.
- Some acquired shunts are modifications of congenital shunts—a balloon septostomy can enlarge a foramen ovale, PFO, or ASD.
- Mechanical shunts are used in some cases of CHD to control blood flow or BP. One example is the modern version of the Blalock–Taussig shunt. These women may be asymptomatic and may have relatively normal intracardiac pressures and blood flow patterns.
- Antibiotic prophylaxis may be recommended.
- The presence of a paediatrician at delivery is warranted because of the high incidence of congenital cardiac lesions in the offspring.

Left to right shunts

A left to right shunt is a cardiac shunt, which allows, or is designed to let blood flow from the left to the right heart. This occurs when:

- There is an opening or passage between the atria, ventricle and/or great vessels and the pressure on the left side of the heart is higher than in the right side.
- Or if the shunt has a one-way valvular opening.

Aetiology

- ASD.
- VSD.
- PDA.
- Coarctation of aorta is frequently associated with ASDs and VSDs.

Pathophysiology

- Pulmonary blood flow is increased. The magnitude of this increase is dependent on both the size of the defect and the pressure gradient. It also depends upon the impedance of the systemic and pulmonary circulations, which are the systemic and pulmonary vascular resistance (SVR and PVR).
- Drugs that increase SVR or decrease PVR will increase the shunt.
- If flow is high enough over a period of time, right ventricular hypertrophy develops and reverses the shunt (Eisenmenger syndrome).

Atrial septal defect (ASD)

ASDs account for ~10% of congenital heart disease.
There are four types of ASD:
- Ostium secundum defects (70–80%).
- Ostium primum defects (20%).
- Sinus venosus defects (10%).
- Coronary sinus defects (<1%).

Pathophysiology
- Left to right shunt—the size of the shunt depends upon the ventricular compliance and the size of the defect.
- The shunt results in right ventricle (RV) diastolic overload and increased pulmonary blood flow.
- The left to right shunt worsens after the first few weeks of life due to a fall in PVR and an increase in SVR.
- Chronic volume overload eventually results in increased left atrial, right atrial, and RV sizes, atrial arrhythmias, RV dysfunction, and, rarely, congestive cardiac failure.
- An age-related reduction in LV compliance augments the left to right shunt and is one of the reasons for the progression of symptoms with age.
- In addition, modest pulmonary arterial hypertension increases with age, so the RV is exposed to increased pressure as well as volume overload and may eventually fail.
- LV dysfunction due to CAD and systemic hypertension may increase the left to right interatrial shunt, resulting in a more rapid clinical deterioration than would be expected.
- Eventually ~10% of ASDs develop a right to left shunt secondary to pulmonary vascular disease.

Interaction with pregnancy
- An ASD is usually well tolerated in pregnancy; the major risk is of paradoxical embolism causing embolic stroke.
- Increased shunting in pregnancy is counterbalanced by the decreased SVR, but patients with ostium primum ASD with cleft mitral or tricuspid valves and insufficiency are at increased risk of LVF or RVF.
- Haemorrhage may cause a significant increase in a left to right shunt due to reduced systemic venous return and an increase in SVR.
- Women older than 30 years are at higher risk of developing atrial arrhythmias and right ventricular dysfunction as a result of the increased blood volume during pregnancy.
- Any degree of pulmonary hypertension may worsen due to an increase in CO and the associated shunt.

Ventricular septal defect (VSD)

With the exceptions of bicuspid aortic valve and mitral valve prolapse, VSD is the most common congenital cardiac malformation. It occurs in around 3 per 1000 live born babies. Defects may exist in isolation, in association with other lesions such as coarctation of the aorta, or as an integral part of lesions such as tetralogy of Fallot.

Pathophysiology
- Depends on the size of the VSD and PVR.
- 50–70% of small defects close spontaneously.
- A large VSD permits a large left to right shunt if there is no pulmonary stenosis or increased PVR.
- Large defects allow the ventricles to function as a single chamber with two outlets.
- Resistance to LV emptying will increase the size of any left to right shunt.
- There is a high risk of endocarditis in small VSDs due to a high velocity jet, particularly if the jet is directed towards the tricuspid valve.
- An adult with an isolated uncorrected restrictive VSD is acyanotic with normal arterial and jugular venous pulses.

Interaction with pregnancy
- In small to moderate sized defects, pregnancy is usually well tolerated, but there is a risk of developing endocarditis and heart failure.
- Any degree of pulmonary hypertension may worsen due to the increase in CO and associated shunt.
- Pulmonary hypertension may worsen in subsequent pregnancies–every pregnancy must be monitored, even if previously asymptomatic.
- With large defects, there is a risk of shunt reversal (Eisenmenger syndrome), ventricular arrhythmias, and aortic insufficiency.

Patent ductus arteriosus (PDA)

The ductus arteriosus is a vessel leading from the bifurcation of the pulmonary artery to the aorta distal to the left subclavian artery. Normally, this vascular channel is open in the fetus to allow most of the blood from the RV to bypass the fluid filled non-functioning lungs, but closes immediately after birth.

Pathophysiology
- The consequences of a patent arterial duct in an adult depend on the size of the shunt and the pressure gradient between the pulmonary and systemic circulation.
- The size of the shunt is proportional to the size of the PDA.
- Small ducts have no haemodynamic consequence and are associated with a low risk of infective endocarditis.
- Moderate sized ducts may cause left sided volume overload and the left ventricle compensates with hypertrophy. This may lead to atrial fibrillation and ventricle dysfunction.
- A large non-restrictive duct may cause pulmonary vascular disease (Eisenmenger syndrome).
- If a duct is clinically detectable, i.e. there is a machinery murmur in the left sub-clavicular area, closure is recommended to avoid long-term haemodynamic complications.
- Severe pulmonary vascular disease results in reversal of flow through the ductus and deoxygenated blood is shunted to the descending aorta and toes become cyanosed (differential cyanosis) and clubbed.

Interaction with pregnancy
- Small to moderate sized defects is usually well tolerated.
- Any degree of pulmonary hypertension may worsen due to an increase in CO and associated shunt.

Anaesthetic management

General principles
- These women are at increased risk of infective endocarditis.
- If there is no RVF there are few problems.
- Women with small defects can be treated as normal.
- Avoid hypercarbia and acidosis as it increases PVR.
- Guard against tachycardia and an increase in SVR as this will increase the left to right shunt.
- IV equipment should have filters as there is a risk of paradoxical embolism.

Labour analgesia
- For large or symptomatic defects, early administration of epidural anaesthesia is indicated, as effective analgesia will reduce sympathetic stimulation and a rise in SVR.
- Slow onset epidural anaesthesia is preferred as a rapid decrease in SVR could result in shunt reversal and an asymptomatic left to right shunt may become a right to left shunt with maternal hypoxaemia.
- Patients with a large defect should receive supplemental oxygen, and oxygen saturation should be monitored during labour as even mild hypoxaemia can result in increased PVR and shunt reversal.

Caesarean section with regional anaesthesia
- Women with small asymptomatic shunts can be treated as normal.
- A low dose incremental CSE is a good choice to provide a dense sacral block with a gradual onset of sympathetic block.

Caesarean section with general anaesthesia
- There is a rapid uptake of anaesthetic gases in the lungs due to increased pulmonary blood flow and an acceleration of the equilibrium of gases between tissue and arterial blood, but alveolar concentration/partial pressures are lowered by the high uptake and leads to slow onset of GA (lower Fa/Fi ratio = slower induction).
- A fall in SVR, caused by volatile agents, reduces the shunt.

Right to left shunt

A right to left shunt is a cardiac shunt that allows, or is designed to cause, blood to flow from the right heart to the left heart. This occurs when:

- There is an opening or passage between the atria, ventricles and/or the great vessels.
- Right heart pressure is higher than left heart pressure, and/or the shunt has a one-way valvular opening.

Aetiology
Right to left shunts can be broadly classified as occurring due to:
- Increased pulmonary blood flow.
  - Truncus arteriosus
  - Single ventricle
  - Transposition of great arteries
  - Total anomalous pulmonary venous drainage
  - Hypoplastic left ventricle.
- Decreased pulmonary blood flow.
  - Tetralogy of Fallot
  - Pulmonary atresia
  - Ebstein's anomaly
  - Hypoplastic RV
  - Truncus arteriosus.
- The most common of these abnormalities is tetralogy of Fallot, which consists of tricuspid atresia, pulmonary atresia, transposition of great arteries with large ASD, and Ebstein's anomaly.
- Patients with these abnormalities are strongly advised against pregnancy. If pregnancy does occur, specialist care and further counselling from an experienced obstetrician and cardiologist is essential.
- Termination of pregnancy may be advised, although this also carries significant risks.

Eisenmenger syndrome

Pathophysiology
A chronic, uncorrected, left to right shunt may produce right ventricular hypertrophy, elevated pulmonary artery pressures, right ventricular dys-function, and ultimately the syndrome described by Eisenmenger in 1897 when the right sided pressure exceeds the left sided pressure.
- The primary lesion may be an ASD or VSD or an aorto-pulmonary communication, such as PDA or truncus arteriosus.
- The pulmonary and RV musculatures undergo remodelling in response to chronic volume overload. High, fixed pulmonary arterial pressure gradually limits flow through the pulmonary vessels.
- A shunt reversal occurs when pulmonary arterial pressure exceeds the level of systemic pressure and the primary left to right shunt becomes a right to left shunt.
- At first the shunt may be bidirectional with acute changes in the PVR or SVR influencing the primary direction of blood flow.
- Pulmonary vessel occlusive disease ultimately leads to irreversible pulmonary hypertension and at this point the correction of the primary lesion is not helpful.

Interaction with pregnancy
- These women are often unable to respond to the increase in demand for oxygen during pregnancy.
- Maintenance of satisfactory oxygenation requires adequate pulmonary blood flow. The decrease in PVR seen in normal pregnancy does not occur because the PVR is fixed.

- The decrease in SVR in pregnancy tends to exacerbate the severity of right to left shunt.
- The pregnancy-associated decrease in functional residual capacity of the lung further predisposes to maternal hypoxaemia.
- There is also an increased risk of thromboembolic episodes.

Anaesthetic implications

General principles
- An early multidisciplinary approach with close communication between obstetrician, cardiologist, and anaesthetist is required.
- A senior anaesthetist should be involved in the delivery of any form of anaesthesia during any stage of pregnancy.
- Operative delivery is frequently required because of maternal decompensation in the third trimester.
- SVR must be maintained.
- Aorto-caval compression must be avoided and the intravascular volume optimized to maintain venous return.
- Blood loss must be treated promptly.
- Prevent pain, hypoxia, hypercarbia, and acidosis, which may increase PVR and increase the shunt, causing further hypoxaemia.
- Supplemental oxygen must be provided at all times during labour, CS, and post-delivery.
- Pulse oximetry is very useful in detecting early acute changes in shunt flow.

Labour
- Epidural for pain relief to prevent sympathetic stimulation can be considered if not contraindicated due to anticoagulation.
- There should be a very slow induction of epidural anaesthesia minimizing any fall in SVR.

Caesarean section
- GA can be very challenging and dangerous.
- Rapid sequence induction causes decreased CO and reduced SVR, which increases right to left shunt flow and should be avoided.
- Myocardial depression during a GA should also be avoided.
- A controlled slow induction of GA is the preferred option, despite being associated with an increased risk of aspiration.
- Intermittent positive pressure ventilation (IPPV) reduces venous return, which reduced CO.
- Regional anaesthesia has been described, but the fall in SVR associated with extensive regional anaesthesia will increase the shunt.
- A very low dose CSE and small incremental epidural boluses should be used.
- Phenylephrine infusion should be used to control the SVR.

Blalock–Taussig shunts

Characteristics

Used to palliate cyanotic heart defects with shunts between the subclavian artery or carotid artery to the right pulmonary artery or from the RV to the pulmonary artery.

Key points

- Increased risk of thrombosis during pregnancy, so often on LMWH.
- Need early cardiology assessment and echocardiography.
- No pulse in left arm.
- Can be hypoxic and polycythaemic.
- May need early delivery because of cardiac failure.
- Avoid hypotension and decreased SVR, as these will dramatically decrease pulmonary perfusion.
- Use very careful slow incremental low dose epidural, CSE, or a cardiac GA with arterial monitoring.
- Use phenylephrine as vasopressor.

Fontan's procedure

Characteristics

Palliative procedure for patients with a functional or anatomical single ventricle permitting diversion of systemic VR to the pulmonary arteries. There is no functional RV, therefore pulmonary flow is entirely passive.

- Improves cyanosis and volume overload, but patients have a limited capacity to increase their CO.
- Patients are at risk of arrhythmias and thromboembolism.
- At risk of paradoxical thromboembolism if fenestrated.
- Progressive decrease in ventricular function.
- Hepatic dysfunction and cyanosis will eventually occur.
- Usually anticoagulated.

Key points

- Will require meticulous cardiac, obstetric, and haematological supervision during pregnancy.
- Most will be anticoagulated with warfarin.
- Vaginal delivery is possible.
- Invasive arterial monitoring may be useful.
- Anticoagulation needs to be stopped for shortest time possible.
- Epidural can be used with care and with good fluid preloading, provided anticoagulation reversed.
- Air and particulate filters essential on all IV lines in patients with intracardiac shunts.
- Labour best in left lateral position because pulmonary flow entirely reliant on passive VR.
- Postpartum will require critical or coronary care monitoring.

Truncus arteriosus

Characteristics

Rare congenital cardiac malformation in which only one artery arises from both ventricles. Four types are described. Type IV is agenesis of pulmonary arteries where pulmonary perfusion is provided by the bronchial arteries. It is associated with VSD, right-sided aortic arch, and truncal valve, and the clinical manifestations depend on pulmonary blood flow.

Key points

- Haemodynamic changes during pregnancy, labour, and puerperium cause impairment of balance between pulmonary and systemic blood flows.
- Right to left shunt progressively worsens due to decrease in SVR. Net effect is deterioration of arterial oxygenation.
- During delivery avoid a reduction in SVR (due to histamine release or vasodilator drugs), rise in PVR (due to hypoxia, hypercarbia, acidosis, or high inflation pressures), fall in CO (due to reduced VR).

Transposition of great vessels

Characteristics

- A congenitally corrected transposition: discordant atrioventricular and ventriculoarterial connections. Associated with VSDs, pulmonary outflow obstruction, tricuspid valve (systemic) deformity, and rhythm disturbances. The anatomical RV with the tricuspid valve is the systemic ventricle; the anatomical LV becomes the pulmonary ventricle thus producing a physiological blood circulation.
- The surgically palliated transposition (Mustard's or Senning's) operations used baffles to redirect venous blood into the LV and pulmonary veins to the systemic RV. The systemic ventricle is the RV and is prone to failure. Patients are prone to arrhythmias, baffle leak with cyanosis, and baffle obstruction with SVC obstruction.
- Since the early 1990s the arterial switch operation has largely been performed. The pulmonary and aortic roots are switched so the LV is the systemic ventricle. Patients are still prone to arrhythmias and ischaemia.

Key points

- Regular review by cardiologist looking for early signs of cardiac failure, ischaemia, or new arrhythmias.
- Palliated women may need early delivery, an early epidural analgesia to decrease catecholamine release and decrease cardiac work.

Stenotic and regurgitant cardiac lesions

Mitral stenosis

Aetiology
Chronic rheumatic heart disease is the most common cause of mitral stenosis, which limits blood flow across the valve to a variable extent.

Incidence
It is more common and presents earlier in the Middle East, Indian subcontinent, and the Far East compared with the West. It is twice as common in females as in males.

Pathophysiology
- The cross-sectional area of a normal mitral valve is 4–5cm^2. When the mitral valve area falls to ~ 2.5cm^2, peak early diastolic ventricular filling rate falls and diastasis is lost.
- The main disturbance in mitral stenosis is of LV filling. This has little impact when the heart rate is slow and the filling period relatively long.
- During exercise when the heart rate increases, flow is only maintained by a pressure gradient between the atrium and the ventricle.
- As stenosis increases, the pressure gradient becomes present at rest and the mean left atrial pressure (LAP) rises.
- Patients with symptomatic mitral stenosis have a valve area of 0.75–1.25cm^2 and a pressure gradient as high as 20–30mmHg across the valve during diastole.
- CO falls and PVR usually increases.
- The sub-valvular apparatus may interfere with LV filling by restricting wall movement, reducing SV, and increasing LAP in the absence of any diastolic pressure gradient across the valve itself.
- LV cavity size is usually normal in young patients, but increases with age and end-diastolic pressure may rise.
- Factors that contribute to left ventricular disease include restriction of filling, coronary emboli, distortion of the septum by right ventricular hypertrophy, and overload.

Classification
According to the valve orifice assessed by echocardiography.
- Mild >2cm^2.
- Moderate 1–2cm^2.
- Severe <1cm^2.

Interaction with pregnancy
- Mitral stenosis limits the patient's ability to increase CO during pregnancy and can be poorly tolerated if the woman is symptomatic prior to pregnancy.
- Women who are asymptomatic tolerate pregnancy well.
- The increased heart rate of pregnancy limits the time for the filling of the left ventricle and results in increased left atrial and pulmonary arterial pressures, increasing the likelihood of pulmonary oedema.

- Atrial fibrillation (AF) increase the risk of maternal morbidity and mortality. Both the loss of atrial systole and increased ventricular rate, decrease CO and increases the risk of pulmonary oedema.
- There is an increased risk of systemic embolism.
- Women with previous pulmonary congestion have an increased risk of mortality during and after pregnancy.
- The risk of maternal death is greatest during labour and the postpartum period. The sudden increase in preload after delivery may cause severe pulmonary oedema.
- Hypovolaemia and a sudden decrease in venous return secondary to haemorrhage or the supine position are poorly tolerated and should be avoided.

Anaesthetic implications

General principles

- These women are at increased risk of infective endocarditis.
- Anticoagulation should be discussed with the obstetricians, anaesthetist and cardiologist.
- Perioperative complications include:
  - Acute pulmonary oedema.
  - RVF.
  - AF.
  - Systemic embolization.
  - Subacute bacterial endocarditis.
  - Pneumonia.

The main areas for consideration are **rate, rhythm,** and **preload**:

- Tachycardia decreases ventricular filling time and thus CO. It also increases LAP that could cause pulmonary oedema.
- Bradycardia tends to cause a decrease in CO due to a fixed SV. AF, which may be induced by anaesthesia, will decrease the ventricular filling by ~ 30%.
- Preload: hypovolaemia may result in reduced LAP and reduction in left ventricular filling. Excessive fluid, on the other hand, will cause pulmonary oedema.
- Afterload: a large decrease in SVR may cause severe hypotension as a result of a relatively fixed CO.
- Patients with mitral stenosis have decreased lung compliance, increased airway resistance, an elevated alveolar–arterial oxygen (A-a O_2) gradient with an increase in the work of breathing. Give supplemental oxygen during labour and delivery.
- Invasive BP monitoring during delivery is essential in mothers with moderate to severe mitral stenosis.
- Regardless of the method of delivery or anaesthetic technique, the patient is at risk of developing pulmonary oedema during the postpartum period. These patients require high dependency care during the immediate postpartum period.

Labour
- It is important to provide adequate analgesia with the onset of painful contractions. Give epidural analgesia during labour and maintain it during the immediate postpartum period to reduce preload and prevent pulmonary oedema.

Caesarean section with regional anaesthesia
- Regional technique is preferred for CS. Epidural has traditionally been the preferred method because it is easier to maintain haemodynamic stability with a slow induction of anaesthesia.
- Good haemodynamic stability can be achieved with a low dose incremental CSE.

Caesarean section with general anaesthesia
- If GA is required, avoid drugs that produce tachycardia (e.g. atropine, ketamine). A β-adrenergic receptor blocker and a modest dose of opioid should be administered before or during the induction of anaesthesia.
- Small doses of phenylephrine ensure haemodynamic stability.

Aortic stenosis

Aortic stenosis (AS) represents a fixed obstruction to LV ejection into the aorta. The obstruction is most commonly at the level of the valve itself—aortic valvar stenosis, but may also be immediately above the sinuses—supra-valvar stenosis, or within the left ventricle—sub-valvular stenosis.

Aetiology
- Congenital: A valve with a single commissure, most frequently presents in infancy or childhood. A congenital bicuspid valve due to fusion of one of the three commissures is more common.
- Rheumatic AS develops as the result of commissural fusion and may subsequently become calcified.
- Very rarely vegetations in infective endocarditis cause significant LV outflow tract obstruction.

Structural and functional changes
- The normal adult aortic valve area (AVA) is 2.6–3.5cm^2. Haemodynamic significant obstruction occurs as the AVA approaches 1.0cm^2.
- Blood flow across a stenotic aortic valve causes a pressure gradient between the LV cavity and the aorta, which in symptomatic cases may be > 60mmHg at rest and reach >200mmHg on exertion.
- Stroke work is increased and left ventricular hypertrophy develops. Wall thickness increases. Cavity size remains normal or decreases due to the concentric hypertrophy.
- Hypertrophy initially allows for the generation of high interventricular pressures, necessary to maintain CO through the stenosis, without dysfunction (compensated AS).

Classification
- Grade 1 AVA = 1.2–1.8cm^2 and mean gradient of 12–25mmHg.
- Grade 2 AVA = 0.8–1.2cm^2 and mean gradient of 25–40mmHg.
- Grade 3 AVA = 0.6–0.8cm^2 and mean gradient of 40–50mmHg.
- Grade 4 AVA< 0.6cm^2 and mean gradient >50mmHg.

The classification of AS by gradient rather than by area will underestimate disease severity once the LV starts to fail.

Interaction with pregnancy
- Women with severe aortic disease should undergo corrective surgery before pregnancy.
- Symptoms early in pregnancy may warrant termination, although valvotomy has been described.
- The increased blood volume of pregnancy allows women with mild AS to tolerate pregnancy well, although they are at risk of developing infective endocarditis after delivery.
- AS is well tolerated if the following are present:
  - Peak gradient < 80mmHg and mean < 50mmHg before pregnancy.
  - Normal LV function.
  - Absence of symptoms.
- The increased CO associated with pregnancy will increase the apparent gradient across the valve. The severity and progression of AS in pregnancy should be determined by the AVA.
- Women with severe AS have a limited ability to compensate for the cardiovascular demands of pregnancy. These patients develop angina, dyspnoea, and syncope.
- As AS becomes more severe, the aortic root immediately distal to the aortic valve may start to dilate. This may be associated with pregnancy and should be monitored.

After pregnancy infective endocarditis may develop with persistent pyrexia and/or sudden aortic insufficiency.

Anaesthetic implications

General principles
- The objective is to maintain the basic haemodynamic state by carefully managing heart rate, filling pressure, and systemic BP.
- Tachycardia reduces CO by increasing the dynamic impedance of stenosis. It can also cause myocardial ischaemia and LVF.
  - Treat the cause (depth of anaesthesia, hypovolaemia, etc.).
  - DO NOT GIVE a β-adrenoceptor blocker.
- Moderate bradycardia is normally tolerated as it reduces the dynamic impedance of the stenosis. If severe, use tiny doses of glycopyrronium bromide to avoid overcorrection and a tachycardia.
- Preload must be maintained to ensure adequate filling of the hypertrophied ventricle. CVP or pulmonary capillary wedge pressure (PCWP) should be maintained at high normal levels.
- Afterload reduction will reduce coronary perfusion and can cause myocardial ischaemia.

Labour
- Careful titration of a low dose epidural is beneficial as it reduces maternal tachycardia and avoids excessive straining in the second stage of labour. It can also facilitate an instrumental delivery.
- Any mother with symptomatic, moderate, or severe AS should have an arterial line.
- Maintain an adequate preload by avoiding aorto-caval compression, dehydration, and hypovolaemia secondary to haemorrhage.

Caesarean section with regional anaesthesia
- Moderate to severe aortic stenosis is a contraindication to single-shot spinal anaesthesia.
- Slow induction with an epidural allows titration of appropriate IV fluids and allows the patient to develop compensatory vasoconstriction above the block.
- A low dose CSE with small incremental epidural top-ups gives good haemodynamic stability and a more predictable block.
- Invasive BP monitoring is essential when managing mothers with moderate to severe AS. BP should be controlled with a phenylephrine infusion.
- A CVP or long line is useful.

Caesarean: general
- Thiopental may result in unwanted myocardial depression and should be avoided. Etomidate and a modest dose of opioid is the preferred choice for induction of general anaesthesia.

Pulmonary stenosis
- This is generally well tolerated, although in severe cases it may precipitate right heart failure, tricuspid regurgitation, and atrial arrhythmias.
- Women with severe disease may be asymptomatic, but the increased haemodynamic load of pregnancy can precipitate heart failure.
- Patients with a peak catheter gradient of > 50mmHg should be considered for balloon valvuloplasty or surgery preconception.
- Even during pregnancy, balloon valvuloplasty may be feasible if symptoms of pulmonary stenosis progress.
- Anaesthetic management of delivery follows the same principles as that for other stenotic valve lesions.

Tricuspid stenosis
- Functional tricuspid stenosis may occur with increased flow through the right heart, as in an ASD.
- Organic tricuspid stenosis is nearly always the result of chronic rheumatic heart disease.
- Rheumatic tricuspid stenosis nearly always co-exists with rheumatic mitral valve disease, although its incidence is about 1 in 10. The two conditions are similar with respect to their pathology and the functional disturbance they cause.

- The primary functional abnormality is obstruction to RV filling associated with a diastolic pressure gradient across the valve. In clinically severe tricuspid stenosis this drop is smaller than it would be with severe mitral stenosis and is usually within the range of 3–10mmHg.
- This causes a corresponding increase in right atrial pressure, which leads to ascites and peripheral oedema.

Anaesthetic implications

- Considerations are similar to those for mitral stenosis.
- Fluid overload in right-sided stenotic lesions does not lead to early pulmonary oedema.

Mitral regurgitation

Aetiology

- There are many causes of mitral regurgitation (MR). Any of the components of the mitral valve apparatus may be involved.
- Infective endocarditis is a major cause of MR.
- Systemic lupus erythematosus (SLE) can affect both mitral and aortic valves, causing thickening of the cusps and sterile vegetations (Libman–Sachs endocarditis). They rarely give rise to significant haemodynamic disturbance, but may predispose to emboli and infective endocarditis.

Pathophysiology

- MR results in volume overload of the LV at the end of diastole due to an increase in preload as well as a reduction in afterload due to the regurgitation of blood into the left atrium.
- Pure MR increases LV output. Since the pressure in the left atrium is lower than that in the aorta, the net force opposing LV ejection is reduced. SV may be up to 3 times normal.
- Ejection into the left atrium begins almost immediately after the start of LV contraction. By the time the aortic valve opens, up to a quarter of the SV may already entered the left atrium. CO is therefore decreased despite increased SV.
- LAPs are increased, with the v or systolic wave sometimes reaching 50—60mmHg. These high pressures shorten the phase of isovolumetric relaxation and greatly increase the velocity of early diastolic LV filling, causing a third heart sound.
- Resting LV output is maintained by a sinus tachycardia that is always present when MR is severe.
- Decompensated MR develops when systolic dysfunction prevents effective ventricular contraction.
- Untreated decompensated MR rapidly progresses to pulmonary oedema and congestive cardiac failure.

Interaction with pregnancy

- MR is typically well tolerated in pregnancy. Pregnant women with rheumatic MR tolerate the increase in blood volume and heart rate if in sinus rhythm. The physiological offloading of the LV due to systemic vasodilation is beneficial.

- There is an increased risk of AF during pregnancy, which may cause acute decompensation.
- The hypercoagulability of pregnancy increases the risk of systemic embolism.
- A raised SVR is poorly tolerated by parturients with regurgitant valvular lesions. During labour, an increase in SVR is caused by labour pain, expulsive efforts (Valsalva manoeuvre) and aortic compression by the uterus.

Anaesthetic management
General principles
- These women are at increased risk of infective endocarditis.
- The aim of management is as follows:
  - Prevent an increase in SVR (pain).
  - Maintain a heart rate that is normal or slightly increased.
  - Maintain sinus rhythm. Treat acute AF aggressively; unstable AF should be treated with prompt cardioversion.
  - Avoid aorto-caval compression and maintain venous return, but guard against an increase in central venous volume.
- In contrast to MS, patients with MR may benefit from the chronotropic effects of ephedrine if a vasopressor is required.

Labour
- Low dose epidural analgesia is preferred. It decreases SVR, which assists the forward flow of blood and helps prevent pulmonary congestion. Epidural anaesthesia also prevents the increase in SVR associated with pain.
- Careful administration of crystalloid and left uterine tilt are necessary to maintain venous return and LV filling as an epidural may decreased venous return.

Caesarean section with regional anaesthesia
- A regional technique is preferred for CS. Epidural has traditionally been the preferred method because it is easier to maintain haemodynamic stability with a slow induction of anaesthesia.
- Good haemodynamic stability can also be achieved with a low dose incremental CSE.

Caesarean section with general anaesthesia
- A careful IV induction with thiopental with opioids should be administered to minimize myocardial depression and maintain heart rate and SVR.

Mitral valve prolapse
- Mitral valve prolapse (MVP) is also called floppy valve syndrome, systolic click–murmur syndrome and Barlow's syndrome.
- Myxomatous degeneration affects the cusps, chordae tendinae, and annulus, which causes the valve to bellow into the left atrium during systole. Involvement of the chordae tendinae can lead to chordal rupture and subsequent MR.

- MVP is associated with many medical conditions including von Willebrand's disease, Ehlers–Danlos syndrome, kyphoscoliosis, pectus excavatum, osteogenesis imperfecta, myotonic dystrophy, and Marfan's syndrome—all of which can have implications in pregnancy.

Aortic regurgitation

Aortic regurgitation (AR) increases SV and when severe and uncorrected, irreversible LV disease.

Aetiology

- Pathology of any components of the aortic valve can lead to AR. These include reduction in leaflet mobility, shortening of free leaflet edges, perforation of leaflets, and annular dilatation.
- Chronic rheumatic involvement leads to an aortic valve whose cusps are thickened, with rolled edges and fused commissures. There may be superimposed calcification or thrombosis.
- Infective endocarditis may lead to cusp destruction or perforation.
- Marfan's syndrome, syphilitic aortitis, ankylosing spondylitis, rheumatoid arthritis, Reiter's syndrome, and relapsing polychondritis all can cause dilatation of the aortic ring, which can lead to AR. They all are associated with other problems in pregnancy.
- A dissecting aortic aneurysm involving the aortic root may separate the cusps from the valve ring and the presence of a high VSD as part of the tetralogy of Fallot, may leave the cusps unsupported.

Pathophysiology

- AR is associated with an increase in LV SV. Volume overload results in eccentric hypertrophy and ventricular dilatation.
- Due to the increased volume of blood ejected, there is pressure overload. This results in concentric hypertrophy.
- Ventricular mass is therefore increased, but wall thickness is usually within normal limits.
- In moderately severe AR, the SV is twice normal and in severe cases up to 3 or even 4 times normal.
- The characteristics of ejection are altered in that the end-diastolic pressure in the aorta is low. The resistance to ejection of blood by the LV is reduced and ventricular systole is prolonged.
- These factors together with the large SV, explain the characteristic rapid upstroke and large pulse volume.
- Peripheral vasodilatation also contributes to the large forward SV. All these are features of compensated AR.
- In long-standing cases the LV cavity increases out of proportion to the SV, with loss of the normal myocardial architecture, in that the cavity becomes more spherical, the walls become stiffer and the end-diastolic pressure increases.
- Eventually, LVEDP and LAP begin to increase.
- Pulmonary hypertension and congestive cardiac failure are features of decompensated AR.

Interaction with pregnancy

Aortic regurgitation is tolerated well during pregnancy for 3 reasons:

- Increase in maternal heart rate decreases the time for regurgitant blood flow during diastole.
- The fall in SVR favours the forward flow of blood and decreases the amount of regurgitant blood flow.
- Increased blood volume in pregnancy helps maintain adequate filling pressures.

Anaesthetic management

General principles

- The goals of anaesthetic management are as follows:
  - Maintain normal or slightly raised heart rate.
  - Bradycardia should be treated promptly.
  - Prevent any increase in SVR.
  - Avoid aorto-caval compression.
  - Avoid myocardial depression during GA.
- Epidural or low dose CSE anaesthesia decreases the afterload and therefore regurgitant flow. It is preferred early in labour if a vaginal delivery is planned or for CS.
- The analgesic effects of an epidural during labour prevent undue sympathetic stimulation. This helps in reducing afterload and prevents LV fluid overload.

Tricuspid regurgitation

- Isolated tricuspid regurgitation is well tolerated in pregnancy.
- When associated with other cardiac lesions, the degree of toleration depends on the pathological process involved.
- The tricuspid valve is much more likely to develop functional regurgitation than the mitral valve. It often occurs in association with dilatation of the right ventricular cavity.
- It is particularly common in patients with pulmonary hypertension in mitral valve disease, but may also occur with primary pulmonary hypertension or in the terminal stages of many types of congenital heart disease, particularly those with a significant left to right shunt.
- Severe, non-rheumatic tricuspid regurgitation is being increasingly recognized after mitral valve replacement, in the absence of significant left-sided disease or pulmonary hypertension.
- Organic tricuspid regurgitation may be congenital, as an isolated abnormality or in association with the Ebstein anomaly. See A–Z in Chapter 25, p. 629.
- Acquired tricuspid regurgitation may be rheumatic in origin or result from infective endocarditis of a previously normal valve, which commonly occurs in IV drug users.
- Mid-systolic prolapse of the tricuspid valve can occur in the same way as that of the mitral valve prolapse and is common in Marfan's syndrome.
- The anaesthetic management of the mother with tricuspid regurgitation is the same as for MR.

Valve replacements

Characteristics

- The need for anticoagulation with metallic valves presents a dilemma in pregnancy. The use of warfarin is still recommended despite the risk of warfarin embryopathy (especially with doses >5mg daily to maintain INR (international normalized ratio) in the therapeutic range).
- The practice of substituting heparin for warfarin in the first trimester potentially eliminates the risk of fetal embryopathy, but increases the risk of thromboembolism and the long-term problems of unfractionated heparin (UFH) use, e.g. thrombocytopenia and osteoporosis.
- The use of LMWH is associated with an increased risk of valve thrombosis and is not currently recommended.
- Very close monitoring of INR and antiXa levels (for women who choose LMWH) is essential.

Key points

- The American Heart Association/American College of Cardiology Task Force report in 1998 recommended the use of warfarin until week 35, following which UFH should be substituted in anticipation of labour and delivery.
- Percutaneous mitral balloon valvuloplasty is currently recommended for mitral stenosis, when pharmacological therapy is ineffective during decompensated valvular disease in pregnancy.

Ross procedure

- Replacement of diseased aortic valve with own pulmonary valve and replacement of pulmonary valve with an aortic cadaver homograft.
- It circumvents anticoagulation-related fetal loss, valve deterioration etc., which are associated with other valve replacement options.

Key points

- With a successful procedure, pregnancy can be uncomplicated, but management requires an understanding of the original valvular defect and corrective cardiac surgery procedure sequelae to that procedure.
- Patients with significant multivalvular heart disease require careful preoperative, multidisciplinary assessment, and anaesthetic planning before delivery, to optimize cardiac function during the peripartum period and make informed decisions regarding mode of delivery and anaesthetic technique.

Pulmonary hypertension

Pulmonary circulation

- The pulmonary circulation is unique because of its high blood flow, low pressure (normally 25/8, mean 12mmHg), and low resistance (normally 200–250dynes/s/cm^5).
- It can accommodate a large increase in blood flow with only a modest increase in pressure, because of its ability to recruit and distend lung blood vessels.
- The normal pulmonary circulation is largely passive with its pressures mainly determined by the function of the RV and LV.
- The precapillary arteries of the lungs are sensitive to falls in both alveolar and capillary oxygen partial pressure. At a partial pressure <7.2kPa their vascular smooth muscle cells contract, due to the activity of voltage-dependent potassium channels, aiming to match perfusion of the capillaries to ventilation of the alveoli.

Aetiology

- Primary pulmonary hypertension is a rare disease affecting young women of child-bearing age.
- Secondary pulmonary hypertension:
  - Cardiac diseases: left to right shunt (ASD, VSD, PDA), LVF, and mitral valve disease.
  - Respiratory disease: chronic obstructive, chronic parenchymal.
  - Pulmonary thromboembolism.
  - Pulmonary vasculitides: SLE, rheumatoid.
  - Infection: HIV, schistosomiasis.
  - Hyperviscosity syndrome: myeloma.
  - Drugs: oral contraceptives, amphetamines, crotalaria teas.

Pathophysiology

- Pulmonary hypertension is present when pulmonary artery pressure rises to a level inappropriate for a given CO.
- The hallmark of pulmonary hypertension is an increased PVR with increased work placed on the right side of the heart.
- Pulmonary hypertension is defined as a mean pulmonary artery pressure (MPAP) ≥25mmHg at rest or 30mmHg on exercise.
- Once present, pulmonary hypertension is self-perpetuating. It induces secondary structural abnormalities in the pulmonary vessels, including smooth muscle hypertrophy and intimal proliferation. These may eventually stimulate atheromatous change and in situ thrombosis, leading to further narrowing of the arterial bed.
- Up to 60% of the pulmonary vascular bed can be obstructed before the symptoms of pulmonary hypertension develop.
- The progressive reduction in number and narrowing of the lumen of precapillary arteries, initially cause a loss of capacity of the pulmonary circulation to accommodate the increased pulmonary blood flow of exercise, with a rapid rise during exercise, while the resting pulmonary artery pressure may not be raised.

- RVF, defined as an inability to sustain the required CO, contributes to the exercise intolerance and breathlessness.
- With disease progression, the PVR increases and so too does the load on the RV. CO subsequently falls and RVF ensues.
- With RVF the right atrial pressure rises and results in the development of peripheral oedema and ascites.

World Health Organization classification of pulmonary hypertension
- Pulmonary artery hypertension.
- Pulmonary hypertension with left heart disease.
- Pulmonary hypertension associated with lung diseases and/or hypoxaemia.
- Pulmonary hypertension associated with thrombotic and/or embolic disease.
- Miscellaneous group.

Clinical features
- Unexplained breathlessness, with no obvious heart or lung disease.
- Symptoms of RVF including: syncope, angina-like chest pain, and peripheral oedema.
- General malaise and cachexia of cardiac failure are end-stage symptoms.
- In 85% of patients a loud second heart sound is heard.
- ECG shows RV strain and right bundle branch block (RBBB).
- Chest radiography shows large pulmonary arteries.
- The screening test is transthoracic echocardiography with Doppler estimation of the tricuspid valve regurgitant flow velocity, which estimates the systolic pulmonary artery pressure.
- Echocardiographic evidence of decompensated right heart failure includes a hypertrophic and dilated RV, tricuspid regurgitation, and right to left septal shift.

Interaction with pregnancy
- Pulmonary hypertension is badly tolerated during pregnancy, because of the poorly compliant pulmonary vasculature and inability of the RV to adapt to the increase in CO.
- Pregnancy increases CO by 30–50%, blood volume by 40–50%, and oxygen consumption by 20%. An impaired RV can be pushed into failure by these increased demands.
- During labour there are further increases with injections of up to 500mL of blood into the circulation with each contraction.
- Postpartum intravascular volume shifts from haemorrhage or diuresis are poorly tolerated.
- The greatest risk occurs in the peripartum period, with most deaths between days 2 and 9 postpartum.
- Mortality remains at 30–50% and pregnancy is not recommended. Death results from irreversible RVF or arrhythmias.

Anaesthetic management

General principles
- The primary goals are similar to those for patients with Eisenmenger syndrome: Prevent pain, hypoxia, acidosis, and hypercapnia, which all increase PVR.
- Maintain intravascular volume and venous return.
- Avoid aorto-caval compression.
- Maintain SVR as close to normal as possible as these patients are unable to increase CO when there is a decrease in SVR.
- Avoid myocardial depression during GA in women with fixed pulmonary hypertension.
- Provide supplemental oxygen throughout labour and delivery.
- Oxytocin can lower SVR and elevate PVR and decrease CO. Care must be taken during administration.
- Pulmonary vascular dilators [e.g. epoprostenol (prostacyclin)] have successfully been used in pregnancy, but their use should be restricted to centres with experience in their use.

Labour
- Low dose epidural anaesthesia can be considered, but slow induction is very important. Hypotension should be actively managed.

Caesarean section with regional anaesthesia
- A single-shot spinal is usually contraindicated.
- A low dose CSE may be an alternative if a subarachnoid block is desired. This can still avoid the rapid reduction in SVR that follows a single-shot spinal with a sympathetic block.

Caesarean section with general anaesthesia
- Pulmonary artery pressure increases during laryngoscopy and intubation. Opioids can help to minimize these effects.
- Inhalation of nitric oxide (NO) might be considered as it causes pulmonary vasodilatation.
- Intensive postoperative management is important as there is an increased incidence of sudden death during this period.

Aortopathy

Characteristics

Dilatation of the aortic root and the ascending aorta is frequently encountered in patients with congenital heart disease. Primary aortic dilatation is associated with coarctation of the aorta, bicuspid aortic valve, tetralogy of Fallot, pulmonary atresia with VSD, or truncus arteriosus. It can be a key feature in genetic syndromes with connective tissue disorders, such as Marfan, Loeys-Dietz, vascular Ehlers-Danlos, aneurysm-osteoarthritis, and Turner syndrome. Secondary dilatation of the aortic root is seen after the Ross operation, modified arterial switch operation systemic outflow tract reconstruction, and after coarctation of the aorta repair.

- All are at high risk in pregnancy due to the increased risk of increasing aortic dilatation with the potential of aortic rupture.
- All should have pre-pregnancy counselling and followed up with regular echo surveillance in a high risk cardiac clinic.

Coarctation of the aorta

Characteristics
- Congenital narrowing of a section of the aorta, usually immediately beyond the origin of the left subclavian artery or just distal to the insertion of the ligamentum arteriosum.
- It is associated with a bicuspid aortic valve and aortopathy.
- Most are surgically corrected in childhood and will not be problematic in pregnancy but patients may still have hypertension and re-stenosis and be at risk of aortic dissection.

Key points
- Early echocardiogram and cardiology review is required.
- If uncorrected, decreases in SVR are not well tolerated.
- Avoid bradycardia and maintain left ventricular filling pressure.
- Carefully titrated epidural with opioids is suitable for vaginal delivery limited 2nd stage approximately 30 minutes.
- CS—GA ± invasive monitoring with remifentanil or other short acting opioids useful to obtund pressor response to intubation. Alternative is carefully titrated CSE or epidural anaesthesia.

Marfan's syndrome

Characteristics
Autosomal dominant disorder of connective tissue.
- Cardiovascular problems causing mitral valve prolapse and regurgitation, aortic valve regurgitation and root dilatation, aortic dissection, and aneurysm.
- Musculoskeletal—tall with long limbs and digits, pectus excavatum, joint laxity, kyphoscoliosis, high arched palate.
- Dural ectasia (ballooning of the lumbosacral dural sac) occurs in 60–90% and can lead to unpredictable spinal block.

Key points
- Regular cardiology assessment with echocardiography to identify early risk of increasing aortic root dilatation.
- Treatment with β-blockers for patients with aortic root dilatation >4cm or dissection to avoid sheer stress.
- CS usually recommended if there is evidence of aortic root dilatation.
- Maintenance of cardiovascular stability with careful titration of regional/general anaesthesia to avoid BP swings.
- Close postpartum haemodynamic monitoring—any degree of bleeding or haemodynamic instability should be promptly treated.
- Dural ectasia can make single-shot spinal unreliable: A CSE is recommended.

Arrhythmias in pregnancy

Characteristics

Arrhythmias in pregnancy are common. For some mothers the arrhythmias may be a recurrence of a previously diagnosed arrhythmia or the first presentation in a woman with known structural heart disease. In most cases there is no previous history of heart disease and the arrhythmias can cause anxiety. The majority of arrhythmias that occur during pregnancy are benign and reassurance is usually all that is required. Tachycardia or bradycardia with fainting can occur with symptomatic aorto-caval compression. A careful history will identify this cause.

- The cardiovascular system undergoes significant changes including an increased HR and CO, reduced SVR, increased plasma catecholamine concentrations and adrenergic receptor sensitivity, atrial stretch, and increased end-diastolic volumes. A combination of these and the heightened visceral awareness experienced in pregnancy may lead a woman to seek advice on symptoms that are within the normal range.
- The pregnant state is unlikely to generate a new arrhythmia but such physiological changes may make pre-existing abnormalities more capable of sustaining an arrhythmia.
- Most tachycardia episodes are initiated by ectopic beats and arrhythmia episodes may increase during pregnancy in line with the increased propensity to ectopic activity.

Diagnosis

- Troublesome arrhythmias require an accurate diagnosis with an ECG during arrhythmia or Holter monitoring for frequent arrhythmias so a reliable opinion about the prognosis and treatment can be given.
- An echo is required to exclude a structural problem.
- Exclude systemic disorders that may present with arrhythmias such as abnormalities of thyroid function, pulmonary embolism, and infections in cases of unexplained sinus tachycardia or atrial fibrillation.

Supraventricular tachycardia

Characteristics

Defined as any tachyarrhythmia with an HR >120bpm, requiring atrial or atrioventricular junctional tissue for its initiation and maintenance. Peripartum oxytocic, tocolytic, and anaesthetic drugs can induce supraventricular tachycardia.

Key points

- Care with the use of oxytocin and ephedrine.
- Reduced atrial filling caused by regional anaesthesia may increase arrhythmogenicity.
- Pharmacological treatment if haemodynamic changes, severe symptoms, or sustained arrhythmias.
- Valsalva manoeuvre and facial ice immersion are well tolerated and aid diagnosis.
- β-blockers, verapamil, and synchronized electrical cardioversion have been used.
- Adenosine is safe in pregnancy and labour.

Long QT syndrome

Characteristics

Rare genetic condition affecting the ion channels in the heart, with risk of Torsades de Pointes, ventricular tachycardia, ventricular fibrillation, and death. Symptomatic patients give a history of syncope, seizures, and cardiac arrest. ECG changes and family history of sudden cardiac death may be present. Prenatal treatment include β-blockers, pacemaker, automatic internal defibrillator, and sympathectomy

Key points

- Ensure all electrolytes are normal.
- Continue β-blockers, avoid class Ia, Ic, and III antiarrhythmics, and minimize catecholamine release.
- Automated defibrillators should be checked in the antenatal period.
- Thiopental, suxamethonium, ondansetron, and ephedrine can all prolong the QT interval.
- Regional anaesthesia for labour is recommended.
- Use bipolar diathermy.
- External defibrillator immediately available.

Brugada syndrome

Characteristics

It is an autosomal dominant disease due to a mutation of sodium voltage-gated channel alpha subunit 5 (SNC5A) gene. It can cause sudden cardiac death and arrhythmia can be provoked by physical activity, fever, or pregnancy. Women prior to pregnancy have usually been investigated because of a history of malignant arrhythmia or sudden arrhythmic death syndrome in the family.

Key points

- Stratified low risk women can be treated normally in pregnancy and delivery.
- Stratified high risk women may have an automated defibrillator that should be checked.
- Large doses of bupivacaine can cause arrhythmias and should not be used. An epidural is contraindicated but the very small dose in a spinal is safe.
- Propofol should be avoided.

Automatic implantable defibrillators

Characteristics

Devices used in the treatment of patients with recurrent tachyarrhythmias unresponsive to conventional drug therapies. Risk of associated fetal arrhythmia is small and direct current (DC) shocks appear to be safe.

Key points

- Need full electrophysiological review.
- Pregnancy does not increase the risk of major implantable cardioverter-related problems or result in a higher number of discharges.
- Leave device on for vaginal delivery.

- Consider turning defibrillator off during caesarean section although it is safe to leave on if diathermy is not used.
- Most have an additional pacing mode, which should be left on. Have external defibrillator pad on the anterior chest wall to provide immediate facility for defibrillator should an arrhythmia occur.
- General or regional anaesthesia is safe.

Further reading

Olsson KM, Channick R. Pregnancy in pulmonary arterial hypertension. *European Respiratory Review* 2016; 25: 431–437.

Greutmann M, Pieper PG. Pregnancy in women with congenital heart disease. *European Heart Journal* 2015; 36: 2491–2499.

Billebeau G et al. Pregnancy in women with a cardiomyopathy: Outcomes and predictors from a retrospective cohort. *Archives of Cardiovascular Diseases* 2018; 111: 199–209.

Nanna M, Stergiopoulos K. Pregnancy complicated by valvular heart disease: an update. *Journal of the American Heart Association* 2014; 3: doi:10.1161/JAHA.113.00712.

Francois K. Aortopathy associated with congenital heart disease: A current literature review. *Annals of Pediatric Cardiology* 2015; 8: 25–36.

Sato H et al. Changes in echocardiographic parameters and hypertension discorders in pregnancies of women with aortic coarctation. *Pregnancy Hypertension* 2017; 10: 46–50.

Tanaka H et al. Maternal and neonatal outcomes in labor and at delivery when long QT syndrome is present. *Journal of Maternal, Fetal and Neonatal Medicine* 2016; 29: 1117–1119.

Adamson DL, Nelson_Piercy C. Managing palpitations and arrhythmias during pregnancy. *Heart.* 2007; 93: 1630–1636.

Respiratory disease

General considerations

- Although minute ventilation increases by 40% during pregnancy, this is trivial in comparison to the marked increase (perhaps 10-fold) that occurs during exercise.
- This considerable reserve in ventilatory capacity is not greatly challenged by pregnancy and respiratory failure due to chronic respiratory disease is uncommon.
- The major problem for women with chronic conditions such as asthma or tuberculosis (TB) is the effect of therapy on pregnancy.
- Breathlessness is a common symptom in pregnancy, presumably associated with the 40% increase in ventilation that occurs in normal women. This cannot be the entire explanation as ventilation increases from before 4 weeks gestation, whereas the maximum incidence of onset of breathlessness is at 28–31 weeks gestation.
- Acute respiratory failure is a major cause of maternal mortality with adult respiratory distress syndrome (ARDS) carrying a mortality of ~70%. Much of the practice of modern obstetrics is directed towards the avoidance of ARDS. For example, the trend towards regional rather than GA reduces the risk of inhalation of stomach contents.
- Regional, rather than GA, is indicated in all patients with significant respiratory disease.

Upper airway obstruction

- The upper airway includes the nose, mouth, pharynx, larynx, and the cervical (extra-thoracic) trachea.
- Signs and symptoms of upper airway obstruction may present acutely (e.g. foreign body), insidiously (e.g. decline in conscious state), or progressively (e.g. laryngeal oedema).

Aetiology

Acute

- Infection (e.g. epiglottitis, tetanus, abscess, diphtheria).
- Trauma (e.g. maxillofacial injury, airway burns).
- Foreign body (e.g. food bolus).
- Loss of airway tone (e.g. residual muscle relaxation, myasthenia gravis, depressant drugs, decreased level of consciousness).
- Equipment related (e.g. occlusion of tracheal tube).
- Allergic reactions.
- Laryngospasm (e.g. post-extubation, hypocalcaemia).

Chronic

- Tumour (e.g. pharynx, larynx).
- Scarr-ing.

Acute on chronic conditions

- Infection and inflammation.
- Haemorrhage.
- Trauma.

Interaction with pregnancy
- Anatomical changes in pregnancy include capillary engorgement and mucosal oedema of the upper airway from the nasal passages down to the pharynx, false cords, glottis, and arytenoids. The presence of pre-eclampsia may make the symptoms worse.
- An increase in minute ventilation and airway oedema will make stridor worse.
- Increasing audible stridor must be differentiated from wheeze associated with asthma. If the diagnosis is in doubt, formal flow/volume loop respiratory function tests are helpful.

Anaesthetic implications
- Oedema of the airway makes upper airway obstruction and bleeding more likely during mask anaesthesia and may make tracheal intubation more difficult.
- A smaller diameter tracheal tube is recommended.
- The increase in chest diameter and enlarged breasts can make laryngoscopy with a standard Macintosh laryngoscope more difficult. A short-handled laryngoscope is often easier to use.
- Failure to intubate the trachea is 7 times more common in the term parturient compared with non-pregnant patients.

Asthma
- Bronchial asthma is a chronic inflammatory disorder of the airways associated with reversible airway obstruction and increased airway responsiveness to a variety of stimuli.
- Bronchial asthma is one of the most common co-existing medical conditions affecting women in the reproductive age group, with a prevalence of 3–5%.
- Asthma occurs in ~1% of pregnant women; 10% of these will need hospital admission for an acute exacerbation.
- Asthma is defined by the presence of three characteristic findings:
  - Reversible airway obstruction.
  - Airway inflammation.
  - Hyper-responsive airway.
- Inflammation produces airway obstruction, with the resultant symptoms of cough, wheeze, and dyspnoea.
- A hyper-responsive airway is marked by an exaggerated response to a variety of broncho-constricting stimuli such as cold, histamine, prostaglandin $F_2\alpha$, etc.

Pathophysiology
- Neural imbalance:
  - The parasympathetic nervous system provides the dominant constrictor input to the airways.
  - Postganglionic fibres release acetylcholine to activate muscarinic receptors to contract the smooth muscle of the airways.
  - The sympathetic nervous system acts to decrease airway tone, but sympathetic innervation of the airway is sparse.

- The process of airway inflammation involves the production of wall oedema and infiltration of the mucosa by a variety of inflammatory cells such as neutrophils, mast cells, macrophages, and eosinophils. These cells produce and release mediators of inflammation including histamine, leukotriene, prostaglandin, thromboxane, and platelet-activating factor. Inflammation is one of the factors modulating the course of asthma.
- The loss of airway epithelium leads to increased exposure to constricting stimuli and enhanced airway responsiveness.

Interaction with pregnancy
- There has always been concern about a possible effect of asthma on the outcome of pregnancy.
- Pregnancy generally has a positive effect on asthma, although in a small number of patient's asthma may worsen.
- Deterioration in symptom control is most frequently associated with failure to take usual preventative medication because of the mistaken belief that the treatment will be harmful to the fetus.
- It is recommended that long- and short-acting β_2 agonists and inhaled steroids should be continued and acute exacerbations treated with oral prednisolone.
- Currently, there is limited data on the use of the relatively new leukotriene receptor antagonists (e.g. montelukast and zafirlukast) in pregnancy. The current recommendation is not to start them in pregnancy but to continue their use in women where symptom control is not achieved with other medications.
- It is unusual for patients to have acute attacks of asthma in labour, probably because of increased production of endogenous steroids.
- Prostaglandins given at delivery can precipitate an asthma attack and should be given with caution.
- Wheeze around delivery must be differentiated from other causes such as pulmonary oedema and upper airway obstruction.

Factors improving asthma during pregnancy
- Progesterone-induced relaxation of airway smooth muscle.
- Increased production of broncho-dilating prostaglandins.
- Increased circulating cortisol.

Factors worsening asthma during pregnancy
- Decreased sensitivity to β-adrenergic agonists.
- Increased production of broncho-constricting prostaglandins.
- Reduced sensitivity to circulating cortisol because of binding of steroid hormone (e.g. progesterone) to cortisol receptors.

Anaesthetic management

- Good preoperative assessment with details of the course of asthma in each individual is very important.
- The medical history should include information about the symptoms of wheeze, dyspnoea, and cough.
- Further information should include the frequency and severity of symptoms, the course of these symptoms during pregnancy, and the date of the most recent flare-up.
- Patients who suffer frequent, severe exacerbations are at increased risk. Look for signs of an acute exacerbation: tachypnoea, pulsus paradoxus, and the use of accessory muscles.
- Chest x-ray, arterial blood gas, and lung function tests should be done routinely.
- The goals of analgesia for labour and delivery in asthmatic women include provision of pain relief, a reduction in the stimulus to hyperpnoea and prevention of maternal stress.
- Optimal analgesia is essential in patients who report exacerbations due to stress and exercise. Epidural for labour during the first stage provides continuous pain relief and reduces the stimulation for hyperventilation. It can also be topped up for a CS.
- Regional anaesthesia has a definite advantage over a GA as it avoids the initiation and exacerbation of a reactive airway during airway instrumentation, reducing the incidence of bronchospasm.
- GA for asthmatic patients undergoing CS requires considerations for preventing aspiration and intraoperative and postoperative bronchospasm.
- Rapid sequence induction may be accomplished using thiopental or propofol. The latter provides better protection against bronchospasm associated with tracheal intubation in asthmatic patients.
- Bronchodilators can be used prophylactically prior to induction or in the event of bronchospasm.
- In the unlikely event of an attack severe enough to require ventilation, maternal hypoxaemia should be avoided because of the associated severe fetal hypoxaemia, as should hypocapnia (PCO_2 <2.3kPa) and alkalosis (pH >7.6) since these have been associated with fetal hypoxaemia, probably due to impaired placental transport.

Chronic bronchitis, bronchiectasis, emphysema

- These conditions are uncommon in pregnancy.
- As pulmonary hypertension is poorly tolerated in pregnancy, cor pulmonale is likely to be the factor limiting maternal safety.
- The presence of arterial hypoxaemia puts the fetus at risk from intrauterine growth restriction (IUGR).

Restrictive lung disease

Restrictive lung disease is characterized by a reduced vital capacity, usually with a small resting volume and normal airway resistance. The reduced lung volume is due either to alteration in lung parenchyma, disease of the pleura, chest wall, or neuromuscular apparatus.

Aetiology
- Intrinsic lung disease or disease of the lung parenchyma is due to infiltration or scarring of the lung tissue (interstitial lung disease) or filling of the air spaces with exudates and debris (pneumonitis). Pulmonary infiltration can be due to:
  - Known causes: asbestosis, radiation, drugs (chemotherapy).
  - Unknown causes: amyloidosis, sarcoidosis, collagen vascular disease.
- Extrinsic or extra-parenchymal lung disease includes:
  - Chest wall or respiratory muscle disease: kyphoscoliosis, myasthenia gravis, Guillain–Barré syndrome, poliomyelitis.
  - Pleural thickening: tumour, inflammation.
  - Space-occupying lesion: tumour, pleural effusion, pneumothorax.
  - Lung resection.

Pathophysiology
- With intrinsic lung disease the main pathophysiological effect is a reduction in all lung volumes due to the excessive recoil of the lungs compared with the outward recoil forces of the chest wall. Expiratory airflow is reduced in proportion to the lung volume.
- Arterial hypoxaemia in these conditions is primarily due to ventilation–perfusion mismatch, with further contribution from intrapulmonary shunts. The diffusion of oxygen is impaired. This contributes little towards hypoxaemia at rest, but is the primary mechanism of exercise induced desaturation.
- Hyperventilation at rest and during exercise is due to reflexes arising from the lungs and the need to maintain minute ventilation with a reduced tidal volume by increasing respiratory frequency.
- In extrinsic lung disorders of the pleura and the thoracic cage, the total compliance of the respiratory system is reduced and hence lung volumes are reduced. Atelectasis results in ventilation–perfusion mismatch. In kyphoscoliosis a Cobb angle >100° is usually associated with respiratory failure.
- Neuromuscular disorders affect an integral part of the respiratory system-ventilation. This can be impaired at the level of the CNS, spinal cord, peripheral nervous system, neuromuscular junction, or respiratory muscles.

Kyphoscoliosis

- Mild degrees of kyphoscoliosis have no effect on pregnancy.
- Successful pregnancy is possible in patients with severe disease and a vital capacity of as little as 1000mL.
- As in other chest diseases, hypoxaemia and pulmonary hypertension are the limiting factors and some women with severe kyphoscoliosis become exhausted and then hypoxaemic in the third trimester.
- Pulmonary function tests should be performed during pregnancy.

- Any suggestion of excessive fatigue or deterioration in serial lung function tests is an indication for hospital admission for rest and nasal IPPV if this is not available at home.
- Progressive hypoxaemia with or without evidence of foetal compromise is an indication for delivery.
- Labour and/or CS are best managed with the assistance of regional anaesthesia, which reduces the risk of atelectasis. If regional anaesthesia is not possible due to spinal deformity, GA must be performed with the backup of critical care facilities for postoperative ventilation.

Cystic fibrosis

- Improved management means that more women with cystic fibrosis are surviving and are having children.
- Pregnancy does not affect mortality if pregnant women with cystic fibrosis are compared with non-pregnant women with cystic fibrosis. However, 24% of all deliveries are preterm.

Pathophysiology

- Cystic fibrosis is an autosomal recessive disorder where there is an abnormality in the epithelial tissues, especially in the respiratory, digestive, and reproductive tracts.
- The defect is thought to lie in the epithelium's cAMP-mediated activation of chloride conductance.
- The viscosity of airway secretions is increased, causing widespread obstruction of small airways with a resultant reduction in lung volumes. This causes ventilation–perfusion mismatch and arterial hypoxaemia.
- Chronic airway obstruction leads to impaired mucus clearance and increased episodes of pulmonary infection. Recurrent infection leads to inflammatory changes and cyst formation.
- Spontaneous pneumothorax may occur.
- Chronic hypoxaemia and lung destruction may produce pulmonary hypertension and cor pulmonale.

Interaction with pregnancy

Factors leading to the deterioration of pulmonary function during pregnancy are:

- Increased airway responsiveness and obstruction.
- Increased work of breathing.
- Cardiovascular changes such as congestive heart failure and pulmonary hypertension associated with the increased blood volume.
- The deterioration of pulmonary function is dependent upon the severity of the disease before pregnancy.
- Poor outcomes were associated with a pregnancy weight gain of <4.5kg and a pre-pregnancy forced vital capacity of <50% of the predicted value. This group is likely to produce a preterm infant and to suffer increased loss of pulmonary function and increased mortality.
- High quality multidisciplinary medical and obstetric care is essential.

Anaesthetic management

- There should be continuous monitoring of maternal oxygen saturation as there is an increased incidence of hypoxaemia.
- Adequate analgesia should be provided to prevent maternal hyperventilation.
- Continuous lumbar epidural analgesia with a sensory block maintained at the level of 10th thoracic dermatome can provide excellent pain relief and reduce the stimulus for hyperventilation.
- High thoracic motor block should be avoided as this would cause respiratory depression that will further increase hypoxaemia.
- Regional anaesthesia is indicated for surgery, but non-invasive positive pressure ventilation (NIPPV) has been described in patients with very poor respiratory function.
- Regional anaesthesia for surgery avoids tracheal intubation and positive pressure ventilation and reduces the incidence of bronchospasm and pneumothorax.
- Considerations for a GA for CS include:
  - Humidification of gases to prevent inspissation of mucus.
  - Frequent suctioning to prevent tracheal tube obstruction.
  - Allow a long expiratory pause to prevent air trapping. This would help reduce pneumothorax secondary to volume trauma.
  - Nitrous oxide should be avoided to prevent worsening of any pre-existing pneumothorax.
  - Active chest physiotherapy should commence as early as possible postoperatively.
  - Antibiotic prophylaxis as per the sputum sensitivity.

Tuberculosis

- Before the advent of anti-tuberculous therapy, TB caused many maternal deaths, particularly in the puerperium.
- A high index of suspicion is necessary to make the diagnosis in pregnancy.
- Most centres in the UK do not screen for TB in pregnancy (Mantoux testing and or chest radiographs).
- Recent evidence from infectious disease surveillance suggests an upsurge in TB prevalence. There is a very strong association between TB and HIV/AIDS in poorer countries where vulnerable women of childbearing age are still highly susceptible to contracting the disease.

Further reading

Linderman KS. Respiratory disease. In: Chestnut DH et al, ed. *Chestnut's Obstetric Anaesthesia, Principles and Practice*, 5th edn. Saunders, 2014, 1179–1194.
Renton M et al. Pregnancy outcomes in cystic fibrosis: a 10-year experience from a UK centre. *Obstetric Medicine* 2015; 8:99–101.

Renal disease

Renal disease in pregnancy can be broadly classified as:
- Renal disease occurring during pregnancy.
  - Urinary tract infection.
  - Urolithiasis.
  - Hypertensive disorders of pregnancy.
  - Acute renal failure.
- Pre-existing renal disease in pregnancy.
  - Chronic hypertension.
  - Chronic renal failure.

Important physiological changes take place in the renal system during pregnancy:
- Increased vascular volume leads to renal enlargement.
- Dilatation of the renal pelvis and ureters due to hormonal changes leads to decreased peristalsis.
- Obstruction to ureteric drainage at the pelvic brim occurs due to pressure by dilated uterine and ovarian veins and the gravid uterus.

Together, these changes predispose pregnant women to vesicoureteral reflux and ascending infection.

Increased CO and decreased intrarenal resistance cause an 80% increase in renal blood flow and a 50% increase in glomerular filtration rate (GFR). Plasma creatinine concentration >73mcmol/L and urea concentration >4.3mmol/L are considered abnormal. Tubular sodium reabsorption and osmoregulation are reset, allowing the physiological hypervolaemia of pregnancy.

Urinary tract infection

- Urinary stasis and increased vesicoureteral reflux lead to increased risk of urinary tract infection (UTI). Untreated UTI will develop into acute pyelonephritis in ~20% of cases.
- Symptoms of acute pyelonephritis include fever, chills, flank pain, and symptoms of a lower UTI. The most common causative organisms found are *E. coli*, *Klebsiella* and *Proteus*.
- Useful antibiotics are nitrofurantoin (not in first trimester), trimethoprim, ampicillin, and the cephalosporins. The choice of antibiotic depends on the sensitivities of the causative organism.
- If mother has been identified as susceptible she should be screened during pregnancy.

Anaesthetic management
- Regional anaesthesia (spinal or epidural) can be considered, provided the patient is receiving antibiotics and are not overtly septic.
- Epidural analgesia may produce a modest increase in maternal temperature in an already febrile patient.
- Local guidelines should be followed.

Urolithiasis

- Urolithiasis is characterized by the abnormal formation of calculi within the renal calyces or pelvis.
- Supersaturation of minerals, stasis, and acidic urine cause stone formation.
- Most stones are calcium oxalate (70%) or calcium phosphate (10%).
- Pregnancy seems to predispose some susceptible women to multiple and recurrent stone formation.
- Pain can be severe and difficult to manage.

Analgesia and anaesthetic management

- The ureters receive sensory innervation through the renal, ovarian, and hypogastric plexus (T11 to L1 spinal segments).
- NSAIDs, although effective in the non-pregnant population, should not be used in pregnancy.
- IV paracetamol is safe in pregnancy and can be beneficial.
- Opioids may be required.
- Epidural analgesia provides pain relief and facilitates passage of the stone due to decreased ureteric spasm.

Acute kidney injury

- Acute kidney injury (AKI) is a sudden episode of kidney failure with damage occurring within a few hours or days.
- AKI is often undiagnosed in pregnancy and it is not uncommon (1–2%).
- Oliguria intra and postpartum is common and does not indicate AKI unless there is a rising creatinine.
- AKI is characterized by a rapid rise in serum creatinine (>73mcmol/L) and urea (>4.3mmol/L) and is confirmed by a decreased eGFR (<90ml/min/1.73m^2).
- Creatinine levels roughly double for every 50% reduction in GFR.
- Urine output may fall to <400mL/day.

Causes of AKI

- *Pre-renal:* (Decreased blood flow to the kidney): hypovolaemic states such as haemorrhage, hyperemesis gravidarum, and low CO states such as heart failure, arrhythmias, and other diseases of the myocardium. Inappropriate/overuse of NSAIDs.
- *Renal:* (Direct damage to the kidneys): acute tubular necrosis, septic abortion, amniotic fluid embolism, interstitial nephritis (NSAIDs), acute glomerulonephritis, pyelonephritis, HELLP (haemolytic anaemia, elevated liver enzymes, and low platelets) syndrome, and eclampsia/pre-eclampsia.
- *Post-renal:* (Blockage of the urinary tract): urolithiasis, ureteral obstruction.

AKI is unusual in pregnancy and reflects severe underlying disease that requires urgent diagnosis and treatment. Many mothers will require urgent referral and transfer for further management.

Chronic kidney disease

- With effective treatments for chronic anaemia and better nutrition, women with chronic kidney disease (CKD) now can become pregnant.
- The outcome depends on pre-pregnancy:
  - Degree of renal dysfunction.
  - Hypertension.
  - Proteinuria.
  - The underlying renal condition.
- What is considered a normal creatinine in a non-pregnant woman can indicate significant renal impairment in a pregnant woman.
- Pregnancy in a parturient with CKD is associated with.
  - Increased rate of decline of renal function.
  - Increased risk of significant proteinuria.
  - Worsening hypertension.
  - Increased risk of pre-eclampsia.
  - Increased risk to the foetus (IUGR and premature delivery).

Management is complex and a multidisciplinary approach is required with significant input from renal physicians and dieticians.

Renal transplant recipients

- Pregnancy is increasingly common after renal transplantation.
- Outcome is generally good if pregnancy is deferred until 1 year after transplantation.
- The new immunosuppressive drugs are well tolerated and most are thought to be safe in pregnancy.
- If the graft is not functioning well prior to pregnancy, the result tends to be the same as for chronic renal impairment, with renal function decline and increased risk of complications.

Anaesthetic management

This is influenced by the extent of renal dysfunction and hypertension. Uraemic patients may be hypovolaemic or hypervolaemic, depending on the time of last dialysis. Close observation of fluid balance must be undertaken.

Regional anaesthesia

- Hypovolaemia and autonomic impairment may cause profound hypotension following regional blockade.
- Proper rehydration and slow establishment of epidural anaesthesia will minimize the impact of the autonomic impairment.
- Coagulation should be checked before regional anaesthesia is considered.
- Ephedrine and other vasopressors may have a potentiated effect.
- Care should be continued on an HDU/ITU.

General anaesthesia

- If required, the patient should be medically optimized, if possible.
- Airway assessment is important due to facial oedema.
- Fibre-optic intubation should be considered in severe pre-eclampsia.

- Obtund the hypertensive response to laryngoscopy with opioids. The paediatricians should be informed of the potential for fetal respiratory depression.
- An arterial line should be considered for close monitoring and to avoid wide swings of BP.
- Delayed gastric emptying and increased gastric acidity increases the risk of aspiration pneumonitis. Proton pump inhibitors should be administered routinely along with sodium citrate.
- Suxamethonium causes an increase in potassium levels in an already hyperkalaemic patient. Potassium levels should be checked prior to any elective procedure. Have a low threshold to use rocuronium to facilitate endotracheal intubation, especially if there is sugammadex available for reversal of neuromuscular blockade.
- Assess neuromuscular function with a nerve stimulator if magnesium has been used as this may prolong the duration of action of muscle relaxants.
- The sleep dose of thiopental required may be reduced due to decreased protein binding.

Further reading

Bateman BT, Polley LS. Hypertensive disorders. In: Chestnut DH et al. *Chestnut's Obstetric Anaesthesia, Principles and Practice*, 5th edn. Saunders, 2014, 825–859.

Beilin Y. Renal Disease. In: Chestnut DH et al. *Chestnut's Obstetric Anaesthesia, Principles and Practice*, 5th edn. Saunders, 2014, 1165–1178.

Diabetes

Aetiological classification of diabetes mellitus

- *Type 1:* (autoimmune/non-immune) Early onset β-cell destruction, genetic susceptibility and environmental factors are implicated. Ketosis occurs with absolute lack of insulin. Previously known as 'insulin-dependent diabetes mellitus (IDDM)'.
- *Type 2:* Previously known as 'non-insulin-dependent diabetes (NIDDM)' or 'maturity-onset diabetes'. Encompasses a spectrum of insulin hyposecretion and insulin resistance. Ketosis is rare. Risk factors include obesity, reduced exercise, and racial origin.
- *Others:* where the cause is known, such as gestational diabetes, drug-induced diabetes, pancreatic disease, and endocrinopathies such as acromegaly/Cushing's disease.

Metabolic changes in pregnancy

- Pregnancy induces substantial alterations in carbohydrate, lipid and amino-acid metabolism, which have been described as a combination of 'facilitated anabolism' and 'accelerated starvation'.
- These changes appear to ensure the optimal availability of nutrients for both fetus and mother.

Carbohydrate metabolism

- Fasting plasma glucose concentrations gradually decline during pregnancy by ~0.5mmol/L, reaching a nadir in the third trimester.
- Postprandial glucose concentrations increase, despite a rise in both basal and stimulated insulin secretion. This appears to be due to peripheral insulin resistance induced by placental hormones and to the effects of oestrogen and progesterone on the maternal pancreas.

Lipid metabolism

- Plasma concentrations of triglycerides, cholesterol, phospholipids, and free fatty acids all increase during pregnancy.
- The increase in circulating free fatty acids is thought to have an important influence on maternal metabolism, providing an alternative source of fuel at a time when fetal and maternal glucose needs are maximal.

Gestational diabetes

- Gestational diabetes may be defined as 'carbohydrate intolerance of variable severity with onset or first recognition during the present pregnancy'.
- This definition includes not only those women in whom diabetes occurs transiently during pregnancy and regresses after delivery, but also those in whom type 2 diabetes arises de novo during pregnancy and persists long term. Some may have had undiagnosed diabetes for some time and are at high risk of fetal and maternal complications.

Obstetric complications of diabetes in pregnancy

- Early fetal loss and congenital abnormalities occur 3–5 times more than in the background population.
- Proteinuria and hypertension occurs approximately twice as often in diabetics compared with normal women. Serum urate and creatinine concentrations should be measured at every antenatal visit and 24h urine protein concentrations from 24 weeks gestation.
- Although the reason for the increased incidence of pre-eclampsia in diabetics is unknown, a link with glycaemic control has been established and the incidence is reduced with optimal diabetic control.
- Diabetic nephropathy is associated with a rapid decline of renal function.
- Cardiovascular disease must be investigated.
- Retinopathy can rapidly deteriorate.
- Type 1 diabetes is associated with other autoimmune problems, such as hypothyroidism and should be screened for.
- Diabetics are at increased risk of wound infection following surgery and instrumental delivery and antibiotics should be given.
- Diabetic mothers are at an increased risk of operative delivery because of a large baby and other obstetric complications such as pre-eclampsia.

Treatment of diabetes

- Tight glycaemic control is recommended to reduce the risk of macrosomia and other complications.
- Insulin therapy is recommended for all but the mildest gestational diabetic where diet control may be adequate.
- Insulin requirements increase in pregnancy although in the last few weeks of pregnancy this may decline.
- Fasting glucose should be between 3.5 and 5.5mmol/L, and a 2h postprandial level should be no more than 7mmol/L.
- Hypoglycaemia is a common problem because of fluctuating insulin requirements and tight glycaemic control.

Management of ketoacidosis in pregnancy

- Diabetic ketoacidosis in pregnancy is a medical emergency which is best treated by a multidisciplinary approach in particular a diabetologist with an interest in pregnancy.
- It can progress rapidly and usually occurs at a lower glucose levels compared with non-pregnant patients.
- Management principles include aggressive volume replacement, initiation of intravenous insulin therapy, correction of acidosis, correction of electrolyte abnormalities, and management of precipitating factors.
- If starvation, usually from intractable vomiting, is the precipitating cause then IV glucose is required with a titrated increase in insulin and potassium.
- Non-reassuring fetal heart patterns are frequently present and it is imperative to correct the maternal metabolic abnormalities first, because both maternal and fetal conditions will usually improve.

Starvation ketosis in non-diabetic pregnant woman

- Is well described and is caused by the increased glucose requirements as pregnancy progresses.
- The initial presentation is similar to ketoacidosis in a diabetic mother and can cause a diagnostic dilemma.
- There can be a very severe ketoacidosis with a marked metabolic acidosis, usually with a normal lactate.
- Fluid and glucose resuscitation is urgently required.

Anaesthetic management

- Clinical decisions must be guided by logical extensions of studies of non-pregnant diabetic and non-diabetic pregnant patients.
- A good preoperative multisystem evaluation should be carried out.
- Autonomic cardiovascular dysfunction should be ruled out and if present treated with vasopressors. BP should be monitored more frequently during labour and delivery.
- Autonomic neuropathy increases gastroparesis and hence increases the risk of aspiration. There is also a decreased cough reflex threshold and possible obstructive sleep apnoea. The anaesthetist should ensure proper perioperative positioning and padding of the extremities during administration of anaesthesia.
- Epidural anaesthesia has been preferred over a single-shot spinal for CS because of the slower onset of sympathetic block. However, a low dose CSE is a good alternative option.
- Epidural analgesia during labour reduces sympathetic stimulation. This prevents hyperglycaemia and increased insulin requirements.
- Diabetic stiff joint syndrome is common in type 1 diabetics. Limited atlanto-occipital joint movement may predispose to difficult intubation. Look for the prayer sign during airway assessment.
- The stiff joint syndrome is also associated with a non-compliant epidural space. Smaller volumes of LA might be sufficient.
- Strict aseptic technique should be followed during administration of central neuraxial blockade as these patients are more prone to infections.

Further reading

Wissler RN. Endocrine disorders. In: Chestnut DH et al. *Chestnut's Obstetric Anaesthesia, Principles and Practice*, 5th edn. Saunders, 2014, 1003–1032.

Bryant SN et al Diabetic ketoacidosis complicating pregnancy. *Journal of Neonatal and Perinatal Medicine* 2017; 10: 17–23.

Sibai BM, Viteri OA. Diabetic ketoacidosis in pregnancy. *Obstetrics and Gynecology* 2014; 123: 167–178.

Patel A. et al. Acute starvation in pregnancy: a cause of severe metabolic acidosis. *International Journal of Obstetric Anesthia* 2011; 20:253–256.

Coagulation disorders

- Normal pregnancy is accompanied by major changes in the coagulation and fibrinolytic systems. There are significant increases in the procoagulant factors (V, VIII, and X) and a very marked increase in plasma fibrinogen.
- In uncomplicated pregnancy, there is no change in antithrombin concentrations during the antenatal period. There is a fall during delivery and then an increase 1 week postpartum. Protein C levels appear to remain constant or increase slightly, but protein S activity falls significantly during normal pregnancy.
- These physiological changes alter the usual balance between the procoagulants and anticoagulants in favour of the factors promoting blood clotting.
- Fibrinolytic activity appears to be reduced during healthy pregnancy but returns to normal rapidly after separation of the placenta and completion of the third stage of labour. This effect is mediated by placental derived plasminogen activator inhibitor type II.
- These changes in the haemostatic systems, together with the increase in blood volume, help to reduce the chances of abnormal haemorrhage at delivery, but also convert pregnancy into a hypercoaguable state that may carry special hazards for both the mother and foetus.
- These hazards include a spectrum of haemostatic disorders, from thromboembolism through to the many conditions associated with disseminated intravascular coagulation (DIC).

Classification

The coagulation disorders can be broadly classified into:
- Thrombocytopenic coagulopathies.
- Congenital coagulopathies.
- Acquired coagulopathies.
- Hypercoaguable disease.

Gestational thrombocytopenia

- As pregnancy advances, there is a progressively small, but significant, fall in the platelet count, probably due to haemodilution.
- Approximately 8% of healthy pregnant women have thrombocytopenia at term, with platelet counts between 90 and 150×10^9/L.
- These women have no history of pre-eclampsia or immune thrombocytopenia and there is no increased incidence of thrombocytopenia in their offspring.
- Platelet counts below 90×10^9/L should raise suspicion of other causes of thrombocytopenia and should be actively looked for.

Idiopathic thrombocytopenia purpura

- There is no test to definitively diagnose idiopathic thrombocytopenia purpura (ITP). Women who are asymptomatic outside pregnancy can develop persistent thrombocytopenia which requires immunosuppression.
- Antibodies directed against platelet antigens are produced primarily in the spleen where phagocytosis by macrophages occurs, and also in the liver and bone marrow.
- The binding of complement to platelets can facilitate their clearance and antibody binding to megakaryocytes can lead to ineffective production of platelets.
- Antiplatelet antibodies (immunoglobulin G) attack platelet membrane glycoproteins and destroy platelets at a rate that cannot be compensated for.

Interaction with pregnancy

- If ITP is diagnosed during pregnancy conservative management is usually sufficient.
- Corticosteroids are administered if the platelet count falls below 30×10^9/L before the onset of labour or $<50\times10^9$/L at the time of delivery.
- Immunoglobulin can be administered if the patient fails to respond to corticosteroid therapy.
- The baby will be affected and delivery must be atraumatic.

Other causes of thrombocytopenia in pregnancy

- Pre-eclampsia/HELLP.
- Thrombotic thrombocytopenia purpura (TTP) (Chapter 25, p. 668).
- DIC.
- Drug induced.

Anaesthetic management

- If the platelet count has been stable then a full blood count (FBC) within 6 hours can inform decision making over neuro-axial analgesia.
- In rapidly changing situations, such as PET, then a FBC within 2 hours should be performed.
- Close liaison with a haematologist is important for all cases of significant thrombocytopenia of $<80\times10^9$/L.
- No single coagulation test has been established as a reliable predictor of haematoma after neuraxial block.
- Platelet number of 80×10^9/L is considered reasonable for an epidural, possibly as low as 50×10^9/L for spinal anaesthesia although local policies should be followed.
- Viscoelastometric haemostatic assays (VHAs) will identify global abnormalities in the coagulation system but are not sensitive to a low platelet count alone and should not be used to inform decision making around neuro-axial choices.
- A platelet count below 50×10^9/L at delivery will need to be supported by a platelet transfusion and prophylactic tranexamic acid. Close liaison with a haematologist is essential.

Congenital coagulopathies: Overview

The common congenital coagulopathies are:
- Von Willebrand's disease.
- Haemophilia A and B.
- Other single factor deficiencies.

> All women with a significant congenital clotting disorder should be de-
> livered in a maternity centre associated with a comprehensive care
> haemophilia centre, as the management of the mother and baby is likely
> to be complicated.

Von Willebrand's disease

Von Willebrand's disease is the most frequent of all inherited haemostatic abnormalities and is therefore the most likely coagulopathy to affect
women in pregnancy. In normal pregnancy a rise in both factor VIIIC and
von Willebrand factor (vWF) is observed in most cases.

Pathophysiology

vWF plays two primary roles in coagulation:
- It facilitates platelet adhesion by binding to platelets and collagen.
- It forms a complex with factor VIII, which decreases the excretion of
  factor VIII.

vWF helps platelet binding to sites of vascular damage. The symptoms of
deficiency therefore mimic disorders of platelet function (bleeding from skin
and mucosa). A deficiency can also result in decreased factor VIII levels and
patients with severe disease can present with haemorrhage into muscles
and joints, similar to that seen in classical haemophilia.

Classification
- Type 1—partial deficiency of vWF, mild—moderate bleeding disorder.
- Type 2a—qualitative defect in vWF.
- Type 2b—qualitative defect in vWF, with increased binding to platelets
  causing thrombocytopenia and can mimic ITP.
- Type 3—complete absence of vWF and reduced levels of factor VIII,
  with severe bleeding disorder.

Interaction with pregnancy
- Pregnancy causes a 3 to 4-fold rise in vWF. As a result, patients with
  type 1 disorder improve during pregnancy as the vWF increases to
  normal levels.
- Levels at 32 weeks are usually adequate to confirm this.
- Women with types 2 and 3 disorders do not improve during pregnancy
  and their care should be at a specialist centre under the care of a
  haematologist with an interest in bleeding disorders.

Anaesthetic management
- DDAVP (desmopressin) and vWF concentrates are used to increase the levels of vWF.
- Vaginal delivery is considered safe if vWF is >40IU/dL.
- If operative delivery is necessary, the level has to be >50IU/dL.
- PPH is not more common than normal but if it occurs it is likely to be severe as vWF falls to pre-pregnancy levels.
- Regional anaesthesia is generally safe in patients with type 1 disease after levels in pregnancy have been checked.
- vWF falls rapidly after delivery and the epidural catheter should be removed early.
- An epidural is not recommended for women with types 2 and 3 disease; however, a spinal anaesthetic could be sited for operative delivery if there is an interval of up to 20min between the administration of vWF concentrates and DDAVP.
- A haematologist's input in the care of this patient is essential.
- Tranexamic acid should be given at delivery and into the postnatal period.

Haemophilia

Haemophilia A and B are X-linked disorders due to a deficiency of factor VIII and IX respectively. Females are usually carriers of this disease as they have only one affected chromosome. The clotting factor level is usually ~50% of normal. The risks in pregnancy for the female carrier of haemophilia are 2-fold:
- She may have very low factor VIII or IX levels and be at risk of excessive bleeding due to lyonization (random deletion of the X chromosome). Haemorrhage can follow surgical or traumatic delivery. These women have the same risk of bleeding as affected males. Delivery must be in a hospital with a haemophilia centre.
- Half male offspring will inherit haemophilia. This has important implications and prenatal diagnosis of this condition.
- A male baby of a haemophilia carrier must be delivered in a maternity unit with a comprehensive care haemophilia centre. The baby is at risk of cerebral haemorrhage and a clear delivery plan is essential.

Clinical classification of either haemophilia A or B
- Mild 5–50% factor level.
- Moderate 1–5% factor level.
- Severe <1% factor level.
- It is important to identify carriers prior to pregnancy, not only to provide appropriate management for the rare mother with pathologically low coagulation activity, but also to provide genetic counselling.
- Changes in factor VIII complex may make the identification of carriers more difficult during pregnancy.

Anaesthetic management
- Most female carriers have normal VIII levels and can have routine neuro-axial analgesia. A woman with normal VIII levels and a female baby can deliver at her local hospital.
- 10–20% of women will have reduced factor VIII (<40U/dL) and are at risk of bleeding during pregnancy and delivery. Factor VIII increases in pregnancy, thus uncomplicated vaginal delivery with levels >40U/dL may not require blood product replacement. For CS, factor VIII concentrate required to achieve >50U/dL. Levels need to be maintained for 4–5 days postoperatively.
- The factor VIII level should be checked during pregnancy, and levels <25% or any signs of bleeding should be treated.
- Delayed PPH is the most common complication in obstetric patients as factor levels fall quickly in the postpartum period.
- Treatment for haemophilia A is factor VIII concentrate, desmopressin, and tranexamic acid.
- Treatment for haemophilia B is factor IX concentrate and tranexamic acid.

Acquired haemophilia
- Causes prolongation of activated partial thromboplastin time (APTT).
- Is a rare acquired bleeding disorder and can occur in pregnancy.
- It is caused by antibodies against factor VIII.
- It can present with severe bleeding in pregnancy and the puerperium with abnormal clotting studies.
- It requires urgent referral to haemophilia centre for immunomodulation therapy.

Other single factor deficiencies: Factor XI deficiency
- Factor XI deficiency (plasma thromboplastin antecedent deficiency) is the most common and can cause PPH.
- History of increased bleeding with dental extractions, trauma, surgery and menorrhagia.

Key points
- Needs early review by haematologist and clear delivery plan in place. Ideally this should be at a delivery unit with a comprehensive care haemophilia centre.
- Regional techniques contraindicated.
- For labour analgesia, avoid IM injections. Use IV opioids ± Entonox®.
- Factor XI concentrate or fresh frozen plasma will be needed to cover operative delivery.
- Tranexamic acid should be used prophylactically.

Acquired coagulopathy
Acquired coagulopathy is uncommon in pregnancy and around delivery but when it occurs can lead to severe PPH and morbidity. If the APTT or pro-thrombin time (PT) is prolonged (above the normal range) and the Clauss fibrinogen <2g/L then urgent investigation for the underlying cause should

be instigated and correction of clotting factors undertaken with the advice of a haematologist. Causes include:

- Pregnancy-induced hypertension.
- Sepsis.
- Placental abruption.
- Retained dead fetus.
- Amniotic fluid embolus.
- Liver disease.
- Therapeutic anticoagulation.

Hypercoagulable disease: Overview

Effective coagulation is maintained by a balance of pro-coagulant and anti-coagulant activity. Pregnancy is a hypercoagulable state and certain diseases increase the risk of thrombosis. Venous thromboses are more common than arterial thromboses and their incidence increases with surgery, pregnancy, use of oral contraceptives, and immobility.

Protein C deficiency

- Protein C is a vitamin K-dependent physiological inhibitor of coagulation with a short half-life (8h).
- Heterozygous protein C deficiency associated with increase in thrombotic tendency especially in pregnancy.
- It acts by inhibiting activated factors V and VIII. Protein C levels increase by 35% during normal pregnancy.
- Thrombosis occurs in 25% of pregnant patients with the deficiency, unless anticoagulation therapy is administered.
- Heparin should be administered during the first and third trimester and either heparin or warfarin can be given during the second trimester.

Protein S deficiency

- Heparin should be administered during the first and third trimester and either heparin or warfarin can be given during the second trimester.
- Protein S is also a vitamin K dependent protein synthesized in the liver. Levels of protein S decrease in normal pregnancy.
- It acts as a cofactor for protein C.
- The treatment of protein S deficiency is identical to that of protein C deficiency.

Antithrombin III deficiency

- Antithrombin III is synthesized in the liver and endothelial cells, and its primary action is the inhibition of activated factor IIa (thrombin) and factors IXa, Xa, XIa, and XIIa.
- Antithrombin deficiency may be congenital or arise secondary to acquired disorders, e.g. liver dysfunction or sepsis.
- It is the most clinically important of the inherited thrombophilias, resulting in venous thromboembolism in the majority of affected individuals, which may be life-threatening during high risk periods such as pregnancy.

Key points
- Prophylactic anticoagulation is indicated during pregnancy and is best provided with LMWH ± low dose aspirin. Heparin acts by potentiation of antithrombin III; therefore, more heparin may be required for the desired effect if levels of antithrombin III are low.
- At the time of delivery, IV antithrombin III concentrate may be substituted or used with LMWH.
- Keep patient warm and well hydrated.
- Regional anaesthesia is possible, but needs to be timed carefully with anticoagulation therapy. Continue with aspirin, as it is not a contraindication to regional anaesthesia.
- Close liaison with the haematologist is essential.

Factor V Leiden mutation

- This is the most common hypercoagulable disorder affecting 5% of the white population.
- This mutation leads to a form of factor V, which when activated is resistant to degradation by activated protein C, thereby increasing pro-coagulant activity.
- Personal history of thrombosis is the most important factor when considering thrombosis risk.
- If had deep vein thrombosis (DVT)/pulmonary embolism in the past, needs to be treated with LMWH in pregnancy.
- Best managed in a joint haematology/high risk obstetric clinic.
- As with the other hyper-coagulant disorders careful management of LMWH is required to facilitate the possibility of regional analgesia, TED (thromboembolism deterrent) stocking in labour.
- Early mobilization and good hydration.
- Consider changing to IV unfractionated heparin around 38th week gestation to allow flexibility if recent thrombosis needing full anticoagulation has occurred.

Anaesthetic implications
- Depending on the mother's personal thrombosis history she will be on prophylactic or therapeutic LMWH during pregnancy.
- Guidelines for the management of mothers with a risk of thrombosis can be found on the Royal College of Obstetrics and Gynaecologists website.
- Many women want to receive regional analgesia or anaesthesia and the timing of anticoagulation is important.
- Information on anticoagulants and regional anaesthesia can be found in Chapter 7.

Further reading

Sharma SK, Mhyre JM. Haematological and coagulation disorders. In: Chestnut DH et al. *Chestnut's Obstetric Anaesthesia, Principles and Practice*. 5th edn. Saunders, 2014, 1033–1052.

Sankaran S, Robinson SE. Immune thrombocytopenia and pregnancy. *Obstetric Medicine* 2011; 4: 140–146.

Mumford AD et al. On behalf of BCSH Committee. Guideline for the diagnosis and management of the rare coagulation disorders: a United Kingdom Haemophilia Centre Doctors' Organization guideline on behalf of the British Committee for Standards in Haematology. *British Journal of Haematology* 2014; 167:304–326.

Ormesher L et al. Management of inherited thrombophilia in pregnancy. *Womens Health (London)* 2016; 12: 433–441.

Antenatal assessment and pain management

Rachel Collis, Lucy De Lloyd, and David Hill

Aims of antenatal anaesthetic assessment in high risk pregnancies

Advances in medical care have resulted in an increasing number of women with concomitant diseases becoming pregnant. Antenatal anaesthetic assessment plays a vital role in the successful management of such patients, as highlighted by successive confidential enquiry reports. Lack of timely intervention by an anaesthetist can contribute to sub-optimal care. Although it is not possible to predict in the antenatal period all mothers who will require an anaesthetic, those considered at high risk and with other medical problems should be assessed.

The benefits

- Avoids the need for short-notice and suboptimal anaesthetic plans being put in place for delivery.
- Enables a detailed history and appropriate physical examination of the patient, which is often difficult or impossible in labour or in an emergency situation.
- Allows review of appropriate information or to prearrange special investigations, e.g. magnetic resonance imaging (MRI) of the lumbar spine.
- The effects of physiological changes in pregnancy on the disease can be given due consideration in patient evaluation and management.
- Enables multidisciplinary input and meetings—anaesthetists, obstetricians, haematologists, cardiologists, immunologists etc.
- Enables the formulation of a management plan tailored to the individual's needs. This plan must be possible on any day and at any time because of the unpredictable nature of labour and delivery, even if an elective CS is planned.
- Explanation of issues to the patient, increasing her ability to make informed choices and decreasing anxiety when labour pain or emergency anaesthesia makes it difficult to communicate complex information.
- Avoids disappointment, especially if the patient's expectations are very different from those of her physicians.
- Highlights special requirements, especially if additional monitoring or senior help is required.

Clinic set-up

- Depending the size of maternity unit, this may vary from *ad hoc* calls to the antenatal clinic, to regular formal clinics which are more popular in larger units and tertiary referral centres, because of the volume of work and complexity of the cases.
- Senior anaesthetic input and continuity is vital to ensure optimal outcome. Many units will now have a regular consultant anaesthetic session dedicated to a clinic.
- Attention is generally targeted at high risk pregnancies due to limitation of resources.

- A formal clinic environment with clerical support is important. A room in an antenatal clinic is appropriate, and most women feel comfortable with this arrangement.
- It is usual that obstetric and medical notes are separated. It is important that every effort is made to have the medical notes available.
- Regular communication of appropriate referrals to obstetricians and midwives is important. Good communication and clear lines of referral should exist between professionals.
- It is important that referrals can be made from midwifery and consultant obstetric clinics and that everybody is aware of the mechanism of referral.

Timing
- Most high risk women benefit from a review at 32–34 weeks gestation.
- An appointment >8 weeks from delivery, where details of likely anaesthetic input are discussed, will have been forgotten or will often not seem relevant to the patient.
- An appointment after 34 weeks will miss some mothers because of premature delivery, and will not allow enough time to communicate with other professionals and organize special investigations.

Any patient with significant medical conditions, especially cardiac disease, should be referred at 24–26 weeks gestation and are likely to need regular review every 4–6 weeks after this because of the changing physiological demands of the pregnancy on the disease.

Documentation
- Date of assessment.
- Patient details.
- Expected date of delivery and current gestation.
- Previous obstetric history and anaesthetic involvement.
- Current delivery plan.
- History of medical problem requiring referral.
- Findings of examination and appropriate investigations.
- Management plans to include suitable anaesthetic techniques and seniority of anaesthetist required.
- Communication of the management plan is important. The attending anaesthetist should have immediate access to such information when the mother is in labour.
- A designated page in the maternity notes or a specific coloured clinic sheet in the main notes will make it immediately clear to midwives, obstetricians, and anaesthetists that the patient had been designated high risk in some way and that there is an anaesthetic plan.
- Notes are not always immediately available and it is useful if a copy of the plan is also stored in a folder on the delivery suite or electronically on the Patient Management System. All anaesthetists and labour ward staff must be aware of the process.
- A delivery suite ward folder is also useful to warn anaesthetic staff of potential problems. There should be a flagging process for alerting staff that the patient has been seen antenatally and that the anaesthetist should be informed on admission.

Suggested referrals to high risk obstetric anaesthetic clinic

Cardiac
- Congenital or acquired heart disease, even if the patient is asymptomatic.
- Significant history of dysrhythmias.

Haematological
- All patients on heparin, LMWH or warfarin in pregnancy.
- Any patient under regular review in a haematology clinic, e.g. idiopathic thrombocytopenia purpura (ITP), thrombotic thrombocytopenia purpura (TTP), antithrombin III deficiency, von Willebrand's disease.
- Sickle cell disease.

Respiratory
- Severe asthma, especially requiring hospital or ICU admission.
- Other significant history of respiratory disease, e.g. cystic fibrosis, sarcoidosis, fibrosing alveolitis, pneumothorax, restrictive chest wall deformities.

Neurological
- History of or current intracranial pathology.
- History of neuro-inflammatory disease, e.g. multiple sclerosis.
- Poorly controlled epilepsy.

Spinal
- All patients with any degree of spina bifida.
- Any patient with a history of back surgery.
- Patients with back problems with specific concerns.
- Patients with neck problems or possibility of difficult intubation.
- Severe kyphoscoliosis especially if causing restrictive lung disease.

Endocrine
- Significant endocrine disease, with the exception of diabetes mellitus or treated thyroid disease.

GIT/liver
- Any patient with a history of major abdominal surgery.
- Chronic liver disease of any cause.

Renal
- Any patient with chronic renal failure.
- All renal transplant recipients.

Anaesthetic
- Previous history or family history of anaesthetic-related problems, e.g. suxamethonium apnoea, malignant hyperthermia.
- Previous history of airway or intubation difficulties.

Drug reactions
- Severe reactions on previous exposure especially to LA and GA drugs.

Obstetric
- Risk of major PPH, e.g. major placenta praevia with a previous CS scar.

Miscellaneous
- Morbid obesity, i.e. BMI>45kg/m^2.
- Substance abusers especially if poorly managed and/or poor venous access.
- Patients who refuse blood transfusion, e.g. Jehovah's Witnesses.
- Patients with severe anxiety or phobias.
- Patients with a previous history of inadequate epidural or spinal anaesthesia who are concerned about their experience.
- Pregnant patients with chronic pain, e.g. symphysis pubis dysfunction.

Specific antenatal problems

Cardiac

All mothers with a history of cardiac disease should be assessed, even if they are asymptomatic.

- Ideally women with known cardiac disease should have attended cardiology clinic for pre-pregnancy counselling, optimization, and preparation for pregnancy.
- Where there a history of heart disease but lack of clarity regarding the diagnosis, echocardiogram or Holter monitor should be arranged as indicated early in the pregnancy.
- Any abnormality should prompt cardiology review to help stratify cardiac risk and inform appropriate antenatal care.
- An accurate understanding of cardiac risk is important to inform where and how the mother should be looked after, both during pregnancy and for delivery, and how often key members of a multidisciplinary team should see her.

The New York Heart Association (NYHA) classes 1–4

- Describing functional status is also very useful, with women with less functional capacity being at higher risk of deterioration in pregnancy.
- It is also worth considering that cardiovascular risk needs to be contextualized for each patient, as the presence of significant co-morbidities will increase predicted maternal risk.

Assessment

- Functional New York Heart Association (NYHA) class.
  - NYHC 1: no limit during ordinary activity.
  - NYHC 2: slight limitation during ordinary activity.
  - NYHC 3: marked limitation of ordinary activity.
  - NYHC 4: no physical activity without symptoms.
- An accurate assessment of the level of physical activity pre-pregnancy and how this has changed. Ask about ordinary daily activities.
- Raised respiratory rate, persistent tachycardia, chest pain, and orthopnoea in the lateral position may reflect deterioration in cardiac function and should be fully investigated.

Data from The Criteria Committee of the New York Heart Association. *Nomenclature and Criteria for Diagnosis of Diseases of the Heart and Great Vessels.* 9th ed. Boston, Mass: Little, Brown & Co; 1994:253–256.

Modified World Health Organization (WHO) classification scoring system

Classifies women into four groups, from I to IV, with associated cardiovascular risk.

- Patients with cardiac lesions in WHO group 1 have minimal increased cardiac risk,
- WHO group II have a small increased risk of mortality and moderately increased risk of morbidity.
- WHO group III are at significantly increased risk of mortality and morbidity.
- Women falling into WHO group IV have an extremely high risk of mortality and severe morbidity, and pregnancy is considered contraindicated.

WHO I
- Uncomplicated, small or mild pulmonary stenosis, patent ductus arteriosus, or mitral valve prolapse.
- Successfully repaired simple lesions (atrial or ventricular septal defect, patent ductus arteriosus, anomalous pulmonary venous drainage).
- Isolated atrial or ventricular ectopic beats.

WHO II (if well and uncomplicated)
- Un-operated atrial or ventricular septal defect.
- Repaired tetralogy of Fallot.
- Most arrhythmias.

WHO II–III (individualized risk)
- Mild left ventricular impairment.
- Hypertrophic cardiomyopathy.
- Native or tissue valvular heart disease not considered WHO I or IV.
- Marfan's syndrome without aortic dilatation.
- Aorta <45 mm in aortiopathy associated with bicuspid aortic valve
- Repaired coarctation.

WHO III
- Mechanical valve.
- Systemic right ventricle (Senning's or Mustard's corrective procedure for correction of transposition of the great vessels).
- Fontan circulation.
- Cyanotic heart disease (unrepaired).
- Other complex congenital heart disease.
- Aortic dilatation 40–45 mm with Marfan's syndrome.
- Aortic dilatation 45–50 mm in aortopathy associated with bicuspid aortic valve.

Conditions in which pregnancy risk is WHO IV (pregnancy contraindicated)
- Pulmonary arterial hypertension of any cause.
- Severe systemic ventricular dysfunction (LVEF <30%, NYHA III–IV).
- Previous peripartum cardiomyopathy with any residual impairment of left ventricular function.
- Severe mitral stenosis, severe symptomatic aortic stenosis.
- Marfan's syndrome with aorta dilated >45 mm.
- Aortic dilatation >50 mm in aortic disease associated with bicuspid aortic valve.
- Native severe coarctation.

Adapted from *Heart*, Thorne S., MacGregor A., and Nelson-Piercy C. Risks of contraception and pregnancy in heart disease. 92(10): 1520–1525, Copyright 2006, with permission from BMJ Publishing Group Ltd.

Multi-disciplinary clinic planning

- Patients identified with cardiac disease associated with increased risk should be seen in a specialist cardiac obstetric clinic. A multidisciplinary team comprising an obstetrician, obstetric anaesthetist, and cardiologist with an interest in pregnancy should assess these mothers early in pregnancy, and at specified intervals throughout the pregnancy, determined by the individualized needs of the patient.
- Usually a patient would be assessed in the first, second, and third trimester for evaluation and optimization, and to plan for the peripartum period.

Peripartum plan

- A clear description of the cardiac pathology and any previous corrective surgery.
- An outline of special precautions required and the principles of management to apply when delivering patient care; the plan may need to change according to circumstances that were not anticipated, but principles of management should still apply.
- Instructions for cardiac and other medications peripartum.
- Planned anaesthesia for labour and operative procedures.
- Grade of anaesthetist who should be directly involved in anaesthetic care. This may vary with the procedure and situation.
- Appropriate monitoring (invasive/non-invasive).
- Guidance for the use of uterotonic medications, e.g. oxytocin bolus/ infusion, suitability of ergometrine.
- Level of care indicated post delivery and recommended duration of stay for observation postpartum.

Low risk cardiac disease: WHO Modified risk I (no increased risk)
- These mothers should have a normal pregnancy and are frequently perplexed as to why they have been asked to attend an anaesthetic clinic. All mothers with cardiac disease should be seen antenatally so that analgesia and anaesthesia can be planned and then given without delay once in labour, if required.
- Assessment by the obstetric anaesthetist can occur at any gestation but in a well mother the ideal time is 32–34 weeks gestation.
- A home delivery or delivery in a midwifery-led unit may be possible for some women.
- In extreme situations, e.g. major obstetric haemorrhage, she may not tolerate the physiological insult as well as a mother with an entirely normal heart, and this should be discussed with the mother prior to delivery.
- Options for labour analgesia or anaesthesia for CS can usually be discussed and planned.

Moderate risk cardiac disease
These patients may present with deteriorating parameters during pregnancy or delivery, but usually tolerate the physiological demands of pregnancy well without major problems.

- A vaginal delivery with appropriate limits set upon it is the mode of delivery associated with the lowest physiological stress, and as such is appropriate for most women with cardiac disease. Sympathetic stress should be minimized, usually with early epidural pain relief, and the time spent in the active second stage may have a limitation placed upon it, before obstetric intervention is employed to assist the delivery.
- In most situations, a routine low dose epidural for labour analgesia is a safe and appropriate choice, with pulse oximetry and non-invasive BP monitoring.
- There are rare exceptions to this, where caesarian section is advised for cardiac reasons; e.g in the mother with a dilated aortic root >4cm, when associated with Marfan's syndrome, In most situations, a caesarean delivery is required only for obstetric indications.
- Patients are best looked after in a hospital that can offer 24h specialist care in case of sudden cardiac problems and obstetric emergencies.
- All mothers in the medium risk group should be seen at regular intervals by a specialist cardiac obstetric multidisciplinary team, including an obstetric anaesthetist. At 32–34 weeks gestation the obstetric anaesthetist can discuss and make a plan for delivery, and more detailed description of anaesthetic plans given to her.

High risk cardiac disease

- These mothers have many complex problems and will need regular review with a high risk cardiac obstetric and anaesthetic clinic to optimize and plan their care at intervals determined by their risk status and clinical progress.
- They may need to be admitted to a high dependency area in hospital (Coronary Care Unit) for monitoring and bed rest at any time during their pregnancy.
- The mother may present in the first or the early part of the second trimester with heart failure, where termination of pregnancy may be necessary, or she may need delivery early in the third trimester once the baby is viable. Multidisciplinary planning and delivery in an environment where complications occurring in the perinatal period can be managed by experienced staff in appropriate specialties, is mandatory in this group.

Haematological

Referrals should include those on anticoagulant medication for previous thromboembolism or thrombophilia, and patients with an abnormality of coagulation, e.g. idiopathic thrombocytopenia, von Willebrand's disease, factor deficiencies, etc.

- A history of the condition needs to be taken together with current haematological input.
- The appropriateness of regional anaesthesia needs to be determined. If contraindicated, alternative methods of pain relief should be discussed, particularly patient-controlled IV opioid analgesia.
- An assessment of the patient's airway is important in case GA is required for operative delivery.
- Close liaison with a haematologist is generally required.

Plan to include

- If regional anaesthesia is considered.
  - Absolute contraindications in bleeding disorders.
  - Timing of regional techniques relating to anticoagulation administration.
  - Timing of epidural catheter removal.
- Requirement for investigations on admission in labour/for CS.
- Documentation of the level of haematological support required on admission.
- Requirement for IV access.
- Assessment of the increased risk of PPH.
- Plan for postpartum oxytocin infusion.
- Whether NSAIDs are contraindicated.

Respiratory

The most common respiratory problem is severe asthma, but with advances in treatment more women with cystic fibrosis are becoming pregnant. It is important to obtain:

- A detailed medication history.
- The level of activity prior to pregnancy.
- Admissions to hospital/ICU.
- Pulmonary function tests may be useful and should be arranged in good time.

Patients should be encouraged to take maintenance medications as some will avoid taking drugs whilst pregnant.

Plan to include

- Continuation of regular medications. May need extra steroid cover for labour where appropriate.
- Benefits of regional analgesia and anaesthesia. Epidurals to be encouraged, particularly in severe asthmatics. GA for operative delivery may be poorly tolerated.
- Explain the relative problems of Entonox® use—it has a drying effect on bronchial secretions if taken over a prolonged period.

Neurological

Women with ongoing or quiescent neurological disease should be assessed, so that a detailed description of the problem can be obtained and full documentation of any neurological deficit made.

- Many women and anaesthetists are fearful that regional anaesthesia is contraindicated or may make the condition worse. A detailed discussion with documentation is required.
- Where there is evidence of current or previous space-occupying lesions, intracranial haemorrhage or infarction, an assessment for evidence of raised intracranial pressure must be undertaken.

- Results of recent investigations, e.g. computed tomography (CT) or MRI brain are essential with a history of recent intracranial pathology.
- Input from a neurologist or neurosurgeon may be required before a decision regarding anaesthetic management is made.

Multiple sclerosis
- Patients with a history of multiple sclerosis frequently present to the obstetric anaesthetist.
- The history should elicit medication, respiratory compromise, and details of any episodes of relapse.
- A detailed neurological examination is required.
- The patient should be counselled regarding the risks and benefits of regional anaesthesia, together with the chance of relapse with or without an anaesthetic procedure.
- There is no convincing evidence that either general or regional anaesthesia has any influence on the incidence of relapse.
- An informed choice with full documentation of what is discussed is important.

Spinal disease

Spina bifida
- History, neurological examination, and documentation are required.
- The level of the defect can be assessed by examination, but the level of the termination of the spinal cord cannot be known without an MRI scan; it may be low due to tethering even in occulta.
- An MRI scan is the gold standard investigation and can be performed in pregnancy. It should be carried out in the second trimester, if possible, because the mother may not be able to lie comfortably and safely on her back in the scanner as pregnancy progresses.
- An MRI scan may be appropriate if the mother is very anxious about pain relief in labour or if she is at high risk of GA.
- A decision regarding appropriateness of regional anaesthesia is dependent on the above. The airway should be assessed in case GA is required.
- Patient-controlled analgesia (PCA) should be discussed with her if regional techniques are contraindicated.

Lumbar disc surgery
- At what spinal level was surgery carried out?
- Was any metal work inserted?
- Previous investigations such as X-rays or MRI.
- Examination to reveal level of scar and neurological deficit.
- Are there any ongoing pain problems?

Plan to include
- Is regional anaesthesia contraindicated?
  - Spinal anaesthesia can usually be performed through a scar if necessary.
  - Epidurals should be inserted away from a visible scar, i.e. one or preferably two interspaces above the site of surgery. This avoids dural puncture as there is a risk of tethering of the dura to the ligamentum flavum due to scar formation.
- Patients should be warned of the increased difficulty of insertion and potential failure due to inadequate spread of LA in the epidural space.
- There is an increased risk of dural puncture with epidural insertion.
- Spinal anaesthesia is generally easier and usually works well, and the patient should be reassured.

Scoliosis
- Assess degree of thoracic and lumbar curvature.
- Determine position of the midline and the presence of palpable spaces.
- Check for neurological dysfunction.
- Is there any respiratory compromise?
- What is the extent of surgery (thoracic/lumbar), and are there anterior or posterior fixation devices?
- Old scans/X-rays are useful.

Plan to include
- Whether regional anaesthesia is contraindicated.
- Ultrasound can help determine anatomy.
- May require a senior, experienced anaesthetist.
- Documentation of any increased risk of inadequate block/failure.
- Controversial: epidural may be contraindicated with metal work because of the theoretical risk of introducing infection.

Obesity

The prevalence of obesity is increasing in developed countries, and many patients do not understand the reasons for their attendance at an anaesthetic clinic. This needs to be discussed with care.

- The history should determine any associated antepartum medical disease, e.g. diabetes, hypertension, pre-eclampsia, and whether there has been a history of previous regional anaesthesia.
- Examination should focus on:
  - Venous access.
  - Airway assessment.
  - Anatomy of the back with attention to fat distribution.

It should be explained to the mother:
- Why regional techniques can be difficult and may take time to establish.
- Why GA should ideally be avoided. (The mother should not be frightened into thinking that GA is absolutely contraindicated, as technical failure of regional anaesthesia is common and GA is then the only option.)
- Many women with a high BMI are now advised to take prophylactic LMWH. Discussion around timing of injection and timing of regional analgesia/anesthesia is required.

Plan to include

- Epidural analgesia is strongly encouraged.
- Epidural may be more difficult to insert with an increased failure rate.
- A written reminder to the on-call anaesthetist that the epidural block should be regularly assessed, re-sited early if inadequate, and kept topped up to reduce the risk of GA.
- Early call for senior help if GA is anticipated.
- Non-invasive BP measurement may be unreliable: consider placing cuff around forearm or siting an arterial line for high risk procedure.
- Risk of PPH is increased.
- Thromboprophylaxis post delivery is important, and an increased dose may be needed.

Further reading

ESC Guidelines on the management of cardiovascular diseases during pregnancy. The Task Force on the Management of Cardiovascular Diseases during Pregnancy of the European Society of Cardiology (ESC)Patel JP, Roberts LN, Patel RK, Arya R. European Heart Journal (2011) 32, 3147–3197

Pregnancy outcomes in women with mechanical prosthetic heart valves—a prospective descriptive population-based study using the United Kingdom Obstetric Surveillance System (UKOSS) data collection system. BJOG. 2018 Jan;125 (1):96. doi: 10.1111/1471-0528.1491

Yucel E, DeFaria Yeh D. Pregnancy in Women with Congenital Heart Disease. Curr Treat Options Cardiovasc Med. 2017 Aug 22; 19 (9):73

Amato MP et al. Management of pregnancy-related issues in multiple sclerosis patients: the need for an interdisciplinary approach. Neurol Sci. 2017 Oct; 38 (10):1849–1858

Principles of pain management during pregnancy

Overview

- Pain may be as a result of pregnancy. It may also arise from acute conditions or be secondary to underlying medical conditions.
- Analgesics are among the most commonly used drugs in pregnancy.
- Analgesic agents almost always cross the placenta but reassuringly most are safe in therapeutic doses.
- Periods of concern are organogenesis (weeks 4–10) and just before delivery.
- Established fetal risk categories exist to guide drug prescribing in pregnant/lactating patients.
- Poorly controlled pain during pregnancy is associated with self-medication behaviour, requests for early caesarean section, and induction of labour, and untreated may induce preterm labour.

General principles

- Adopt a multimodal and multidisciplinary approach.
- Expect different pains to vary in their opioid responsiveness.
- Concomitant use of physiotherapy, psychology, and complimentary medicine are encouraged.
- Aim to prevent progression to chronic pain.
- Control acute pain adequately; escalate doses.
- Treat any neuropathic component if present.
- Logical use of analgesics, reviewing dosages and their response as pregnancy advances.
- Use slow release analgesics if pain is constant.
- Use quick release analgesics for activity related pain prior to aggravating activity.
- Treat psychological vulnerability (poor coping strategies).
- Address sleep disturbance.
- Make realistic goals.

Minimize fetal risk

- Use non-pharmacological options if possible.
- Consider local anaesthetic infiltration or nerve blocks.
- Avoid drugs during organogenesis and before delivery.

Generic pathway for pain management in pregnancy

Step 1. Assessment

- Review onset of pain: If acute or injury related, establish specific diagnosis.
- If it is a flare up of a chronic condition—escalate usual medication.
- If it is associated focal tenderness—consider suitability for injection.
- Spinal or pelvic related pain—consider suitability for physiotherapy.
- If pain is activity or incident related—use short acting analgesia.
- If pain is constant—use slow release analgesia.
- If a neuropathic component is present e.g. burning, shooting, stabbing features—go to step 5.

Step 2. Physiotherapy

- The role of concomitant physiotherapy to address pain in pregnancy is invaluable. Physiotherapists interested in obstetric problems are particularly helpful in the multidisciplinary management of the common musculoskeletal pains associated with pregnancy.

Step 3. Local anaesthetic +/- steroid injection

The use of local anaesthesia +/- steroid injections is indicated for:

- Focal areas of tenderness, e.g. myofascial pain, trigger points, abdominal nerve entrapment.
- Spinal pain, e.g. facet joints, paravertebral muscles, sacroiliac joints, coccyx pain.
- Pelvic pain, e.g. pubic symphysis.

Step 4. Systemic analgesia

Short acting

First level

- Paracetamol 1g 6hrly (max 4g/day),

Second level (combine with weak opioid)

- Codeine/paracetamol combination (co-codamol 8/500mg) 6hrly.
- Tramadol/paracetamol combination (37.5/500mg) 6hrly.

Third level (escalate weak opioid)

- Tramadol 50mg–100mg 6hrly.
- Codeine/ paracetamol (co-codamol 30/500) 6 hrly.

Slow release

First level (weak opioid)

- Buprenorphine 5–10 micrograms/hr 7 day patch.
- Tramadol MR 50mg BD.

Second level (moderate opioid)
- Buprenorphine 20 micrograms/hr 7 day patch.
- Buprenorphine 35 micrograms/hr 3 day patch.
- Fentanyl patch 12 micrograms/hr every 3 day.

Third level (strong opioid)
- Fentanyl 25–50 micrograms/hr 3 day patch.
- Oxycontin 10–20 micrograms 12hrly.

Step 5. Neuropathic medication

First level
- Gabapentin 100mg TDS escalate up to 600mg TDS.
- Combine with paracetamol and weak opioid.
- Consider topical capsaicin 0.025% or 0.075%.
- Consider lidocaine patch 5%.

Second level
- Add in amitriptyline (2nd & 3rd trimesters only).

Third level
- Add in strong opioid (slow release).
- Consider methadone (long half-life).
- Consider lidocaine infusion.

Non-pharmacological techniques

Heat & cold

Local application of heat or cold can be effective in muscular and myofascial pain. Cool gel pads have been found effective in perineal pain post delivery.

Transcutaeous electrical nerve stimulation (TENS)

There is little evidence to support its use in pregnancy. TENS has been shown to reduce analgesic consumption in chronic pain patients and retrospective studies have reported benefit in 70% who purchased TENS units. Pregnant women as a group are very motivated and may be satisfied with its moderate effect. TENS may be useful in:

- Spinal pain.
- Myofascial pain.
- Nerve entrapments.
- Pelvic arthropathy.
- Uterine pain.

Most pain management services offer Clinical Nurse Specialist TENS clinics, who will advise on the appropriate settings for the TENS unit.

Acupuncture

It is prudent to avoid acupuncture in the 1st trimester when pregnancy loss is high. Acupuncturists are cautious in pregnancy although widely used in China. There are studies and case reports to support the use of acupuncture for low back pain and pelvic pain in pregnancy: six or more treatments are required. There is no consensus about the exact 'forbidden points' in pregnancy as different schools and authors vary. These are the general principles of use:

- Avoid direct trauma over the gravid uterus.
- Needling depth and orientation are critical.
- Avoid increasing sympathetic tone by excess stimulation.

Acupuncture during pregnancy is a specialist area and should only be carried out by a qualified and experienced acupuncturist.

Physiotherapy in pregnancy

Physiotherapy has been reported mainly for low back and pelvic pain. Effective reported therapies include:

- Exercise programmes—land and water based.
- Back care classes.
- Postural feedback.
- Massage & relaxation
- Sacroiliac belts.
- Uterine support pillows.

Physical therapy is effective for pain associated muscle spasm and maintaining core stability.

Psychology in chronic pain management

Plays a key role in improving coping strategies and maintaining function.
Effective techniques include:
- Coping strategies.
- Goal setting & pacing.
- Relaxation.
- Cognitive therapy (negative thoughts).
- EMDR (Eye movement desensitization and reprocessing).

Patients suitable for referral have poor coping skills, pain behaviour, and
disproportionate suffering.

Drug use in pregnancy

Categorizing fetal risk

The following categorization of drugs according to fetal risk is adapted from the Australian Drug Evaluation Committee (ADEC) recommendations in Table 5.1.

Table 5.1 ADEC Fetal risk classification

Category	Classification of fetal risk
A	Drugs that have been taken by a large number of pregnant women without proven fetal harm
B	Drugs taken by limited number of pregnant women without proven fetal harm:
	B1 Animal studies have not proven fetal harm
	B2 Animal studies lacking, but available data does not suggest fetal harm
	B3 Animal studies have proven fetal harm, but significance in humans uncertain
C	Have caused harmful fetal effects (pharmacological) but not malformations
D	High risk of fetal damage, only use in exceptional circumstances
X	Very high risk of fetal harm. Do not use in pregnancy

Reproduced from Australian categorisation system for prescribing medicines in pregnancy, 2011, Therapeutic Goods Administration, used with permission of the Australian Government. © Commonwealth of Australia 2011.

https://www.tga.gov.au/australian-categorisation-system-prescribing-medicines-pregnancy

The drugs commonly used in pregnancy are categorized below according to the Australian prescribing medicines in pregnancy database. However, there are international differences between the designated categories.

Local anaesthetics and depo-steroids

Bupivacaine/lidocaine (Category A)
- Usual dose range for injection in pain management is 2–5ml of 0.25% levobupivacaine or 1% lidocaine.

Depo-steroid (Category A)
- Usual dose for methylprednisolone is 5–10mg per injection combined with local anaesthetic.
- Usual total dose of methylprednisiolone per treatment is 40mg.
- Treatment intervals usually 4–6 months.
- The analgesic effect can outlast the duration of the local anaesthetic.

Oral analgesics in pregnancy

Paracetamol (Category A)

- Paracetamol has been used since 1893 and it is the analgesic of choice in pregnancy.
- At therapeutic doses there have been no known teratogenic effects and is considered safe.
- When maternal toxic levels are reached facial cleft, spina bifida, and pyloric stenosis have been reported.
- The fetus is also at risk of toxicity as paracetamol crosses the placenta, as does the antidote, acetylcysteine.
- Adverse effects have also been observed in mothers with pre-eclampsia.

Aspirin (Category C)

- Aspirin has been found to be problematic in pregnancy; however, it is commonly self-administered.
- Consumption during pregnancy may produce anaemia, haemorrhage, prolonged gestation and labour, stillbirth, and pre-eclampsia.
- There is conflicting evidence of the safety of fetal exposure. First trimester use may be associated with increased risk of gastroschisis.
- Low dose aspirin (40–150mg/day) is used to treat thrombophilia syndromes to reduce the incidence of fetal loss. No fetal abnormalities have been reported after chronic low dose exposure.
- The use of high dose aspirin (rheumatological conditions) in the second half of pregnancy is more controversial. The main concerns are:
  - Bleeding during delivery (maternal and fetal).
  - Premature closure of the ductus arteriosis.
  - Oligohydramnios.

NSAIDs (Category C)

- Indometacin, ibuprofen, naproxen, diclofenac, or ketoprofen are not considered teratogenic in humans, although their use in early pregnancy has been associated with increased risk of miscarriage.
- These drugs are used for their anti-prostaglandin effects in both rheumatological and myofascial pain syndromes.
- Ibuprofen has been studied the most in pregnancy. Its use has been reported in over 100 pregnancies without congenital abnormalities. In usual doses (300–600 mg/day) ibuprofen is considered safe in pregnancy. However, persistent pulmonary hypertension has been reported in neonates following fetal exposure.
- Higher does (ankylosing spondylitis, rheumatoid arthritis) during the third trimester may cause premature closure of the ductus arteriosis, particularly in preterm labour. It is recommended they are discontinued in the 32nd gestational week.
- Topical usage generally results in negligible blood levels and may be considered safe.

Opioids (Category C)
- The experience of opioids, e.g. tramadol, oxycodone, fentanyl, and buprenorphine in pregnancy arises from opioid abuse patients who become pregnant. Animal teratogenicity and fetal loss has been reported.
- Overall opioids are considered safe in pregnancy.
- Opioid use has been linked with low birth weight and strabismus in babies, and possibly associated with schizophrenia in adult life.
- Prolonged antenatal exposure risks neonatal withdrawal syndrome. This requires treatment in 60–90% of infants.
- Neonatal outcome appears to be better when mothers require opiates for chronic pain rather than addiction although other environmental factors may be relevant.

Codeine (Category A)
- Codeine phosphate is commonly self-administered.
- Cautious use in first trimester.
- Prolonged use of codeine has caused codeine withdrawal in neonate.
- Up to 9% of adults and 40% of children cannot metabolize codeine to morphine and it is therefore an ineffective analgesic in these patients.

Tramadol (Category C)
- Tramadol has been shown to be embryotoxic and fetotoxic in mice, rats, and rabbits at maternally toxic doses, i.e. 3 to 15 times the maximum human dose or higher.
- No harm to the fetus due to tramadol was seen at doses that were not maternally toxic.

General advice on opioid use
- Pregnant women on long term opioids should not have them abruptly stopped.
- During labour and delivery opioid treatment should be maintained.
- If operative delivery arises, post-operative doses should be increased.
- In opioid-maintained mothers, neonatal withdrawal treatment with morphine (mean 10 days) is preferred to phenobarbital (mean 17 days).

Neuropathic drugs

Anticonvulsants general advice
- Women who remain on anticonvulsants should be counselled on the fetal risk.
- Monotherapy reduces fetal risk.
- Folic acid supplements (5mg) should be taken 4 weeks prior to and 12 weeks after conception.
- Regular abnormality scans are recommended if therapy is continued through pregnancy.

Gabapentin (Category B1) and pregabalin (Category B3)
- There is limited human data, but no reports of teratogenicity.
- Usually dosing is prescribed 3 times a day—start at 100mg 8hrly, and escalate over several weeks to reach 600mg 8hrly.
- Somnolence, nausea, and weight gain can occur.

Carbemazepine (Category D)

- Associated with 0.5–1% incidence of neural tube defects and also associated with craniofacial and coagulation defects in fetus.
- Often used as main therapy in trigeminal neuralgia or post herpetic neuralgia at high doses of 1200–2400mg/day.
- Should be stopped in 1st trimester and replaced with opioids (often high dose required), gabapentin or lamotrigine could be introduced from 2nd trimester.

Lamotrigine (Category D)

- Not a first line drug for neuropathic pain.

Other therapies

Amitriptyline (Category C)

- Use in first trimester is associated with limb reduction abnormalities; 2nd & 3rd trimester have no reports of excess abnormalities.
- Prolonged use has led to neonatal withdrawal symptoms and overdose is harmful to both mother and fetus. Dry mouth and somnolence can be a problem.
- Usual dose is 10mg at 8pm, may be escalated up to 70mg, which is an optimum dose.
- Good at addressing sleep disturbance associated with pain.

Baclofen (Category B3)

- Teratogenicity in animals has been reported.
- Useful as second line in trigeminal neuralgia and as muscle relaxant in myofascial pain/fibromyalgia.
- Usual dose 10mg 8hrly and avoid abrupt withdrawal.

Methadone (Category C)

- Methadone has a long half-life and should be initiated as an inpatient.
- It is used off licence for resistant neuropathic pain.
- Usual dosing starts at 5mg once a day and escalated to 8hrly.

Capsaicin ointment

- Fetal risk has not been categorized, but no human teratogenicity has been reported.
- Available in 0.025% and 0.075% for topical use in diabetic neuropathy and post herpetic neuralgia.
- May also be useful in myofascial pain.

Common pain problems

Low back pain

Low back pain (LBP) or pelvic girdle pain is common throughout pregnancy, with ligamentous laxity (relaxin) as the main precipitating factor. Other risk factors are smoking, obesity, and previous back pain. Note that epidural analgesia for labour pain is not associated with long term back pain.

Table 5.2 Red and yellow flags in lower back pain

Red flags: investigation required	Yellow flags: psychosocial factors indicative of long term chronicity
• Features of cauda equina syndrome	• A negative attitude that back pain is harmful
• Significant trauma	• Fear avoidance behaviour
• Weight loss	• An expectation that passive treatment is necessary
• History of cancer	• A tendency to depression, low morale and social withdrawal
• Fever	• Social or financial problems
• Possibility of HIV	
• Steroid use	
• Under 20yrs of age	
• Severe night pain	
• Pain worse when lying down	

Adapted from New Zealand Acute Low Back Pain Guide: INCORPORATING THE GUIDE TO ASSESSING PSYCHOSOCIAL YELLOW FLAGS IN ACUTE LOW BACK PAIN. New Zealand Guidelines Group. Licensed under a Creative Commons 4.0 International Attribution.

Non-specific LBP
- The majority of acute LBP has no cause (non-specific LBP) and improves within 6–8 weeks.
- Non-specific LBP is associated with radiation to buttocks and/or knees.

Degenerative disc disease
- This will manifest as LBP with radiation below the knee, neurogenic claudication, intermittent numbness, and/or weakness of the legs. Severity varies from 'leaking disc' to annular tear to frank prolapse.
- Red flags suggesting serious spinal pathology and referral for investigation, and yellow flags identify barriers to early recovery suitable for psychology referral are detailed in Table 5.2.

Management
- Maintain mobility (no more than 2 days bed rest).
- Maintain normal activity and remain at work.
- Physiotherapy: manipulation +/- therapeutic exercise (limited during 1st week).
- Injections: trigger points, ligaments and facet joints, epidural steroid injection if nerve root pain present via pain clinic referral.
- TENS may be useful.
- There is some weak evidence to support the use of acupuncture for back pain associated with pregnancy whilst the use of lumbar support garments may reduce pain on movement and analgesic use.
- Specific strengthening exercises reduce back pain.

Systemic analgesia
- Use slow release if pain is constant.
- If activity related, use short acting analgesia.
- Escalate as per generic pathway.
- Diazepam 2mg 8hrly (Category C) for short periods only for pain associated muscle spasm.

Acute prolapsed disc
- This is rare in pregnancy ~ 1:10,000.
- Most patients can be treated conservatively, but those with incapacitating pain, progressive neurological deficits, or bowel or bladder dysfunction may require MRI and surgical treatment.

Chronic back pain
- Chronic back pain +/- leg pain is managed with a combination of opioids, LA/steroid injections, physiotherapy, and psychological support.
- Postpartum assessment for invasive pain interventions should be considered.

Headache (migraine)
- Worst in 1st trimester, but often improves in 2nd & 3rd trimesters.
- Prevention with acupuncture and biofeedback are useful.
- Metoprolol & propranolol use only in exceptional circumstances.
- Analgesia is limited to paracetamol +/- codeine and ibuprofen for short periods but avoid NSAIDs in 3rd trimester. If severe consider moderate opioid.
- Nausea can be managed with ondansetron (category B1) or prochlorperazine (category C).
- Triptans and ergot derivatives are contraindicated.

Management
Acute attacks can be managed using a combination of:
- Acupuncture.
- Relaxation & sleep.
- Massage.
- Ice packs/gel pads.
- Biofeedback.

Abdominal nerve entrapment
A rapidly enlarging uterus can lead to pain and paraesthesia from cutaneous nerves that traverse the rectus muscles or inguinal ligaments, leading to skin sensitivity and irritating sensations.

Common problem sites
- Abdominal wall (tender points along costal margins).
- Ilioinguinal nerve.
- Genitofemoral nerve.
- Lateral cutaneous nerve of thigh (meralgia paraesthetica).

Symptomatic relief
May be achieved with:
- Local anaesthetic injections—tender points around course of nerves should be sought and these injected. Addition of steroid may be of benefit but sometimes can make pain worse.
- TENS.
- Ice packs/gel pads.
- Gabapentin +/- amitriptyline (not 1st trimester).

Carpal tunnel syndrome
- Compression of either median or ulnar nerves can occur.
- Paraesthesia is common and pain is experienced in 50%.
- Exclude pre-eclampsia and heart failure as a cause.

Management
- Remove rings and bracelets.
- Elevate hand at night.
- Night time splint.
- Paracetamol (NSAIDs worsen fluid retention).
- Rarely surgical release (under regional block).

Pelvic arthropathy
A common problem and can present during or after pregnancy. Ligament relaxation allows widening of pubic symphysis gap and lumbosacral joints. Ultrasound can measure symphysis gap.

Management
- Bed rest.
- Acupuncture.
- Physiotherapy, especially hydrotherapy if available.
- Pelvic binders.
- Walking aids.
- Short acting analgesia prior to walking (reduces muscle spasm).
- Treat associated neuropathic pain (common).
- Rarely surgery postpartum.

Ureteric obstruction
Often manifests in 2nd & 3rd trimesters as the enlarging uterus compresses ureters as they cross pelvic brim.

Management
- Adopting hand knee position.
- Paracetamol/ibuprofen/weak opioid.

Neuropathic pain (NeP)
There are over 100 causes of NeP, with varying degrees of neuropathic and nociceptive components. Table 5.3:
- Patients with NeP complain of burning or shooting pain, usually unresponsive to usual pain killers.
- Skin sensitivity may be present or there areas of numbness that are painful.
- Sleep disturbance is common as are depressive thoughts.

Table 5.3 Causes of NeP

Purely neuropathic pain	Partially neuropathic pain	Neuropathic component to pain
Post herpetic neuralgia	Atypical facial pain	Fibromyalgia
Diabetic neuropathy	Postlaminectomy pain	Chronic fatigue syndrome
Trigeminal neuralgia	CRPS	Chronic daily headache
Phantom limb	Postoperative neuralgia	Whiplash injury

Management

Management is usually a combination of:

- *Opioids*: high doses are usually required.
- *Amitriptyline*: 10mg at night escalated to 70mg over 6 weeks.
- *Anticonvulsants*: Try and avoid in 1st trimester. Monotherapy only, gabapentin or pregabalin considered safest. Folic acid, and abnormality scans recommended if used.
- *Topical agents:* Can be used in post-herpetic neuralgia and painful diabetic neuropathy.
- Lidocaine 5% patch.
- Capsaicin ointment.

Further reading

Shah S et al. Pain management in pregnancy: Multimodal approaches. Pain Research and Treatment 2015: 987483.

Australian government Department of Health: Prescribing medicines in pregnancy database Dec 2018—https://www.tga.gov.au/prescribing-medicines-pregnancy-database#searchname

Non-regional labour analgesia

Matthew Turner and Graeme Lilley

Pain in labour

Labour presents a physiological and psychological challenge for women. The latter stages of pregnancy can be a difficult time emotionally. Fear and apprehension are experienced alongside excitement. These emotions, both positive and negative, will affect the woman's birth experience.

Pain associated with labour has been described by Melzack as one of the most intense forms of pain that can be experienced. However, removing pain completely from labour does not necessarily mean a better birth experience for the mother. Women need to be included in the decisions regarding their individualized pain management plan. Providing clear information about the types of pain relief available has been found to increase feelings of control.

Women may now choose to deliver their baby in different places, e.g. consultant-led units, midwife-led units, or at home, depending on their risk assessment and the mother's own wishes. This ultimately means that not all options will be immediately available for all women. Information regarding the options for pain relief offered at each site should be made readily available to all expectant mothers during pregnancy and discussed in detail during the third trimester.

Pain pathways

- Pain during the first stage of labour is initially due to contraction of the body of the uterus, leading to dilatation of the cervix and lower uterine segment, and their subsequent distension and tearing during uterine contractions.
- The pain is visceral in nature and is therefore diffuse or poorly localized, often referred to another area, e.g. the back, and can be associated with profound nausea or vomiting.
- The intensity of pain is related to the speed of cervical dilatation and the strength of uterine contractions.
- Pain impulses during the first stage of labour are transmitted via afferent A and small C fibres from the uterus and cervix to the thoracolumbar sympathetic chain through T10, T11, T12, and L1 spinal nerves, and enter the dorsal horn of the spinal cord through their posterior roots.
- Pain during the latter part of the first stage and the second stage of labour results from continuing uterine contractions, and, in addition, pain and pressure related to stretching of the vagina and pelvic floor to accommodate the presenting part.
- This pain is more somatic in nature and is therefore well localized, often sharp, definite, not referred, constant, and not usually associated with nausea.
- Pain impulses during the second stage are transmitted via the pudendal nerve and into the spinal cord via S2, S3, and S4 spinal nerve roots. See Fig 6.1 Pain pathways of labour.

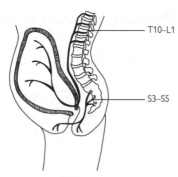

Fig. 6.1 Pain pathways of labour.

Effect of pain on maternal physiology

- Labour places massive physical demands upon both mother and fetus. Some of these demands are directly related to pain and can therefore be lessened by effective analgesia.
- The CO increases by 25–50% in labour, as a result of tachycardia secondary to pain and increased circulating catecholamines.
- Epidural analgesia has been shown to reduce cardiac index by 3–6%, and MAP by 1–9% (not influenced by fluid preload).
- This is of particular importance to the parturient with cardiac disease.
- The increased minute ventilation associated with labour pain results in a decrease in maternal $PaCO_2$, i.e. <3kPa, which is below the already physiologically low levels of late pregnancy. Hypocapnoea leads to maternal alkalosis with a shift in the haemoglobin A (HbA) oxyhaemoglobin curve to the *left*, i.e. less O_2 is released to fetal haemoglobin (HbF) and less CO_2 taken up by HbA. The fetus is at risk of becoming hypercapnoeic and hypoxic in this environment.
- Effective analgesia aims to return the maternofetal acid–base balance to the term status quo.

Factors influencing the pain of childbirth

For most women, childbirth is associated with very severe pain, often exceeding all expectations. However, the threshold at which women perceive differing intensity of pain varies greatly and is influenced by many physical and psychological factors (see Table 6.1).

Table 6.1 Factors influencing pain experience

Physical	Psychological
Age	Knowledge/preparation for childbirth
Parity	Expectation of pain
Size of infant/birth canal	Prior pain experiences
Abnormal fetal presentation	Fear and anxiety
Speed of cervical dilatation	Confidence to cope
Frequency of contractions	Supportive birthing partner
Stage of labour	Education and social class
Maternal position in labour	Culture and beliefs

Pain during dysfunctional labour

- Increased intensity of pain may indicate that the labour is not progressing as expected.
- Dysfunctional labour or dystocia in labour is associated with increased pain and therefore the woman should be reassessed for evidence of cephalopelvic disproportion, a macrosomic baby, or an abnormal presenting part, e.g. brow or face presentation.
- Women with dysfunctional labour are more likely to request an early epidural.
- Uterine rupture should be excluded if a woman suffers continuous abdominal pain or breakthrough pain despite an adequate epidural analgesic block.

Information

- Women need comprehensive information about the various analgesic choices that are available in their place of delivery.
- Not having their choice of analgesia available to them causes maternal dissatisfaction.
- Many women will attend local midwifery-run classes and analgesic options will be discussed. The midwives running these classes need up to date information on locally available epidural services and protocols.
- OAA's Labour Pains or locally produced leaflets can be made available in the antenatal clinic which describe in detail the pros and cons of the different analgesic techniques and their local availability. These are particularly useful for those mothers not attending antenatal classes.
- Many women will now use the Internet to supplement information from midwives. Reliable and accurate information on all forms of pain relief can be found on the Obstetric Anaesthetists' Association (OAA) website labourpains.com.

Non-pharmacological options

The Complementary Medicine Field of The Cochrane Collaboration defines complementary medicine as 'practices and ideas which are outside the domain of conventional medicine in several countries' and is defined by its users as 'preventing or treating illness, or promoting health and well being' (Cochrane Collaboration, 2003).

- The use of complementary and alternative medicine has become popular with consumers worldwide, often with little or no evidence to support their use.
- Complementary therapies are more commonly used by women of reproductive age, with almost half reporting use. It is possible that a significant proportion of women are using these therapies during pregnancy.
- Many women would like to avoid pharmacological or invasive methods of pain relief in labour. This may contribute towards the popularity of complementary methods of pain management.
- It is important for the obstetric anaesthetist to be familiar with complementary techniques and therapies in order that the efficacy and limitations of therapies might be discussed.

Categories of therapies

- Psychological support, e.g. partner/midwife continuous support, doula.
- Mind–body interventions, e.g. breathing, hypnosis, yoga, relaxation therapies.
- Biofeedback, e.g. changes in thoughts/emotions affecting physiology
- Alternative medical practice, e.g. homeopathy, traditional Chinese medicine.
- Manual handling methods, e.g. massage, reflexology.
- Physiological and biological treatments, e.g. TENS, water blocks.
- Bioelectromagnetic applications, e.g. magnets.
- Water immersion.

Mind–body interventions

- This was popularized by Grantly Dick-Read after publication of his books *Natural Childbirth* in 1933 and *Childbirth without Fear* in 1944.
- He postulated that the pain of childbirth was largely a product of modern living, leading to a cycle of fear, tension, and pain.
- Relaxation, meditation, visualization, and breathing are commonly used for labour and are widely accessible through teaching during antenatal classes.
- Yoga, meditation, and hypnosis may have a calming effect and provide a distraction from pain and tension.

Biofeedback

- Describes a therapeutic technique where individuals receive training to improve their health and well-being by responding to signals from their own bodies, such as muscle tension, heart rate, and temperature.
- Electronic instruments identify the stimuli, and patients gain control of physiological responses under expert supervision.

Aromatherapy

- Essential oils are used, drawing on the healing power of plants. The oils may be massaged into the skin or inhaled using a steam infusion or burner.
- The mechanism of action of aromatherapy is unclear. Studies have demonstrated psychological improvement in mood and anxiety levels.

Acupuncture

- Fine needles are inserted into different parts of the body. The points used to reduce labour pain are located on the hands, feet, and ears.
- Acupressure involves applying pressure on the acupuncture point. The aim is to treat illness and soothe pain by stimulating the specific points.

Homeopathy

- Works on the principle that 'like cures like'. Remedies are prescribed as potencies as a result of tiny and highly diluted amounts of the substances from which they are derived. The more times the substance is diluted, the greater the potency. Remedies are derived from herbs, minerals, and other natural substances.
- The principle of treatment is that the substance will stimulate the body and healing functions, so achieving a state of balance with relief of symptoms. It is proposed that homeopathy enables the woman in labour to cope, to soothe, and relax her, which may reduce her pain.

Massage

- Massage is commonly used to help relax tense muscles and soothe and calm the individual.
- Massage may help to relieve pain in labour by inhibiting pain signals or by improving blood flow and oxygenation of tissues. Different massage techniques may help different women.

Reflexology

- Reflexologists propose that there are reflex points on the feet corresponding to organs and structures of the body.
- Pain may be reduced by gentle manipulation on certain parts of the foot.
- Pressure applied to the feet has been shown to result in an anaesthetizing effect on other parts of the body.

Cochrane 2012, Authors Conclusions

- 'Most methods of non-pharmacological pain management are noninvasive and appear to be safe for the mother and baby, however their effectiveness is unclear due to limited high quality evidence.'

Transcutaneous electrical nerve stimulation (TENS)

- Widely accepted by mothers and midwives for pain relief during labour, because of its lack of side effects for both mother and fetus.
- Often used in late third trimester to treat LBP or in early labour.
- Four pads are positioned over the lower back and a low voltage electrical current is transmitted constantly to the underlying skin with a 'boost' during uterine contractions.

- Mechanism of action is based on the 'gate theory of pain'.
- Probably most effective in the latent or early phase of labour.
- Allows the mother to mobilize, which may be beneficial and increase its acceptability.
- Meta-analysis failed to demonstrate its efficacy as an analgesic.

Water blocks

- Popular in Scandinavian countries.
- 0.1mL of sterile water is injected intradermally in four spots over the sacrum.
- Intense burning seems to induce pain relief.
- The mechanism is probably similar to TENS.

Water immersion

- The sensation of warm water may soothe the pain of labour and has a long history in lay and clinical care.
- Birthing pools are now widely available on midwifery-led and obstetrician-led delivery units and may be utilized at any stage of labour.
- The water supports the weight of the gravid uterus and aids movement, facilitating the neuro-hormonal interactions of labour, easing pain, and possibly optimizing progress. Fetal position may be optimized by maternal movement, encouraging flexion.
- Water immersion may be associated with improved uterine perfusion and shorter labour with fewer interventions.
- Blood pressure is reduced in shoulder depth water due to vasodilatation.
- Water immersion may increase maternal satisfaction and sense of control, whilst it has been postulated that in the relaxed mother the release of endogenous opioids is optimized.
- Evidence suggests that water immersion during the first stage of labour reduces the use of epidural or spinal analgesia.
- There is no evidence of increased adverse effects to the fetus/neonate or woman from labouring in water or waterbirth.

Further reading

Jones L et al. Pain management for women in labour: An overview of systematic reviews. *Cochrane Database of Systematic Reviews* 2012; 14: CD009234.

Cluett ER, Burns EE. Immersion in water in labour and birth. *Cochrane Database of Systematic Reviews* 2009; 5:CD000111.

Levett KM et al. Complementary therapies for labour and birth study: a randomised controlled trial of antenatal integrative medicine for pain management in labour. *BMJ* 2016; 12;6.

Non-pharmacological—summary

The advantages and disadvantages of non-pharmacological options are summarized in Table 6.2.

Table 6.2 Non-pharmacological options—advantages and disadvantages

Therapy	Advantages	Disadvantages
TENS	Non-invasive, easy to use. Good for back pain	Useful only in early labour. Availability
Immersion	Popular. Backed by government initiative	Availability. Cannot be used with many other methods
Massage	Perceived as highly effective	Labour intensive
Acupuncture	Drug free	Invasive. Needs trained therapist
Biofeedback		Not widely used. Needs expert supervision and monitoring equipment
Water blocks	Easy to perform. Good for back pain	Temporary relief only (<90min). Initial burning
Continuous support	Almost universal use. Useful at any stage	None
Hypnosis	Non-invasive	Not all susceptible. Time consuming
Aromatherapy	Non-invasive	Oils need to be tested
Homeopathy	Few	Needs individual prescription

TENS = Transcutaneous electrical nerve stimulation.

The mechanism of action and supporting evidence for the use of non-pharmacological options are summarized in Table 6.3.

Table 6.3 Mechanism of action and evidence

Therapy	Mechanism of action	Evidence
TENS	Based on gate theory	Systematic review of 8 RCTs failed to demonstrate analgesic effect
Immersion	Sensation of warm water inhibits pain transmission. Supports gravid uterus	Cochrane review of 11 trials. Single trials showed lower pain intensity, reduced BP and better satisfaction
Massage	Inhibits pain transmission. Provides support and distraction	Four trials showed reduced pain intensity in massage groups
Acupuncture	May inhibit pain transmission by neural method (gate theory) or by release of endorphins or endogenous opioids	Two RCTs comparing acupuncture/acupressure with control showed better pain relief satisfaction
Biofeedback	Gain control of physiological responses	Four studies examining assisted vaginal birth and section showed no benefit
Water blocks	Injection of 0.1mL sterile water in 4 spots over sacrum. Action similar to TENS	Two double-blind RCTs showed reduction in labour pain, but other work showed they were not rated by women as effective as other methods
Continuous support	Presence of a trained support person can improve the physiological and psychological aspects of labour, e.g. partner, friend, or doula (a doula is a professional non-medical support and advocate)	Cochrane review of 15 RCTs involving 12,791 women. Those with continuous support, as opposed to conventional care, were less likely to have intrapartum analgesia, operative birth, or be dissatisfied with their experiences
Hypnosis	Hypnotic state has better control over pain	Cochrane review of 7 RCTs, >1000 women. No significant improvement in satisfaction or any other parameters
Aromatherapy	Essential oils for therapeutic effect	Two RCTs found no difference in benefit
Homeopathy	Minute amount of substance to relieve symptoms	No research

TENS = Transcutaneous electrical nerve stimulation; RCT = Randomized controlled trial.

Systemic opioids

The use of IM or IV opioids to reduce the pain of labour is common and widely accepted by mothers. When regional analgesia is contra-indicated, it is important that alternative pain relief methods, e.g. systemic opioids, are offered to women who request them. The choice of IM opioid used in delivery units is largely historical. Pethidine and diamorphine are the most widely used in the UK.

In recent years, administration of IV opioids via a patient-controlled analgesia (PCA) device has gained increasing popularity. It has the benefit of giving the mother a degree of control over her pain relief, which may improve satisfaction.

Remifentanil is the opioid that comes closest to the ideal drug profile when used via IV PCA to manage the pain of labour, without neonatal respiratory depression being a major problem.

All opioids share the same side effect profile to differing extents:

- Dose-dependent respiratory depression of mother and neonate.
- Delayed gastric emptying, increased gastric volumes, nausea, and vomiting.
- Sedation, dysphoria, euphoria, and amnesia.
- Hypotension.

Pethidine

- Pethidine (meperidine) is a synthetic phenylpiperidine derivative, related to fentanyl and sufentanil. It is 28 times more lipid soluble than morphine. It is metabolized to the active metabolite norpethidine, which has convulsant properties and is contra-indicated in those with severe pre-eclampsia, epilepsy and other causes of renal impairment.
- Pethidine is bound to A_1-acid glycoprotein but readily crosses the placenta by passive diffusion and reaches equilibrium within 6min. Peak plasma concentrations in the fetus occurs 2–3h following IM injection in the mother. In the acidotic environment of the fetal circulation, the weak base is more ionized and thus accumulates due to ion trapping.
- Pethidine was made legally available in the UK to midwives for independent use in 1950 and remains the most widely used IM opioid in labour.
- It is usually administered in two divided doses of 75–100mg, up to a maximum dose of 200mg.
- Despite widespread use, its efficacy as an analgesic has been questioned. Many obstetric anaesthetists believe that its use as a labour analgesic should be stopped.
- It does however seem to help the parturient cope better, by means of dysphoria, sedation, amnesia, etc.
- Several studies have found it inferior to other IM opiates (e.g. diamorphine) in terms of analgesia and its adverse effects on mother and baby.
- Respiratory depression is more common in the neonate than the mother. The babies of mothers who received pethidine have been shown to be sleepier and slower to establish feeding.

- About 10% of neonates will have a 1min Apgar score of <6 if pethidine is given 2–3h before delivery as this coincides with peak fetal concentrations. The incidence is very much reduced if given before or after this.
- The practice of not giving the mother pethidine in the second stage of labour for fear of neonatal sedation is illogical.
- Norpethidine is also found in the neonate and may contribute to sedation for several days.

Diamorphine
- Diamorphine is more soluble and has a more rapid onset of action than morphine or pethidine.
- After administration it is rapidly hydrolysed to 6-monoacetylmorphine and then later metabolized to morphine. It is eliminated rapidly by the placenta.
- When diamorphine and pethidine were compared, patients who received pethidine were more likely to report no pain relief. The incidence of vomiting was lower in the diamorphine group. Pethidine was associated with lower Apgar scores at 1min.
- It has been rated by both mothers and midwives as being subjectively superior to pethidine and Entonox®.

Morphine
- This naturally occurring opioid is bound to albumin in the circulation and rapidly crosses the placenta.
- It is not trapped in the fetal circulation and diffuses quickly back into the maternal circulation due to rapid elimination and subsequent diffusion gradient.
- It is metabolized to an opioid agonist (morphine-6-glucoronide) and an antagonist (morphine-3-glucoronide) in varying quantities.
- It was popular in the 1920s and 1930s, and used with hyoscine to induce 'twilight sleep' for labour and delivery.
- Women frequently had little memory of labour or of being in pain.

Fentanyl
- Fentanyl is a synthetic phenylpiperidine derivative, without active metabolites. It is highly bound to albumin. It has analgesic potencies 100× greater than morphine and 800× greater than pethidine.
- Its high lipid solubility results in a rapid onset.
- A long (78h) terminal half-life (longer than morphine and pethidine) will result in accumulation, in the mother and fetus, after repeated IM doses.
- IV PCA fentanyl has been investigated in two randomized controlled trials:
  - When compared with epidural anaesthesia, satisfaction was similar in the two groups (although 3/10 changed from PCA to epidural). There were no differences in Apgar scores or cord gases, but SpO_2 <90% was more common in babies of PCA mothers. The authors recommend monitoring of the fetus postnatally.
  - When compared with alfentanil, analgesia was described as inadequate in 42% of the alfentanil group and 9% of the fentanyl group.

Traditional opioid analgesia regimes for labour analgesia are summarized in Table 6.4.

Table 6.4 Opioid analgesia—a summary of traditional dosing regimes

Opioid	IM	IV via PCA device
Pethidine	75–100mg 2 doses may be administered by qualified midwife	10mg bolus Lockout time 5min Optional loading dose of 25–50mg
Morphine	5–10mg	1mg bolus Lockout time 5min Optional loading dose of 5mg
Diamorphine	2.5–5mg	0.5mg bolus Lockout time 5min Optional loading dose of 2.5mg
Fentanyl	Rarely used	20 micrograms bolus Lockout time 5min Optional loading dose of 50 micrograms

Remifentanil
- Remifentanil is a μ-receptor agonist that is a derivative of fentanyl, and is described as ultra short-acting.
- It is rapidly hydrolysed by the non-saturatable red cell and tissue esterases. It has a terminal half-life of <10min and a context-sensitive half-life of 73min.
- It was introduced into obstetric analgesia in the late 1990s, which was reflected by a number of case reports of effective analgesia in the literature, and subsequently a substantial body of evidence supporting its use for labour analgesia.
- Remifentanil as analgesia for labour is available in over a third of units in the UK.
- Recent meta-analysis confirms it to be a more effective labour analgesic than parenteral and inhalational alternatives.
- Various IV PCA remifentanil dosing regimes have been described (see Table 6.5).
- The optimal delivery regime has yet to be determined, but the above regimes seem the most successful.
- Modified dosing regime reflects evolving pain stimulus as labour proceeds, demonstrating reduced requests for additional analgesia in one RCT, but requires specialist PCA programming.
- General consensus in the literature is that a dedicated intravenous cannula is required to avoid accidental bolus administration.

Table 6.5 Remifentanil PCA—some examples of dosing regimes

Bolus dose	Lockout	Continuous infusion	Features
0.25–0.5 micrograms/kg	2 min	Nil	Nil
20–40 micrograms	3 min	Nil	Nil
20 micrograms	1 min	50 micrograms/hr	Boluses adjusted to response
18–60 micrograms	1 min	50 micrograms/hr	Bolus dependent on button press duration

- IV PCA remifentanil requires careful monitoring of the mother and fetus.
- Continuous maternal oxygen saturation of the mother is mandatory.
- Supplemental oxygen should be available and may be required.
- The mother requires one-to-one care with a midwife trained in the assessment of the mother using remifentanil.

Adverse effects

- Recent literature review suggests almost a third of patients using remifentanil PCA develop some degree of respiratory depression.
- Patients spend up to 5% of their time whilst using the PCA with oxygen saturations below 90%.
- There are case reports of respiratory arrest associated with remifentanil in labour
- There is one case report of cardiac arrest in labour associated with remifentanil PCA, although the precise aetiology of the incident remains uncertain.
- Extreme caution must be employed when using remifentanil where other opioids have been administered in preceding hours, and departmental protocol should reinforce this.

RESPITE trial

The RESPITE trial, reported in May 2017, investigated the difference between women receiving pethidine IM and remifentanil PCA after requesting opioid analgesia. The primary outcome was conversion to epidural. Secondary outcomes included visual analog scale pain scores, maternal satisfaction, side effects, and neonatal status. A summary of the findings are presented in Table 6.6.

In the abstract accompanying the oral presentation in May 2017, the authors suggest re-evaluating opioid pain relief.

Table 6.6 Respite trial results

	Remifentanil	Pethidine
n	201	199
Epidural conversion	39/201 (19%)	81/199 (41%)
Instrumental delivery	52/199 (26%)	106/199 (53%)
Median VAS scores	Lower	
O₂ saturations	Lower	
Supplemental O₂	More likely	
Maternal satisfaction	Significantly greater	
Respiratory depression	No difference	
Neonatal status	No difference	
Breastfeeding rates	No difference	

VAS = visual analog scale.

Data from Wilson MJA et al, RESPITE Trial Collaborative Group. Intrave-nous remifentanil patient-controlled analgesia versus intramuscular pethidine for pain relief in labour (RESPITE): an open-label, multicentre, randomised controlled trial. *Lancet.* 2018 Aug 25;392(10148):662-672. doi: 10.1016/S0140-6736(18)31613-1. Epub 2018 Aug 13.

Further reading

Wilson MJA et al. RESPITE Trial Collaborative Group. Intravenous remifentanil patient-controlled analgesia versus intramuscular pethidine for pain relief in labour (RESPITE): an open-label, multicentre, randomised controlled trial. *Lance.* 2018; 392: 662–672.

Fairlie FM et al. Intramuscular opioids for maternal pain relief in labour: a randomized controlled trial comparing pethidine with diamorphine. *British Journal of Obstetrics and Gynaecology* 1999; 106: 1181–1187.

Blair JM et al. Patient-controlled analgesia for labour using remifentanil: a feasibility study. *British Journal of Anaesthesia* 2001; 87: 415–420.

Thurlow JA et al. Remifentanil by patient-controlled analgesia compared with intramuscular meperidine for pain relief in labour. *British Journal of Anaesthesia* 2002; 88: 374–378.

Muchatuta NA, Kinsella SM. Remifentanil for labour analgesia: time to draw breath? *Anaesthesia* 2013: 68:227–235

Marr R et al. Cardiac arrest with remifentanil patient-controlled analgesia. *Anaesthesia* 2013: 68:283–287

Wilson MJ et al. A randomized controlled trial of remifentanil intravenous PCA vs pethidine for pain relief in labour (RESPITE). *International Journal of Obstetric Anaesthesia* 2017;31, Supplement 1:S8.

Inhalational analgesia

Inhalational analgesia for childbirth was popularized by the administration of chloroform to Queen Victoria by Dr John Snow for the birth of her 8th child, Prince Leopold in 1853.

Entonox®

- Nitrous oxide in air was first described for labour analgesia in 1880.
- Its use was popular for 80 years, with up to 80% N_2O and <10% oxygen!
- Many portable devices, such as the Queen Charlotte's apparatus, were widely used by obstetricians and midwives for home deliveries.
- Invented by Dr Mike Tunstall in 1961, Entonox® (50% N_2O in O_2) was approved for unsupervised use by midwives in 1965.
- A survey in 1990 found Entonox® available in 99% of obstetric units in the UK and used by 60% of mothers in labour.
- Although it is very popular in Europe, it is not used in North America.
- Distraction, relaxation, and sense of control all increase the subjective benefit of Entonox®.
- Although popular and subjectively approved by mothers, the analgesic effect is probably limited.
- Mothers in the National Birthday Trust 1990 survey thought that Entonox® was generally superior to pethidine.
- Shown in two studies to offer better pain relief than placebo.
- Adverse effects include drowsiness, dizziness, nausea, and vomiting.
- N_2O has a low blood gas solubility coefficient of 0.47, therefore it equilibrates with blood and is washed out of the lungs quickly. There is minimal accumulation with intermittent use in labour.
- There is the theoretical risk of bone marrow suppression with prolonged use.
- There may be an occupational risk to midwives especially if administered in poorly ventilated rooms.

Halogenated agents

- Chloroform was commonly administered via an open face mask or gauze for much of the first half of the 20th century.
- In the 1940s, chloroform-containing glass capsules were introduced so a safer measured quantity could be administered.
- The halogenated agents superseded chloroform after deaths from ventricular fibrillation and oversedation occurred.
- Trichloroethylene and then methoxyflurane were routinely used by midwives through fixed low dose draw-over inhalers until the 1970s.
- Midwives are no longer allowed to administer halogenated agents, and an anaesthetist must now be present.
- Can still be administered via a draw-over inhaler mixed with air or Entonox®.
- Active scavenging in delivery suites is required to comply with Health and Safety occupational exposure standards.

Isofluarne and Desflurane
- Isoflurane and desflurane have been used with limited supporting evidence, but sevoflurane remains the most widely used agent nationally

Sevoflurane
- A study investigated 2–3% sevoflurane in air and O_2, administered intermittently aiming for an end-tidal sevoflurane of 1–1.4%.
- Analgesic properties increased to 0.8%, but increased sedation occurred at higher doses.
- If given 1min prior to contraction, it significantly reduced pain.
- Apgar scores were unaffected.
- 0.8% sevoflurane is more effective than Entonox®.

Further reading

Fortescue C, Wee M. Analgesia in labour: non regional techniques. *Continuing Education in Anaesthesia, Critical Care and Pain* 2005; 5: 9–13.

Yeo ST et al. Analgesia with sevoflurane during labour: I. Determination of the optimum concentration. *British Journal of Anaesthesia* 2007; 981: 105–109.

Yeo ST et al. . Analgesia with sevoflurane during labour: II. Sevoflurane compared with Entonox® for labour analgesia. *British Journal of Anaesthesia* 2007; 98: 110–115.

Regional techniques in pregnancy

Rachel Collis and Sarah Harries

Introduction/benefits

Regional analgesia has provided mothers with enormous benefit since its introduction in the UK in the early 1970s. Since then, the number of procedures has continued to increase, and now the majority of mothers who request regional analgesia can have an epidural for pain relief on request. In addition, the number of operative deliveries and other surgical procedures has continued to rise, and now the majority of CSs are performed with the mother awake.

The provision of these services has had enormous benefits for mother, baby, and partner, on both safety and humanitarian grounds. The avoidance of GA, where possible, has probably contributed to a fall in maternal deaths related to anaesthesia. Allowing the mother to be awake during the birth of her baby by CS has sound medical benefits, but also improves satisfaction for both her and her partner.

Despite the popularity and overall safety of regional techniques: epidurals and spinals that are performed badly, cause injury, or do not work properly have led to an increase in complaints and legal claims against obstetric anaesthetists. Therefore appropriate consent, documentation, and conduct of regional procedures is of paramount importance when performing any regional technique in pregnancy.

Absolute contraindications

Maternal refusal
- The woman's wishes should be respected at all times. However, the woman has the right to change her mind at any time later.
- All decisions and discussions should be accurately recorded in the case notes.

Allergy
- True allergy to amide local anaesthetic is very rare.
- Ascertain the history of the reaction, check the case notes, and enquire about formal allergy testing.
- Is there a MedicAlert® bracelet?
  The majority of epidural packs and kits are latex free.

Sepsis
- Localized infection at the intended insertion site.
- Exaggerated or uncontrollable hypotension may occur in the overtly septic patient, who is already vasodilated, intravascular volume depleted, and has myocardial depression.
- There is the risk of introducing infected blood into a sterile epidural or subarachnoid space.
- Coagulation/platelet abnormalities may be present or developing.

Raised intercranial pressure
- Diagnostic imaging may be required.

Clotting abnormalities
- Platelet count <70×10^9/L (spinal) and <100×10^9/L (epidural). If the platelet count is below these levels, senior anaesthetic advice should be sought to assess the balance of risk vs benefit.
- Evidence of clotting dysfunction.
- Strong history of bleeding tendency, even if tests are normal.

Lack of appropriately trained staff and/or equipment
- Full resuscitation facilities must be available.
- There should be an appropriately trained person to instigate and interpret monitoring for both the woman and fetus for the duration of the epidural.
- Large bore patent IV access must be *in situ* to allow prompt treatment in the event of maternal hypotension/collapse.

Bleeding disorders

Congenital clotting abnormalities
- Usually single factor deficiencies with a personal history of bleeding and family history.

Reduced/absent synthesis of clotting factors and fibrinogen
- 2° to pre-existing liver disease, liver involvement in pre-eclampsia, intrahepatic cholestasis of pregnancy, vitamin K deficiency and drugs.

Increased consumption
- Disseminated intravascular coagulation 2° to sepsis, intrauterine death, severe pre-eclampsia, placental abruption, and amniotic fluid embolism.

Acute loss ± dilution
- Haemorrhage and massive blood transfusion. Packed red cells lack factors V, VIII, XI, platelets, and fibrinogen.

Thrombocytopenia
- Gestational thrombocytopenia of pregnancy (GTP) is clinically indistinguishable from mild immune thrombocytopenia purpura (ITP), both of which are relatively common during pregnancy. GTP resolves postpartum.

Hypertensive disorders of pregnancy
- The second most common cause of thrombocytopenia, with excessive platelet consumption and altered function. HELLP syndrome represents the most extreme end of the spectrum.

Drug-induced thrombocytopenia
- 2° to heparin therapy (HIT), penicillin, H_2-antagonists, thiazide diuretics, hydralazine, and cocaine.

Uraemia
- Alters platelet function detrimentally.

Type 2b von Willibrand's disease
- Associated with persistently low von Willibrand's factor levels and thrombocytopenia in pregnancy.

Relative contraindications

- Hypovolaemia with ongoing haemorrhage.
- Rapidly falling platelet count, e.g. in severe pre-eclampsia or HELLP. Repeat the platelet count if >2h old and check clotting.
- Raised white cell count (WCC) e.g. >25×10^9/L. The level of WCC or C-reactive protein at which it is unsafe to site an epidural in labour has not been determined. A WCC of >25×10^9/L is common in labour and may not be associated with infection. If the WCC is raised and other signs of infection evident, the source of the infection should be sought and treated with appropriate antibiotics prior to placement of an epidural. A minimum of 1×IV dose is recommended.
- Anatomical anomalies, e.g. spina bifida cystica or previous spinal surgery. Check notes for neurosurgical comment regarding regional techniques. Has she had an epidural or spinal previously? Were there any difficulties during the procedure, with the block or after delivery?
- Cardiovascular disease, in particular stenotic valvular lesions and cardiomyopathies, where the patient cannot cope with a sudden reduction in SVR. This is seldom a problem when fractionated low dose bupivacaine/opioid mixture is used. A high level of vigilance and invasive BP monitoring may be required for safe regional analgesia or anaesthesia.
- Active neurological disease. There should be consultation with a neurologist and documentation of current neurological status, along with chronological details of relapses and remission periods.
- If a relative contraindication exists, the medical and obstetric history should be reviewed together with any related laboratory investigations.
- The case notes should be checked for any antenatal anaesthetic clinic alerts and/or input from other specialties sought. For example, neurosurgical referral may prompt an MRI scan to determine the anatomy of the spinal column and epidural space if a spinal anomaly exists.
- Senior anaesthetic input should be sought in these cases and there should be detailed documentation of the delivery plan in the case notes.

The management of the mother on anticoagulants

Low molecular weight heparins (LMWHs)

- Are used during pregnancy for treatment or prophylaxis of venous thromboembolic disease, pro-thrombotic disease such as Factor V Leiden mutation, protein S and protein C deficiency, and antiphospholipid syndrome.
- LMWHs have a good safety profile, with reduced risk of osteoporosis and heparin induced thrombocytopenia (HIT) compared with unfractionated heparin. See Table 7.1 for the safe timing of anticoagulants and regional techniques.

Unfractionated heparin

- Unfractionated heparin (UFH) does not cross the placenta, therefore it is safe during organogenesis in the first trimester compared with warfarin. It may be the preferred agent in late pregnancy when delivery is imminent, as its effects can be rapidly reversed.

Warfarin

- Can be used from the second trimester to near term. It is avoided in the first trimester as it is associated with dose-related developmental abnormalities during organogenesis; these are associated with a larger dose >5mg rather than the INR.

IV heparin infusion

- May also be used in patients at high risk of venous thromboembolism.

Low dose aspirin

- Frequently used as prophylaxis in women at high risk of developing pre-eclampsia or recurrent miscarriage.
- Aspirin use is not a contraindication to siting an epidural catheter. There is little evidence to support an increased risk of vertebral canal haematoma if aspirin or an NSAID is used as a sole agent.
- If used together or in conjunction with LMWH, interaction may occur and senior haematological advice should be sought.

Novel oral anticoagulants

- Novel oral anticoagulants (NOACs) are currently not recommended in pregnancy.

Table 7.1 Safe timings for regional techniques with anticoagulants

Drug	Time to regional insertion after last dose	Time to next dose following insertion	Cautions/other Remember to consider the overall picture
LMWH			
Prophylactic dose (depending on patient weight, dosage ranges from 20–80mg enoxaparin)	12h	4h	Consider waiting longer (up to 24h) if procedure technically difficult or if there is ongoing bleeding
Therapeutic dose (>40mg enoxaparin, dose will be weight and anti-Factor Xa activity dependent)	24h		APTT is normal. Monitoring of anti-Xa levels may be required if regional anaesthesia is considered within these time frames or if the mother has renal impairment
UFH			
Heparin SC (5000IU)	4h	1h	As above
IV infusion	Stop infusion, check clotting after 1h. APTT should be normal and platelet count >100×10⁹/L. Inform senior anaesthetist	Infusion should not be started until 12h after siting an epidural and extended to 24h if there was a bloody tap Catheter can be removed 4h after stopping infusion if APTT is normal and platelet count >100×10⁹/L.	Ideally, heparin should be stopped 4–6h prior to surgery. If delivery imminent, spontaneous or otherwise, discuss with senior anaesthetist and obstetrician Protamine 1mg per 100IU heparin by slow IV injection will reverse the effect. Beware severe hypotension, bronchospasm and flushing. Caution if fish/shellfish allergy

(Continued)

Table 7.1 (Contd.)

Drug	Time to regional insertion after last dose	Time to next dose following insertion	Cautions/other Remember to consider the overall picture
Other drugs which may affect clotting/platelet function			
Aspirin NSAIDs	No wait necessary	No wait necessary	May be synergy with concomitant administration or other antiplatelet agent. Interaction with LMWH may occur Beware in disease states causing alteration of platelet number/function
Warfarin	INR <1.5	Use heparin regimen until INR re-established	After stopping warfarin, INR takes 3–5 days to fall to <1.5 If delivery imminent, discuss with haematologist In an emergency, warfarin can be reversed with vitamin K and prothrombin complex Remember the baby is anticoagulated which may not be reversed with these measures Takes 3–4 days for the INR to rise to >2.0 after warfarin recommenced

The same time frames for placement relate to removal of an epidural catheter.

Further reading

Reducing the Risk of Venous Thromboembolism during Pregnancy and the Puerperium. Green-top Guideline No. 37a April 2015. www.rcog.org.uk/globalassets/documents/guidelines/gtg-37a.pdf

Horlocker TT et al. Regional anesthesia in the patient receiving antithrombotic or thrombolytic therapy: American Society of Regional Anesthesia and Pain Medicine Evidence-Based Guidelines (Third Edition). *Regional Anesthesia and Pain Medicine*. 2010; 35: 64–101.

Leffert LR et al. Neuraxial anesthesia in obstetric patients receiving thromboprophylaxis with unfractionated or low-molecular-weight heparin: A systematic review of spinal epidural hematoma. *Anesthia and Analgesia* 2017; 125: 223–231.

Association of Anaesthetists of Great Britain and Ireland, Obstetric Anaesthetists' Association and Regional Anaesthesia UK. Regional anaesthesia and patients with abnormalities of coagulation. *Anaesthesia* 2013; 68: 966–972. Available online at: http://onlinelibrary.wiley.com/doi/10.1111/anae.12359/abstract

Consent

There is a legal, ethical, and professional requirement to obtain informed consent prior to performing a procedure on any patient.

For consent to treatment to be valid:

- Adequate information must be supplied including the benefits, risks, and complications of the procedure.
- A person should be considered to have the capacity to give consent and to make a balanced decision free from coercion. A person is deemed to have capacity if they are able to understand and retain the relevant treatment information. They must understand the procedure or treatment, and be able to balance the risks and benefits to arrive at a decision before issuing consent.
- Capacity may be compromised by drugs, fatigue, pain, or anxiety, but these would need to be extreme to incapacitate her.
- A woman deemed competent to give consent is free to change her decision at any time.

Special considerations

Birth plans

- If epidural analgesia is requested during labour but refused in the birth plan, the woman's most recent wishes are to be respected and the usual consent procedure followed.
- The change of decision from the original birth plan should be documented in the notes, and the woman should be asked to countersign the record if possible.
- If during labour the woman loses capacity, the decision in the birth plan should be adhered to and treated as an Advance Decision ('advance directive'), and considered legally binding.

Non-English-speaking women

- Information leaflets in a variety of languages regarding analgesia in labour are available from the OAA (labourpains.com).
- An interpreter should be made available, ideally from outside the family group. Every attempt should be made to discuss analgesia in the antenatal period.

Parturients under the age of 18

- 16- and 17-year-old women are considered to be adults with regards to making decisions regarding medical intervention.
- Younger teenagers may be considered competent to give consent; however, the physical and psychological demands of labour may compromise capacity.
- Excessive control by a parent that appears to be against the wishes of the young parturient should be strongly discouraged, as a child is generally thought to be able to give consent from 12 years of age.

Lack of capacity

- If a patient lacks capacity, whether permanent or temporary, and in the absence of an 'Advance Decision' ('advance directive'), treatment can be carried out without consent, directed in the patient's best interests. The Mental Capacity Act Code of Practice should be followed.
- The treatment should be discussed with family or carers, but this is not a legal requirement.

Obtaining informed consent for epidural analgesia during labour

- Women want information and to be brought into the consent process, even if they are distressed or apparently incapable of retaining information.
- Roughly a third of information will be retained accurately.
- Signed consent is not necessary. However, a record of the discussion, including the risks and complications, should be documented in full in the medical case notes with the date and time of the assessment.
- The discussion should ideally be witnessed by the birthing partner or midwife, and the notes countersigned by the attending midwife.
- Talk between contractions—if contractions are fast and furious or the woman is using Entonox® continuously, try to involve the birth partner in the process and keep explanations short and simple.
- Try to confirm their understanding of epidural analgesia initially. Has she received any antenatal education or advice regarding epidural analgesia either from antenatal groups or via other media, e.g. magazines or websites?
- Answers to specific questions should be full, frank, and honest, and recorded in the notes.

What information should you give?

Essential information
- The procedure—the correct position, local anaesthetic infiltration, the need to keep as still as possible, etc.
- The risk of a severe headache following accidental dural puncture, e.g. 1: 100.
- Inadequate or incomplete analgesia and how this can be remedied.
- The increased risk of instrumental delivery associated with epidural analgesia.

Consider also telling her
- The need for intermittent monitoring of BP and continuous CTG.
- Nausea and vomiting.
- Itching associated with opioids.
- Tenderness or bruising at insertion site for 24–48h but no increased risk of long-term backache.
- The risk of neurological complications in 1:10,000.
- The risk of epidural-related infections—very rare.

Further reading

Mental Capacity Act Code of Practice www.gov.uk/government/publications/mental-capacity-act-code-of-practice

Good practice in consent implementation guide: Dept of Health www.health.wa.gov.au/mhareview/resources/documents/UK_DOH_implementation_guide.pdf

Bethune L et al. Complications of obstetric regional analgesia: how much information is enough? *International Journal of Obstetrics and Anesthesia* 2004; 13: 30–34.

AAGBI: Consent for anaesthesia 2017 www.aagbi.org/sites/default/files/AAGBI_Consent_for_anaesthesia_2017_0.pdf

Mahomed K et al. Epidural analgesia during labour—maternal understanding and experience—informed consent. *Journal of Obstetrics and Gynaecology* 2015; 35:807–809.

Monitoring

- A midwife fully trained in the management of epidurals and their complications should remain with the woman once an epidural is sited.
- The anaesthetist should stay in the room after the first test dose and ideally until an adequate analgesic block is established.
- There must be adequate facility for BP, heart rate, and pulse oximeter monitoring in the delivery room.
- Lack of monitoring equipment or appropriately trained personnel is a contraindication to siting an epidural.

Before siting the epidural

- Request a maternal BP prior to commencing the epidural, ideally taken when the woman is not having a contraction, and compare this with antenatal BP recordings. An unexpected elevated BP may indicate pre-eclampsia, warranting further obstetric and anaesthetic investigation.
- Look at a recent CTG tracing to determine the baseline FHR and features indicative of fetal distress. A 10–15min CTG trace is ideal and can be commenced whilst consent is taken and IV access is established.
- Establish patent IV access. There is a lack of evidence that fluid preload is beneficial, but rapid access to IV fluids may be required in an emergency.

After the first test dose

- Maternal BP should be checked and recorded every 5min for 20min.
- After 5min, check for evidence of accidental intrathecal injection. Presence of a motor block should quickly differentiate between an intrathecal and epidural injection of local anaesthetic.
- FHR should be monitored continuously for 20min. Maternal hypotension will reduce uteroplacental perfusion and may lead to sudden fetal distress.
- Reduce aorto-caval compression with careful positioning of the mother.
- Consider more frequent BP monitoring if BP labile or evidence of fetal distress.
- Check maternal heart rate if BP low; the block may be unusually high, causing a bradycardia.

Once the epidural is established

- For continuous epidural infusion and patient-controlled epidural analgesia (PCEA), the BP should be checked and recorded every 30min.
- For an intermittent 'top-up' regime or any additional 'top-ups', the BP and FHR should be checked every 5mins for 15mins after each 'top-up'.
- Any change in the mother's condition, e.g. nausea, dizziness, breathing difficulties, warrants a full set of observations and a review by an anaesthetist. Observations should continue until the problem is rectified.
- Remind the midwife of the importance of ongoing maternal observations as the epidural can migrate intrathecally, subdurally, or intravascularly at any time.

Ambulatory analgesia—'mobile epidural'

Monitor BP and FHR as previously.

In addition

- Measure BP whilst recumbent and again whilst upright to ensure adequate sympathetic response.
- Tests of adequate motor function using the Bromage scale, straight leg raises, and deep knee bends whilst standing should be performed prior to ambulation.
- 'Top-ups' can be given with the woman sitting or reclining. Monitor BP every 5min for 15min and continuous FHR is recommended.
- Motor function should be assessed fully after each 'top-up'.
- Reclining/upright BP should be checked to ensure the absence of postural hypotension after 'top-ups'.

Further reading

Association of Anaesthetists of Great Britain and Ireland and Obstetric Anaesthetists' Association. *OAA/AAGBI Guidelines for Obstetric Anaesthetic Services.* 2013.

Documentation

- Documentation of the epidural procedure should be contemporaneous, legible, and complete.
- Most obstetric units have a dedicated regional analgesia/anaesthesia chart with space for initial anaesthetic assessment, discussion and consent, subsequent recording of top-ups, vital signs, and information relating to complications and/or adverse events. There are a number of good examples on the OAA web-site.
- If such a chart is not available, the relevant information should be recorded in the patient case notes with date and times documented appropriately.
- It is a legal requirement to keep an anaesthetic record. In addition, this information is invaluable to other members of the team, e.g. at handover, for ongoing audit, research, and training.

Documentation should include

- Name and grade of anaesthetist.
- Date and time of procedure.
- Verbal request for epidural or indication for therapeutic epidural with evidence of verbal consent.
- Risks and side effects discussed and incidences quoted, e.g. postdural puncture headache (PDPH) 1%.
- IV access site and gauge of cannula.
- Patient position.
- Full aseptic technique (gloves, gown, hat, mask, drape).
- Level of intervertebral space and approach (midline/paramedian).
- Volume and percentage of local anaesthetic infiltration.
- Tuohy needle gauge.
- Loss of resistance technique (saline/air).
- Presence/absence of paraesthesia.
- Depth of needle to epidural space.
- Presence/absence CSF or blood.
- Length of catheter left in space.
- CSF/blood in catheter.
- Initial bolus dose.
- Subsequent doses including pain scores, block height and deficits, and any remedial action.
- Vital signs.
- Any complications at time of insertion or thereafter.
- In addition, there should be written evidence of a full anaesthetic assessment, including airway assessment and inspection of the spine.

Positioning the mother

- The techniques of epidural, spinal, and CSE analgesia and anaesthesia can be used in labour and for caesarean delivery.
- The problems encountered by the obstetric anaesthetist are unique when compared with other patient groups.
- The mother may find it very difficult to remain still during the procedure because of frequent contractions.
- She may find it difficult to maintain an ideal position during insertion because of her pregnancy.
- A labour room bed is not ideal for the position of both the mother and anaesthetist.
- Because of these difficulties, meticulous care and explanation is required in positioning the mother before commencing any procedure.
- Poor positioning may result in multiple, unnecessary attempts and is responsible for the majority of failures to site an epidural or spinal.
- Ensure the woman is in the correct position and identify the relevant interspace *prior* to scrubbing up and draping.

Sitting position

See Fig 7.1.

- Ensure the woman is sitting on a flat, level mattress (avoiding dips or grooves in the delivery bed).
- Place her feet flat on a high stool with calves close to the side of the bed. Try to prevent her knees falling laterally.
- Always ensure the knees are higher than the hips to reduce the lumbar lordosis.
- Ask her to hold a pillow in front of her chest, place her chin on her chest, and relax her shoulders.
- Her shoulders, hips, knees, and ankles should be in line. Even if it is not obvious to the observer, the mother will frequently feel her spine is twisted and it is worth asking about it.
- If sitting on the operating table, it may be helpful to tilt the table 5° towards the anaesthetist to reduce lumbar lordosis.
- Ask the mother to relax or slouch; when all the other elements are in place the required movement for this is small and easy to achieve for the majority of mothers.

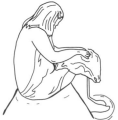

The ideal sitting position
- Knees above hips
- Feet flat and heals close to bed
- Shoulders relaxed
- Pillow close to abdomen
- Back gently curled outwards

Fig. 7.1 The sitting position.

Common errors

Twisting of the spine is caused by:
- The mother is sitting on the uneven detachable end of a delivery bed.
- The bed is not level (head end is tilted up), which tends to encourage the mother to lean sideways.
- The mother is encouraged to maintain her position by an assistant (frequently the partner or midwife) placing their hands on her shoulders.

This can be a helpful manoeuvre, but if the assistant is not directly in front of the mother she can twist towards them.

Leaning forward rather than flexing the spine is caused by:
- Shoulders being hunched and tense.
- Feet are not on a high enough support. The natural flexion of the lumbar spine when the knees are brought above the hips is lost. This commonly occurs when the bed is raised to accommodate the anaesthetist's position. The mother then does not feel secure and leans rather than curls forward.
- The mother's feet are high enough but she slides her feet and calves away from the side of the bed.
- The anaesthetist is not in an optimal position.
- The mother is sitting too far across a wide delivery bed. This can be improved by bringing the mother towards you, but care is required to ensure she is still able to sit with her feet firmly on a stool.

The anaesthetist has learned the technique whilst sitting
- Due to the limitations of a labour room bed, hand position and needle direction are frequently compromised.

Lateral position

See Fig 7.2.

- When the woman is lying on her left side, ensure her back is parallel to and as close to the edge of the bed as possible.
- Her knees should be drawn up in front of her abdomen as far as they will go, and her chin should rest on her chest.
- Place a pillow under her head to level the spine and another between her knees to prevent the pelvis tilting.

Ideal lateral position
- Head on a pillow and chin brought forward
- Back parallel and close to the edge of bed
- Legs brought up as far as possible and together

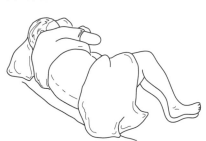

Fig. 7.2 The lateral position.

Common errors
- The back is not parallel to the edge of the bed, making it difficult to identify the perpendicular approach to the spinous processes.
- The knees are not drawn up adequately to facilitate lumbar flexion.
- The knees are not drawn up evenly, resulting in twisting of the spine.

Bring the lower leg to the abdomen first, then bring the upper leg to join it. This improves the degree of hip flexion and reduces the risk of twisting the pelvis and lumbar spine.

Problems common to both positions
- The mother changes her position because of painful contractions.
- The mother changes her position because of the pain of local anaesthetic infiltration or needle insertion.

The anaesthetist has to be constantly aware of these problems. Time spent rectifying any movement may reduce the overall time it takes to insert an epidural or spinal anaesthetic.
- If the midline is difficult to feel and the mother may have moved, remove the needle completely and start again.
- If the epidural is unexpectedly difficult and the spinous process or lamina is encountered more than twice, remove the needle completely and start again.
- If difficulties continue, an experienced anaesthetic assistant can be very helpful. They can optimize the mother's position, encourage her to maintain that position, and move her back into the correct position if she moves a little. In many units it is not usual practice for an ODP to help the anaesthetist in delivery rooms, but as one should be available for theatre, it may be possible to ask for help in case of difficulty.
- It is unacceptable for the anaesthetist to have multiple attempts.
- Re-evaluate the situation.
- Ask for help from someone more experienced.

Skin preparation

- Visual inspection and examination of the back should be undertaken at the preprocedural assessment. Localized infection at or near the proposed site of epidural insertion is an absolute contraindication to its placement. Position the patient and identify landmarks prior to disinfecting the skin.
- Ensure the CTG straps are well away from the area of insertion, but CTG monitoring should continue during the procedure.
- Maximum aseptic technique is mandatory, with gloves, gown, hat, and mask. Scrub up to the elbows with a surgical scrub solution.
- Chlorhexidine is superior to other agents (e.g. povidone iodine) at killing bacteria and reducing the incidence of infection. Alcohol solutions are more effective than aqueous solutions.
- Chlorhexidine (0.5%) in ethanol (80%) is effective within 15s.
- A chlorhexidine and alcohol spray applied directly to the skin should be kept well away from the epidural or spinal tray, reducing the rare complication of chemical meningitis.

Preparation of the skin

- Spraying or painting the skin twice with the chosen disinfectant solution reduces the absolute bacterial count on the skin. The skin must be allowed to dry completely between applications for full effect. It is unclear if double spraying reduces the incidence of rare bacterial infections around epidural sites.
- If the skin is painted, a fresh swab should be used for each application and painted from the insertion site outwards in a circular motion.
- Try to avoid any further rubbing or abrasive pressure to the skin once the skin prep has dried.
- Apply a sterile drape to the back and ensure that it is secure.
- If there is an unsterile area of bed between the anaesthetist and the drape on the patient's back, cover it with another sterile drape.
- If sterility is compromised, you must re-prep the field.

Further reading

Siddiqui N et al. Optimal hand washing technique to minimize bacterial contamination before neuraxial anesthesia: a randomized control trial. *International Journal of Obstetric Anesthesia* 2017; 29: 39–44.

Siddiqui NT et al. The effect of gowning on labor epidural catheter colonization rate: a randomized controlled trial. *Regional Anesthia and Pain Medicine* 2014; 39: 520–524.

Techniques of epidural insertion

Most centres have a fully equipped mobile epidural trolley, which can be moved between delivery rooms as required.

Equipment
You will need the following:
- Stable work surface.
- Sterile dressing pack with swabs and forceps.
- Skin disinfectant.
- Range of syringes and needles for local anaesthetic infiltration.
- Filter needle.
- Sterile drapes—ideally with a window and adhesive sides.
- 16G or 18G Tuohy needle.
- Loss of resistance syringe.
- Epidural catheter with connector and filter.
- 0.9% saline.
- 1% lidocaine (skin infiltration)
- Epidural dressings.
- Epidural drugs.
- Ephedrine 3mg/ml/phenylephrine 12.5–25mg/ml.

Technique

Position
- Both sitting and lateral positions are acceptable. Sitting is easier to identify the midline, but may have a slightly higher incidence of dural puncture and bloody tap.

Interspace
- A mid-lumbar interspace is ideal L2/3 or L3/4. The L4/5 interspace is advocated by some to reduce the risk of accidental spinal cord damage should an accidental dural puncture occur. Even if palpable, this space is frequently difficult to use and may lead to more failures.

Midline vs paramedian
- The midline approach is the most frequently practised technique. A full understanding of the anatomy of both techniques will help if difficulties are encountered.

Midline
- A midline approach is anatomically more straightforward. There may be an increased risk of false loss of resistance due to small deficits in the interspinous ligaments. There may be a midline deficit in the ligamentum flavum with an increased risk of accidental dural puncture.

Paramedian
- Is a successful technique only once the anaesthetist has a strong three-dimensional image of the anatomy of the vertebral column.
- It may be more painful as the vertebral lamina is purposely identified. As a bony landmark is established, advocates feel there is a reduced chance of a false loss of resistance and dural puncture.

Air vs saline

- The incidence of dural puncture is thought to be lower and there is less risk of a patchy block with saline.
- Air makes it easier to identify a dural puncture should it occur as any clear fluid emerging from the needle can only be CSF. Thirty percent of dural punctures are not identified during insertion and the discrepancy may be in part caused by earlier recognition with air.
- Both techniques are acceptable, the skill of the operator being the most important factor.
- A recent survey showed that many anaesthetists use both techniques in different circumstances, and the more experienced the anaesthetist the more likely they are to vary.

Fluid preload

- There is no need to administer a fluid preload unless the woman is hypovolaemic.
- An IV cannula is mandatory and in many units it is still recommended that IV fluids should be connected.

Procedure

- Ensure no contraindications to epidural insertion and that informed consent has been given.
- Full resuscitation equipment is available.
- Confirm patent large bore IV access and IV fluids are available.
- Position the patient.
- Identify the relevant interspace (L3/4) and mark.
- Put on theatre hat and mask, scrub up and put on gown and gloves.
- Prepare the back using scrupulous aseptic technique.
- Assemble equipment and check patency of epidural catheter by flushing with saline.
- Infiltrate the skin with a 25G needle using 2–5mL of 1% lidocaine at and around the midpoint of the interspace (a common problem is failure to anaesthetize the dermis by infiltrating too deeply).
- Insert the Tuohy needle (obturator *in situ*) through the skin and supraspinous ligament so that the needle is held firm. On average this is 2–3cm but may be less in the very slim or considerably more in the obese. If the tip of the needle is not in the interspinous ligament before pressure is put on the syringe there will be a false loss of resistance.
- Remove obturator and observe hub of needle for clear fluid/blood.
- Attach loss of resistance syringe.
- If using saline, exert a continuous pressure on the plunger of the syringe as it is advanced until there is sudden loss of resistance.
- If using air, advance the needle carefully 1mm or less at a time. Each time the needle is stationary, check for loss of resistance by intermittently pushing gently on the plunger of the syringe.
- It is important to keep control of the Tuohy needle so the epidural space is entered slowly. Too fast an approach or lurching into the epidural space from lack of control will increase the risk of dural puncture.
- If air is used, a minimal amount of air (max 1mL) should be injected into the epidural space.

- If saline is used, 2–3mL can be safely used, but more will result in pain and the mother is likely to move, resulting in an increased risk of dural puncture. Saline is more likely to emerge via the Tuohy needle, raising unnecessary concerns of a dural puncture.
- Remove the syringe from the Tuohy needle and observe for clear fluid or blood. If saline is used for loss of resistance, a few drops of clear fluid may emerge from the hub. CSF flow is continuous and brisk. If in doubt, check for the presence of glucose using a glucose indicator strip.
- Note the depth of the space and thread the catheter to around the 15cm mark. Inform the woman that she may feel a slight transient electric shock down her legs as you pass the catheter.
- Remove the Tuohy needle carefully over the catheter, taking care not to pull the catheter out. Pull back the catheter so that 3–5cm remains in the epidural space. Longer lengths may pass through the intervertebral foramen, while shorter lengths may come out of the epidural space altogether.
- Flush the catheter with saline then observe for blood or flow of clear fluid. Lift the catheter up to determine a drop in the saline meniscus. Hold the open catheter below the patient to see if excessive clear fluid or blood drips out. Then gently aspirate.
- Never withdraw the catheter through the Tuohy needle as there is a risk of shearing the catheter. If unable to insert the catheter freely into the epidural space but the tip has already passed through the Tuohy needle, remove the Tuohy needle and catheter as a unit.
- Fix the connector mechanism to the catheter and perform a tug test to confirm that it is secure. Attach the bacterial filter.
- Secure the catheter to the skin such that the depth markings on the catheter can be clearly seen—dressings should ideally be transparent and semi-permeable. Strap the catheter over the shoulder of the non-dominant hand.

- Although continuous saline and intermittent air are often described as separate techniques, many anaesthetists will use a combination of both techniques and different hand positions (see Figs 7.3–7.5).
- Multi-hole epidural catheters are most commonly used because there is a reduced incidence of unsatisfactory or unilateral blocks as the three holes face in different directions.
- Single hole catheters may have the advantage of reducing the risk of a multicompartment catheter (proximal hole in the epidural space and the distal hole in the intrathecal space).
- Figures 7.3–7.5 demonstrate three common methods of holding a Tuohy needle and syringe during insertion. In all techniques, continuous pressure is placed on the plunger with one hand, while the needle is controlled by the other.

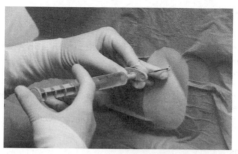

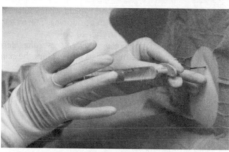

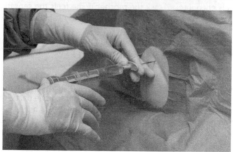

Figures 7.3–7.5 Demonstrates three common methods of holding a Tuohy needle and syringe during insertion. In all techniques continuous pressure is placed on the plunger with one hand, while the needle is controlled by the other.

Further reading

Brogly N et al. Epidural space identification with loss of resistance technique for epidural analgesia during labor: A randomized controlled study using air or saline-new arguments for an old controversy. *Anesthia and Analgesia* 2018; 126: 532–536.

Wantman A et al. Techniques for identifying the epidural space: a survey of practice amongst anaesthetists in the UK. *Anaesthesia* 2006; 61: 370–375.

Antibas PL et al. Air versus saline in the loss of resistance technique for identification of the epidural space. *Cochrane Database Syst Rev*. 18;(7):CD008938

Bahar M et al. The lateral recumbent head-down position decreases the incidence of epidural venous puncture during catheter insertion in obese parturients. *Canadian Journal of Anaesthesia* 2004; 51: 577–580.

Difficulties with insertion

The most common causes for difficulty in siting an epidural
- Suboptimal positioning of the woman.
- Failure to insert the needle in the midline.
- Directing the needle too far laterally even if the insertion point is correct.
- Failure to identify the mid-interspinous point correctly.

Top tips
- Establish a rapport with the mother and explain what you are doing—this will help gain her co-operation with positioning. Talk to her face to face initially, explaining what you want her to do.
- Deep palpation of the back and feeling the iliac crests after deciding on the interspace will cause the mother to move. Mark the skin before prep and concentrate on that space.
- Infiltrate the skin and subcutaneous tissues adequately with lidocaine 1%. An 'orange peel' wheel should be seen. Failure to anaesthetize the dermis adequately is a common reason for the mother to move.
- If bone is encountered on the second attempt, either superficially or deep, STOP and re-evaluate your position.
- It may be helpful, especially in the obese, to ask the mother where the midline is. (They always know!)
- If lamina is encountered, ask the mother if she feels the sensation to the RIGHT or LEFT then redirect the needle slightly cephalad and towards the midline.
- She may be unable to tolerate the sitting position due to pain, especially if the baby is in the occipito-posterior (OP) position. Try the left lateral position.
- The sitting position may be the best to identify the midline in the obese woman.
- Delivery mattresses often consist of several detachable parts—make sure that she is not sitting across a join in the mattress as this will destabilize her position.
- The stool she has her feet on is slipping so she feels unstable and therefore leans rather than bends. Her feet can also slip if she is wearing socks and her feet are on a smooth surface.
- If she is unable to keep still, consider performing a low dose spinal to produce rapid analgesia. The epidural is then performed when she is more comfortable and co-operative.
- In the morbidly obese parturient, it may be necessary to use a long (12 or 15cm) Tuohy needle. The principles are the same; however, senior help or supervision should be sought if you are unfamiliar using it.
- If difficulties continue, call for help early. It is unacceptable to subject a woman to multiple, prolonged attempts at insertion.
- Once the Tuohy needle is in the epidural space, there may be difficulties advancing the catheter through the needle.

- If severe pain is experienced, STOP and remove catheter and needle together.
- If there is no pain, try gently injecting a few more mls of saline and rotating the needle through 45°.
- If the catheter continues not to thread, start again.

Pain on insertion
- Pain may be felt as:
  - The Tuohy needle punctures the skin and subcutaneous tissues.
  - Fluid or air is lost into the interspinous ligaments.
  - The needle hits the periosteum.
  - The needle or catheter hits a nerve root.
  - The spinal cord is damaged.

- If pain is experienced, stop advancing the Tuohy needle and ask if the pain persists. If it does, withdraw the needle until the pain goes.
- Ascertain the location and type of pain.
- Infiltrate more local anaesthetic to the skin and subcutaneous tissues with a 24 or 25G needle. Avoid using a green (19G) needle as there is a risk of accidental dural puncture.
- Try not to 'walk' the needle off the bony vertebrae. The periosteum may feel sore for some days after.
- 'Shooting' or 'electric shock' type pain may be felt down one leg if a nerve or nerve root is accidentally brushed (neuropraxia), as well as tingling or numbness. Withdraw the needle slightly and redirect away from the side that the pain is felt. If the sensation recurs, try a different interspace.
- If the needle pierces the spinal cord, there will be sudden severe pain, paraesthesia, and possibly paralysis. The spinal cord usually ends at L1/2 in adults; however, anatomical anomalies do exist. If there is a suggestion of conus damage, seek senior neurological advice immediately.

On insertion of the epidural catheter
- The epidural catheter should pass freely through the Tuohy needle.
- On advancing the catheter into the epidural space, the woman may experience a transient shooting sensation down either leg. Warn her about this and when it occurs, advance the catheter a little further. If it does not very rapidly disappear, withdraw the needle and catheter together.
- Never force the catheter as it may kink or twist, shedding particles into the epidural space. Similarly, never tug or yank the catheter when withdrawing it.
- If the woman experiences pain on injection through the catheter, stop injecting immediately. Confirm that there is no drug error and remove the catheter. Seek senior advice regarding re-siting at a different interspace.

Bloody tap

The valveless veins of the epidural venous plexus—Batson's plexus—are engorged and distended during pregnancy, and their thin walls make them vulnerable to damage if traumatized by a needle or catheter. There is an increased risk of bloody tap in the obese parturient in the sitting position.

Through the Tuohy needle
• If bleeding occurs through the Tuohy needle once the obturator is removed, it should be withdrawn and inserted at a different interspace.

Through the epidural catheter
• It is essential to ensure that the epidural catheter has not been placed into a vein prior to injecting any drugs through it.
• If blood is seen in the epidural catheter during insertion, continue to insert the catheter and remove the Tuohy needle.
• Pull the catheter back so that the desired length is in the epidural space, i.e. 3–5cm.
• Flush the catheter with saline.
• Lower the catheter to see if blood flows freely.
• Aspirate gently so as not to collapse the delicate vessel walls.
• If blood is aspirated, flush the catheter with normal saline and re-aspirate. If the catheter is blood free, cautiously give the first dose.
• If blood is still aspirated or free flowing, pull back the catheter 1cm at a time, flushing and aspirating until blood is no longer seen. Remember to leave a minimum of 3cm within the epidural space.
• If blood is still seen within the catheter, remove it and re-site the catheter at a different interspace.
• If there is any doubt as to whether the catheter is sited in a vein, it is safer to remove it and start again.

Remember to document events contemporaneously and clearly. Although epidural haematomas are rare, remain vigilant for neurological signs or symptoms.

Accidental dural puncture

The incidence of accidental dural puncture (ADP) in the pregnant woman is quoted as between 0.5 and 2.6%, with ~70% of women subsequently developing a PDPH. There is an increased incidence if loss of resistance to air is used. The dura may be punctured by the Tuohy needle or the epidural catheter.

Practical management

Dural puncture with the Tuohy needle

- Clear fluid will be seen to appear and flow continuously from the hub of the Tuohy needle once the obturator or syringe is removed.
- If saline is used for loss of resistance, it is common for a few drops to appear at the needle hub, but that is all.
- If there is any doubt, check the fluid for the presence of glucose using a glucose indicator strip.
- If ADP is confirmed, there are two ways to proceed:
  - *Either:* Pass the epidural catheter through the needle, aiming to leave 2–2.5cm in the subarachnoid space. Secure and label the catheter clearly as 'SPINAL'. Establish the block with divided doses of 2mg bupivacaine and 5 micrograms fentanyl. All subsequent doses should be given by an anaesthetist ONLY.
  - *Or:* Remove the needle and repeat the procedure at a different interspace. Proceed carefully as there is always the risk of performing another dural puncture. Once sited, the first dose should also be given cautiously as some of the epidural dose may migrate intrathecally through the meningeal tear. Less local anaesthetic may be needed if the epidural is later used for CS. High dose top-ups must be given with great care.

Dural puncture with the epidural catheter

- If the epidural catheter has passed into the subarachnoid space, clear CSF will be aspirated easily.
- If saline has been used for loss of resistance, the presence of glucose will confirm the fluid as CSF and the catheter should be managed as above. See Table 7.2 for the methods of distinguishing CSF and saline solution.

Remember

- Tell the woman what has happened, what to expect and what the treatment options are. Document the complications and ensuing discussion.
- An anaesthetist should perform all epidural or spinal top-ups in the presence of a dural puncture and the resulting block should be carefully documented.
- Ensure that the midwife understands the nature of the block if a spinal catheter is used and is vigilant for the onset of headache in the postnatal period.
- There is no need to prevent the woman pushing during the second stage.
- Inform a senior anaesthetist and complete relevant paperwork, e.g. follow-up book or audit database.
- Consider using a small dose of epidural or intrathecal opiate as it may reduce the risk of PDPH.
- Do not do an early blood-patch, i.e. before the patient develops a PDPH.

Table 7.2 Distinguishing features between CSF and normal saline in suspected accidental dural puncture

	CSF	Normal saline
Dural puncture with needle	Gushing and persistent	Few drops then ceases
Dural puncture with catheter	Ongoing aspiration possible. No falling meniscus if catheter raised above head height	Nil aspirated. Falling fluid meniscus if catheter raised above head height
Temperature	Warm	Cold
Protein	Present	Absent
Glucose	Present	Absent
pH	7.5	<7.5

There is a small physiological leak of CSF into the epidural space which may contribute to a false-positive result.

Techniques of spinal insertion

Spinal anaesthesia is commonly performed for CS, but in addition it can be used as the first part of a CSE technique in labour and as a single shot for other obstetric procedures, e.g. forceps delivery, retained placenta and suturing of the perineum.

Relative and absolute contraindications, consent, monitoring, documentation, positioning the mother, skin preparations, pain on insertion, and difficulties with insertion are as above.

Equipment
You will need the following:
- Stable work surface.
- Sterile dressing pack with swabs and forceps.
- Skin disinfectant.
- Range of syringes and needles for local anaesthetic infiltration.
- Filter needle for drawing up intrathecal drugs.
- Sterile drapes—ideally with a window and adhesive sides.
- 24–27G pencil-point spinal needle.
- Spinal drugs.
- 1% lidocaine for skin infiltration.
- Ephedrine 3mg/mL/phenylephrine 12.5–25mg/mL

Technique
- There is a clear end-point (the appearance of CSF at the hub of the spinal needle, which in health has a sparkling quality).

Position
In general terms a spinal anaesthetic is easier to teach and perform than an epidural anaesthetic (See Figs 7.6 and 7.7), but if the mother is not optimally positioned it may be impossible.

Sitting position
- In general, the midline can be more readily identified.
- CSF pressure is higher and it appears more quickly at the hub of the spinal needle, therefore confirming position.
- 'Heavy intrathecal solutions' will produce a low or saddle block if the mother is not laid down quickly, although this may be useful in some situations.

Lateral position
See Fig. 7.8.

- May be more comfortable for the mother, especially if she is very distressed.
- The end-point of CSF in the hub of the needle can appear very slowly, which can cause some difficulties and sometimes result in multiple unnecessary attempts.
- 'The Oxford position' (See Fig. 7.9) is described for intrathecal injection where the shoulders and head are raised, thus preventing intrathecal solutions from moving too far cephalad. This may cause twisting of the lumbar spine—extra care during positioning and identification of landmarks is needed.

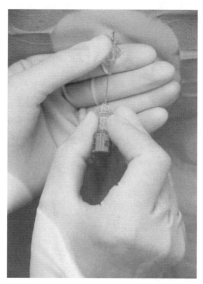

Fig. 7.6 Spinal needle grip. The needle is gripped like a pencil. The advantage is that the subtle differences in the feel of the tissue layers are more easily felt, as well as the 'dural click' as the thecal sac is entered.

Interspace

Much has been written about the safe intervertebral space for spinal injection. The L3/4 interspace is ideal, but the L4/5 interspace is advocated by some to reduce the risk of accidental spinal cord damage.

- The spinal cord (conus) ends most commonly between the L1 and L2 vertebral bodies.
- Tuffier's line is an imaginary line from right to left iliac crest. On plain X-ray it most commonly bisects the body of L4, thus aiding in the identification of the L3/4 (just above) and L4/5 (just below) this line. The hips must be felt with the patient sitting straight up prior to the patient adopting a curled position, if it is to be accurately used to identify the L3–4 interspace.
- The accurate identification of the iliac crests can be very difficult, especially if the bony landmarks are difficult to feel because of adipose tissue.
- A MRI study showed that anaesthetists were frequently unable to identify a marked intervertebral space accurately and more worryingly, were frequently one, two, or even three spaces out, nearly always in the cephalad direction. In other words, the space marked could have been L1/2 and the anaesthetist thought they were at L3/4. This could clearly endanger a normal spinal cord.

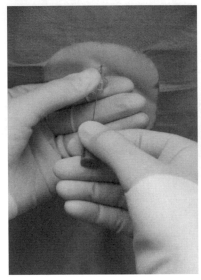

Fig. 7.7 This is a firmer grip—more like a dagger. It is much more difficult to feel subtle changes, but fine needles bend less and can therefore be easier to control.

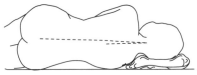

Fig. 7.8 With a pillow under the head and neck only, the spine typically slopes downwards.

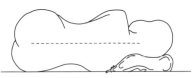

Fig. 7.9 The Oxford position. With the pillow under the lower shoulder, the spine now comes to the vertical.

- Other landmark techniques such as counting down from the 12th rib, counting up from the posterior superior iliac spines and marking an imaginary line 2/3rds of the way down the back from C7 to where the buttocks meet the bed may add additional information.
- Relying on any one technique could lead to inaccuracy, and probably adopting a number together whilst taking an overview of the back is safest.

- It is therefore recommended that the back is examined, landmarks identified, and the interspace chosen before sterilizing the skin and draping the back.
- Choosing the lowest palpable interspace may also help, but this may be as low as L5/S1 where spinal anaesthesia may be impossible, or L4/5, which can be difficult because of the limited flexion of the spine at this level and the shape of the vertebral canal.

Midline vs paramedian
- The midline approach is the most frequently practised technique. A full understanding of the anatomy of both techniques will help if difficulties are encountered.

Midline
- A midline approach is anatomically more straightforward.

Paramedian
- Is a successful technique only once the anaesthetist has a strong 3D image of the anatomy of the vertebral column.
- The approach is different from a paramedian epidural and needs to be taught separately.
- The approach can be useful if the interspinous ligaments are unusually calcified or the vertebra are fixed because of unusual anatomy or surgical fixation.

Procedure
- Ensure no contraindications to insertion and that informed consent has been given.
- Full resuscitation equipment must be available.
- Confirm patent, large bore IV access with crystalloid infusion is available.
- Identify the relevant interspace.
- Position the patient.
- Put on theatre hat and mask, scrub up, and put on gown and gloves.
- Prepare the back using scrupulous aseptic technique.
- Draw up intrathecal drugs using a filter needle.
- Infiltrate the skin with 25G needle using 2–5mL of 1% lidocaine at and around the midpoint of the interspace. (A common problem is failure to anaesthetize the dermis by infiltrating too deeply).
- Insert the introducer of the spinal needle until it is firmly gripped within the interspinous ligament. In most patients insert to its full length as it stabilizes the flexible spinal needle as it is advanced through tough interspinous ligaments.
- Hold the spinal needle with the aperture usually directed cephalad.

- Carefully introduce the spinal needle identifying the anatomical layers during insertion.
- Having identified the ligamentum flavum, push the needle forward a couple more millimetres until a gentle pop is felt.
- Remove the stylet of the spinal needle and confirm placement by the appearance of CSF at the hub of the needle.
- Wait for CSF to appear at the hub, BUT before the hub is completely filled with CSF, attach the syringe containing the intrathecal injection. (If the hub is entirely filled by CSF the contents of the syringe tend to leak during injection even if the syringe has been tightly applied.
- Stabilize the needle and syringe during injection.
- It is usual to confirm CSF by gently aspirating on the syringe just before injection. It may be very difficult to aspirate through a 27G or smaller spinal needle.
- Barbotage is controversial. The advocates claim the spinal block works more quickly. The detractors claim it can more readily lead to spinal needle movement and failure.
- Re-confirming needle position by re-aspirating at the end of injection will confirm that the needle has not moved. Detractors believe this adds nothing as it is in assessment of anaesthesia that will ultimately verify adequate injection.
- Remove syringe, needle, and introducer as one at the end of the injection.

Spinal needles

'Pencil-point' spinal needles which divide the vertically arranged dural fibres are now most widely used rather than the Quincke or bevelled needles which tended to cut the fibres, leaving a trap door cut in the dura. This has caused a huge reduction in the incidence of PDPH and was a major factor in the increasing popularity of spinal anaesthesia in obstetric anaesthetic practice from the late 1980s onwards. The most commonly used sizes are 24 and 25G, although some anaesthetists use as small as 27G. The smaller needles offer a marginal advantage in terms of decreased rate of PDPH, but can be more prone to deformity when passing through more solid tissues and give a slower flashback of CSF.

- The use of 22G spinal needles is more controversial in the obstetric population because of the increased risk of headache, even with a pencil-point tip. This needle can be useful if the interspinous ligaments are unusually tough.
- If the mother is obese. A 22G needle can be used without an introducer, and a standard 90mm needle can be successfully inserted into the CSF ≥9cm from the skin. Although a longer spinal needle can be used in this situation, they are more flexible and difficult to use. Obese mothers have a lower risk of PDPH and a 22G needle is acceptable.

Top tips

- Take as much care with positioning the mother as with an epidural, just because it is fundamentally an easier technique does not mean it will be more successful if the mother is inadequately positioned.
- If probable dural puncture has occurred, take the stillete out quickly. This action draws the CSF down the spinal needle, especially if the needle is of a small diameter, making it easier to confirm correct placement.
- If paraesthesia is more than momentary, do not inject into the CSF and remove the needle.
- If the feeling of dural puncture has occurred but no CSF obtained, rotate the needle through 90°. If CSF is still not seen, withdraw the spinal needle and redirect as it is likely that the ligamentum flavum has been punctured but because of lateral placement the dura has not been punctured.

Continuous spinal anaesthesia

- This is not currently popular in obstetric anaesthetic practice, although there are case reports that have described its successful use in parturients with complex cardiac or other problems. This technique allows controlled and gradual development of a dense regional block while maintaining haemodynamic stability.
- Various microcatheters have been described. A 22G catheter can be inserted over a 27G spinal needle. The risk of headache is acceptably low when used for specific clinical indications, but probably too high for routine use.

Combined spinal–epidural technique

CSE is a technique that has increased in popularity for both labour analgesia and CS. It combines the advantages of rapid complete anaesthesia characteristic of spinal anaesthesia with the flexibility to continue anaesthesia for as long as required. It is described either as a separate technique where the spinal and epidural are inserted at different times and sometimes using a different interspace, or as a needle through needle technique.

- The technique of CSE as a separate technique should follow the description of epidural and spinal anaesthesia above.
- The technique of needle through needle CSE is described below and in Figs 7.10–7.13
- Relative and absolute contraindications, consent, monitoring, documentation, positioning the mother, skin preparations, pain on insertion, and difficulties with insertion are as above.

Equipment

You will need the following:
- Stable work surface.
- Sterile dressing pack with swabs and forceps.
- Skin disinfectant.
- Range of syringes and needles for local anaesthetic infiltration.
- Filter needle.
- Spinal and epidural needle. Either:
  - Separate 80mm Tuohy needle and 120mm spinal needle.
  - Specially designed CSE kit with a locking device for the spinal needle.
- Loss of resistance syringe.
- Epidural catheter.
- Connector and filter.
- 0.9% saline.
- 1% lidocaine.
- Epidural dressings.
- Epidural drugs and/or saline for the epidural space.
- Ephedrine 3mg/ml/phenylephrine 12.5–25mg/ml.

Technique

- The technique for epidural insertion is described above and is not fundamentally different.
- The major difference is that as dural puncture is part of the technique the choice of intervertebral space should follow the spinal technique.

Procedure

- Initially as for the epidural technique.
- Once the epidural space is identified, control the volume of saline injected (1–2ml).

- Remove the stylet of the spinal needle BEFORE inserting it through the Tuohy needle (hastens CSF backflow).
- Gently insert the spinal needle until the end of the Tuohy needle is identified. From this point, continue to advance with care.
- There is frequently a feel of a 'dural click' on entering the CSF.
- If a dural click is felt OR CSF appears at the hub of the spinal needle, STOP advancing the spinal needle.
- The spinal needle is frequently NOT fully advanced at this point but DO NOT advance further.
- With a locking CSE kit, lock the spinal needle and inject intrathecal drugs (See Figs 7.10 and 7.11).
- If a non-locking spinal needle is used, stabilize spinal and Tuohy needle together (See Figs 7.12 and 7.13) and inject intrathecal drugs.
- Remove the spinal needle as quickly as possible and insert the epidural catheter as above. Remove the epidural needle.
- If the CSE has been carried out in the sitting position and the block is required to spread upwards, the mother can be placed in the lateral position before the catheter is withdrawn to the required length, flushed, aspirated, and fixed.
- Injecting saline into the epidural space can increase the spread of the intrathecal drugs. Limit the saline injection during flushing to 2–3ml to minimize this effect unless this is desired.

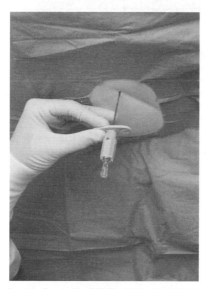

Fig. 7.10 Hand position for a locking CSE: The left hand is stabilized against the patient's back.

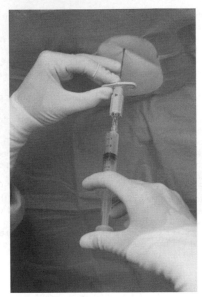

Fig. 7.11 Hand position for a locking CSE: The left hand position does not have to change and the spinal needle is firmly held by the interlocking mechanism during intrathecal injection.

The major problems encountered during CSE are
- 'Dry tap': the epidural space is identified but the spinal needle does not pass into the CSF.
- This can occur if:
  - The Tuohy needle is too lateral.
  - Too low an interspace is chosen. There is some evidence that the thecal sac becomes more triangular in some patients at L4/5 (See Figs 7.14 and 7.15). If this is the case, the needle through needle technique may be less successful. If it is likely that the L4/5 interspace has been used, attempt the technique again at the L3/4 interspace.
- Intrathecal injection fails because of movement of the spinal needle. A locking kit reduces this problem, but not entirely as needle movement can occur during locking. Practice holding, locking, and injecting whatever equipment is available before using it on a patient.

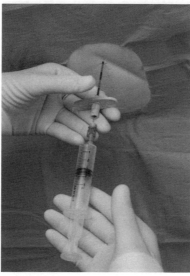

Fig. 7.12 Hand position to stabilize spinal needle for a non-locking CSE: Stabilize spiral needle as it leaving the Tuohy needle with the fingers behind.

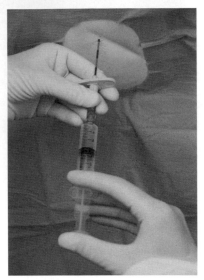

Fig. 7.13 Movement is prevented by gripping the spinal needle with the hub of the Tuohy needle between thumb and fingers.

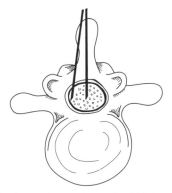

Fig. 7.14 If the thecal sac and bony canal are oval, a slightly lateral approach will be successful.

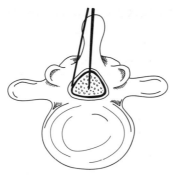

Fig. 7.15 It is common at lower interspaces for the thecal sac and bony canal to become more triangular, with the apex of the triangle posterior. If this is the case, a similar lateral approach with a spinal needle will result in a 'dry trap'.

Removing the epidural catheter

The epidural catheter can be removed as soon as possible after delivery of baby and placenta, unless the following apply:

Platelet or clotting dysfunction

• Await return to normal clotting reference range and platelet count >80×10^9/L

Pre-eclampsia

• Can be associated with decreased platelet count or coagulopathy.
• Await return to normal values as above.

Accidental dural puncture

• If a spinal catheter has been used as first-line management, consider leaving *in situ* for 6–8h post delivery. Label the catheter very carefully with a documented plan around removal

Additional procedures anticipated

• E.g. further perineal suturing, return to theatre for examination or ongoing bleeding.

If difficulties with postdelivery pain management anticipated

• E.g. opioid addiction, chronic pain-related problems. Discuss postdelivery analgesia plan with senior anaesthetist.
• Heparins may be required for postpartum thromboembolic prophylaxis or treatment. They may be given safely 4h after an epidural is removed (See Table 7.1).

Top tip: If the epidural catheter does not come out easily

• Place the mother in the exact position she was in during insertion.
• Don't assume you know if you didn't put it in, ASK HER.
• It is then very unusual for the catheter not to come out easily.
• Never pull hard, as there are many reports of broken catheters.

Ultrasound in obstetric practice

Rafal Baraz

Neuraxial blockade

The use of ultrasound to aid the location of the spinal and epidural space is not a new concept. There is currently enough evidence to support improved outcomes, better patients' experience, and reduced complications when using ultrasound.

The National Institute of Health and Clinical Excellence (NICE) has published interventional procedure guidance in January 2008 (IPG249) stating ultrasound imaging may be used to help identify the epidural space. Despite this publication and established evidence of increased safety, the use of ultrasound in neuraxial blockade remains limited. This could be due to:

- Familiarity of anaesthetists with the landmark technique.
- Lack of technical ultrasound skills.
- Time constraints.
- Urgency to provide analgesia.
- Limited application in real time.

Benefits of using ultrasound

Current evidence supports the use of ultrasound to aid the insertion of spinal and epidural anaesthesia. The routine use of ultrasound:

- Improves the success rate for first insertion and reduces the risk of failed or traumatic spinal or lumbar punctures.
- Reduces the number of attempts, number of needle insertions, and redirections, which cause pain, skin bruising, a delay in providing pain relief for labour or surgical intervention, and potentially increases the risk of dural puncture, nerve damage, and infection.
- Provides best insertion point, level, and angle of insertion in patients with scoliosis, previous back surgery, and morbid obesity.
- Studies have shown that operators using the landmark technique often insert the needle higher than intended.
- Knowing the depth of the epidural space theoretically reduces the risk of dural puncture. It guides the operator in choosing the appropriate needle length before undertaking the procedure. This is especially important in the morbidly obese woman.

Challenges of spinal ultrasound imaging

- Most anaesthetists are familiar with the linear high frequency probe, which is often used for insertion of central venous catheters and most nerve blocks.
- Although this probe produces high resolution images, it has no place in neuraxial imaging due to limited penetration.
- A curvilinear low-frequency probe is required, which uses frequencies between 2 and 5 MHz. This is necessary to visualize the deep structures of the spine, but produces low-quality images.
- The bony structure of the spine contributes further to reduced image quality as bone reflects most of the ultrasound waves back and structures beyond the bone cannot be visualized (Figs 8.1–8.3b).

Scanning views (planes)

There are a number of scanning views which the anaesthetist should be familiar with when using ultrasound.

Longitudinal (sagittal) midline view

- Place the curvilinear probe longitudinally in the middle of the patient's spine.
- Move the probe sideways until the midline of the patient's back is determined by identifying the spinous processes, which appear as hyperechoic structures with their corresponding shadows anteriorly (Fig. 8.1).
- This view is used to identify the midline.
- The acoustic window between the spinous processes in this plane is too narrow to visualize other structures, when compared to the paramedian sagittal oblique view.

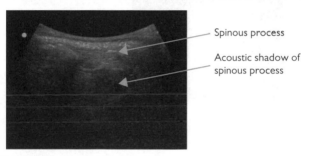

Spinous process

Acoustic shadow of spinous process

Fig. 8.1 Longitudinal (sagittal) midline view.

Paramedian sagittal oblique view

- This view provides accurate spinal level identification and visualization of vital spinal structures such as the lamina, ligamentum flavum, posterior dura, intrathecal space, and anterior dura.
- It also allows measurement of the distance between the skin and the posterior dura.

- Place the curvilinear low frequency probe over the sacrum 1–2cm lateral to the midline with slight medial angulation towards the midline. The sacrum should appear as a long and flat hyperechoic structure with a large shadow anteriorly (Fig. 8.2a).
- Maintaining the same angle mentioned above, move the probe cranially to identify the interlaminar spaces of L5–S1, L4–L5, L3–L4 (Fig. 8.2b).
- In this plane, the first bone identified is the lamina with an acoustic shadow anteriorly.
- If difficulty is experienced during the scanning process, move the probe sideways between the median sagittal and the paramedian sagittal oblique planes until picture is optimized.
- Alternatively start again by scanning the sacrum first and going upwards.

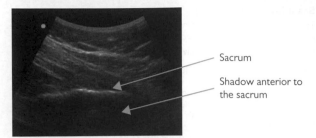

Fig. 8.2a Paramedian sagittal oblique view of sacrum.

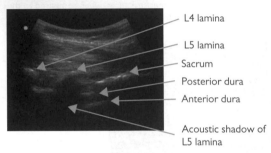

Fig. 8.2b Paramedian sagittal oblique view of L4/L5.

Transverse view
In this view almost all spinal structures can be visualized. It also provides accurate identification of the midline and measurement of the distance between the skin and the posterior dura. There are two planes:

• Through the spinous process and the left and right laminae: In this plane, it is not possible to visualize the dura due to the acoustic shadow produced by the spinous process and the laminae. It allows identification of the midline by keeping the spinous process in the middle of the ultrasound screen (Fig. 8.3a).
• Through the interspinous ligament: This plane allows direct viualization of ligament flavum/posterior dura complex and the distance from the skin. Other structures such as the articular surfaces, transverse processes, intrathecal space, anterior dura, and possibly the posterior border of the vertebral body, also appear in this plane. This is the plane that one should aim for when performing pre-procedure ultrasound scanning for a spinal, an epidural, and a combined spinal-epidural.

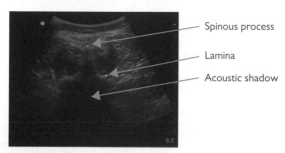

Fig. 8.3a Transverse view through spinous process.

- Spinous process
- Lamina
- Acoustic shadow

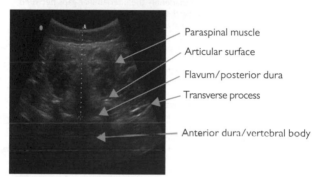

Fig. 8.3b Transverse view through interspinous ligament.

- Paraspinal muscle
- Articular surface
- Flavum/posterior dura
- Transverse process
- Anterior dura/vertebral body

- Place the curvilinear probe in the middle of the patient's back in the transverse plane over the level decided on and identified during the paramedian sagittal oblique view.
- Scanning through the spinous process identifies the midline point of needle insertion (Fig. 8.3a).
- Scanning through the interspinous ligament will directly visualize ligament flavum/dura complex and its distance from skin (Fig. 8.3b).

Ultrasound guided spinal and epidural blocks

The majority of anaesthetists using ultrasound for neuraxial blockade identify the anatomical landmarks pre-procedure and not in real time. Ultrasound guided epidural insertion in real time should only be attempted by highly skilled clinicians with advanced ultrasound skills due to complexity and difficulty in visualizing the needle at all times. The real time technique will not be described in this chapter.

Pre-procedure scanning of the lumbosacral spine
- Position the patient in the sitting or lateral position with maximum flexion of the lumbar spine. Optimize the position before scanning.
- Select the curvilinear low frequency probe with appropriate ultrasound gel.
- Place the probe over the sacrum 1–2cm lateral to the midline with slight medial angulation towards the midline (paramedian sagittal oblique view).
- Identify the sacrum, which appears as a long and flat hyperechoic structure with a large shadow anteriorly (Fig 8.2a).
- Maintain the same angle and move the probe cranially to identify the gap between the sacrum and the lamina of L5 (L5–S1 acoustic window) through which the posterior dura can be visualized (Fig 8.2b).
- Move the probe further up to identify the interlaminar gaps between L4–L5, L3–L4, and L2–L3 (Fig 8.4).
- Maintaining the probe in the paramedian sagittal oblique view with the interlaminar space in the middle of the ultrasound beam (middle point on the screen) and mark the appropriate level along the middle of the probe.
- Rotate the probe at the same interspace into the transverse plane to scan through the interspinous ligament, visualizing the ligament flavum/dura complex.
- Move the probe slightly sideways until the picture is symmetrical and mark the skin vertically at the middle of the probe.
- Move the probe slightly cranially to identify the spinous process of the level above and then slightly caudally to identify the spinous process of the vertebra below—this should help to find the optimal angle of needle insertion.

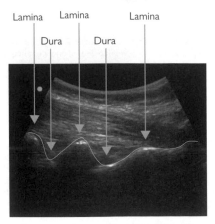

Fig. 8.4 Saw tooth appearance in paramedian sagittal oblique view.

- The angle of needle insertion should mimic the angle at which the best image of the posterior dura is obtained in the transverse plane.
- Draw a transverse line through the 1st skin mark and a vertical line through the 2nd skin mark—your point of needle insertion is where the two lines cross each other (Fig 8.5).
- Once the insertion point has been obtained, do not change the patient's position or the position of the operating table.
- Calculation of the distance between the skin and the posterior dura should establish the safe distance of needle insertion before breaching the dura.

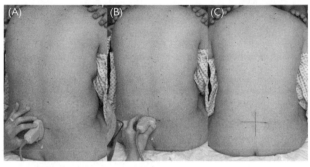

Fig. 8.5 The skin mark in picture A corresponds to the interlaminar space of L3–4 space. The vertical skin mark in picture B represents the midline. Picture C represents the needle insertion point at L3–4 space.

Transversus abdominis plane block

The terminal branches of the anterior rami of T7–L1 lie in the transversus abdominal plane (TAP), which is the plane between the internal oblique and transversus abdominis muscles. Injection of local anaesthetic in this TAP has been shown to provide analgesia and reducing morphine requirement following caesarean delivery for both the landmark and ultrasound guided techniques. The ultrasound guided technique provides direct visualization of the needle and its tip and potentially reduces complications such as bowel perforation and vascular placement. It also has the potential to provide better analgesia due to direct visualization of the deposition and spread of local anaesthetic.

Method

- Perform the block at the end of caesarean section.
- Draw up 2×20-ml syringes of 0.25% levobupivacaine. (Caution in patients who have received near maximum dose of local anaesthetic via the epidural catheter).
- Use an aseptic technique.
- Place the ultrasound machine on the side you are blocking while standing on the opposite side, with the screen facing you.
- Place the linear (38mm) high frequency ultrasound transducer horizontally across the abdomen at the level of the umbilicus. Identify the rectus muscle and move the probe laterally to visualize the three muscles of the lateral abdominal wall (external oblique, internal oblique, and the transversus abdominis muscles) (Fig 8.6).
- Move laterally until the probe is positioned between the iliac crest and costal margin in the anterior axillary line.

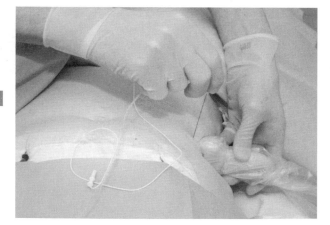

Fig. 8.6 Real time ultrasound guided transversus abdominal plane block. For optimal visualization of the needle shaft, the needle should be parallel to the ultrasound beam.

- Keep the transducer as perpendicular as possible.
- Use an 80–100mm, 21–22 gauge block needle. Insert 5mm away from the edge of the transducer and advance the needle parallel to the transducer (parallel to the ultrasound beam) through the external oblique muscle (first pop).
- Keep the needle parallel to the probe (ultrasound beam) and ensure the needle is visualized at all times. If you are unable to see the needle, move the transducer slightly cranially or caudally until the needle shaft is visualized (Fig 8.7).

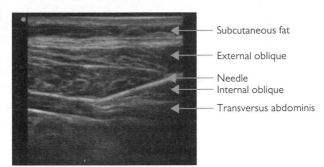

Subcutaneous fat

External oblique

Needle
Internal oblique

Transversus abdominis

Fig. 8.7 Real time ultrasound guided TAP block showing the entire needle shaft with its tip between the internal oblique and the transversus abdominis muscles

- Continue advancing the needle through the internal oblique until the tip of the needle lies between the internal oblique and transversus abdominis muscles (you may feel a second pop).
- Aspirate before injecting the local anaesthetic. Inject 0.5–1ml to confirm injection into the correct plane. Inject a total of 20–25ml of 0.25% levobupivacaine. Aspirate every 5ml to exclude intravascular injection.
- Repeat on the other side.
- Theoretically TAP blocks provide analgesia to the skin, muscles, and parietal peritoneum of the anterior abdominal wall (T7–L1), but in reality, the block is very variable.

Additional uses

Vascular access

The use of ultrasound (in real time) offers the safest option for central venous cannulation in both the obstetric and non-obstetric population.

The most popular approach is the short axis out of plane view as both the internal jugular and the common carotid can be visualized in the same view, but the long axis view has the advantage of viewing the needle shaft during vessel puncture and confirming the guide wire is inside the vein before dilating.

Every maternity unit should have immediate access to ultrasound to assist insertion of central venous lines, especially for women who are:
- Coagulaopathic.
- Hypovolaemic.
- Morbidly obese.

Ultrasound has also proven to be invaluable during insertion of peripheral venous and arterial lines, especially in the obese parturient or those known to be intravenous drug users.

Gastric ultrasound

- Aspiration of gastric contents during anaesthesia is a serious complication, which can lead to significant morbidity and mortality, and is well recognized in the non-fasted, emergency obstetric population.
- Gastric content and volume assessment has been described as a new point-of-care ultrasound application, before induction of anaesthesia, to assess the aspiration risk and guide anaesthetic management.
- The sonographic characteristics of different types of gastric content (empty, clear fluid, solid) have been described, as well as the methods for quantitative assessment of gastric volume.
- Further evidence is needed of its application before its use is adopted in the obstetric setting prior to timely GA.

Further reading

Shaikh F et al. Ultrasound imaging for lumbar punctures and epidural catheterizations: systematic review and meta-analysis. *BMJ* 2013; 346: f1720.

Ultrasound-guided cauterization of epidural space. National Institute for Health and Clinical Excellence. 2008. https://www.nice.org.uk/guidance/ipg249.

Ecimovic P et al. Ultrasound in obstetric anaesthesia: a review of current applications. *International Journal of Obstetric Anaesthesia* 2010; 19: 320–326.

Belavy D et al. Ultrasound guided transversus abdominis plane block for analgesia after Caesarean delivery. *British Journal of Anaesthesia* 2009; 103: 726–730.

Van de Putte P et al. Ultrasound assessment of gastric content and volume. *British Journal of Anaesthesia* 2014; 113: 12–22.

Regional analgesia for Labour

Sarah Harries and Rachel Collis

Introduction

Epidural analgesia

- Epidural analgesia is the most effective form of analgesia during labour.
- It is the only technique which can potentially provide complete analgesia and has a number of physiological maternal and fetal benefits.
- An effective epidural can be extended to provide rapid epidural anaesthesia if urgent CS is required.
- Epidural analgesia was first described as caudal analgesia, then continuous lumbar analgesia from the late 1940s.
- Its use was strictly limited because of a lack of expertise in the techniques and the short-acting local anaesthetics available, which over a few hours became ineffective because of tachyphylaxis.
- Interest and development of epidural analgesia for labour began in earnest in the mid-1960s with the introduction of longer lasting local anaesthetics, e.g. bupivacaine.
- Pharmacological and technological advances, as well as a greater understanding of anatomy and physiology, have contributed to its safety and efficacy, with ~25% of women receiving epidural analgesia during labour in the UK today.

Physiological and psychological benefits of epidural analgesia

- As well as minimizing the sensory component of labour, epidural analgesia confers a number of benefits to both mother and fetus.
- Catecholamines and prostaglandins are released in response to the pain of uterine contractions and cervical distension.
- Epidural blockade can limit rises in CO and SVR associated with increased circulating catecholamines.
- Increased oxygen consumption associated with pain and maternal effort can be reduced by effective epidural blockade.
- Maternal and fetal acidosis is minimized and intervillous blood flow is enhanced by arteriolar vasodilatation.
- Uterine contractions may become more coordinated or may become less frequent.
- These factors are of particular importance in the sick parturient or in those with pre-existing cardiorespiratory disease.

The effect of epidural analgesia on labour and delivery

- Epidural analgesia **does not** increase the likelihood of a CS.
- There are associations between epidural analgesia and a prolonged first and second stage of labour, augmentation of labour, and need for instrumental delivery. However, there is little evidence to suggest that epidural analgesia is the sole causative factor in these cases.
- Epidural analgesia is not the cause of postpartum backache, nor does it increase the likelihood of developing long-term back problems.
- There is a rise in maternal temperature after epidural analgesia for labour. The exact cause is unknown, although alterations in maternal thermoregulation have been implicated, but it is important to distinguish it from infection to prevent unnecessary use of antibiotics.

Indications for epidural analgesia

Maternal request
- There is no circumstance where it is considered acceptable for a person to experience untreated severe pain, amenable to safe intervention, while under a physician's care.
- In early labour <3cm cervical dilatation an epidural can be safely sited if delivery is expected in the next 24-hours.
- A fully dilated cervix is not a contraindication to site an epidural, unless delivery is imminent.

Augmentation of labour
- Oxytocic drug infusions, e.g. oxytocin, can cause painful, forceful contractions and epidural analgesia is often encouraged to aid compliance.

Hypertensive disease
- Sympathetic blockade may aid BP control, e.g. in pre-eclampsia.
- An effective epidural will avoid the hazards of GA if a CS is required.

Morbid obesity
- An epidural should be recommended early in labour, as an effective block may minimize the need for GA in the event of emergency CS.
- It should be reassessed regularly to ensure that it continues to function optimally.

Predicated difficult airway or intubation risk
- To avoid the need for an emergency GA.

History/family history of significant GA problems
- Malignant hyperpyrexia, suxamethonium apnoea, or anaphylaxis.

Cardiac and respiratory disease
- An effective epidural minimizes the increase in CO and minute ventilation associated with labour and delivery.
- It is essential to ensure that changes to preload and afterload are minimized and aorto-caval compression is avoided at all costs.
- In severe cardiac disease, invasive BP monitoring may be indicated.

Cerebrovascular disease
- Pushing and straining will cause a rise in the intracranial pressure, which may be deleterious in the presence of cerebral aneurysms, arteriovenous malformations, or other intracranial disease. Regional analgesia will facilitate an operative delivery in these cases.

Multiple pregnancy and breech presentation
- To facilitate assisted or operative delivery, which is often required.

Further reading

Segal S. Labor epidural analgesia and maternal fever. *Anesthia and Analgesia* 2010; 111:1467–1475.

Jones L et al. Pain management for women in labour: an overview of systematic reviews. *Cochrane Database Systematic Reviews* 2012; 14: CD009234.

Anim-Somuah M et al. Epidural versus non-epidural or no analgesia in labour. Cochrane Database Systematic Reviews 2011; 7: CD000331.

Howell CJ et al. Randomised study of long term outcome after epidural versus non-epidural analgesia during labour. *BMJ* 2002; 325: 35.

Drugs in the epidural space

- The most common class of drugs used to provide epidural analgesia in labour are the amide LAs.
- Addition of an opioid results in a synergistic action leading to superior analgesia as well as reduced overall local anaesthetic requirements.
- There is increased maternal satisfaction, less likelihood of motor block, less cardiovascular instability, and an improved safety profile from low concentration LA mixtures.

Local anaesthetic drugs

- LAs block fast sodium channels, causing a reversible inhibition of neuronal transmission.
- Once injected into the epidural space, the LA diffuses across the dural cuff to gain access to the lumbosacral nerve roots and the dorsal root ganglia.
- It also diffuses directly across the dura into the CSF and thus to the spinal cord and its blood vessels.
- LAs are non-selective in that sensory, motor, and autonomic neurons are blocked. C fibres (pain) are blocked first, followed by the larger Aδ (motor, proprioception) and Aβ (pressure, light touch) fibres.

Racemic bupivacaine
- Still widely used for labour analgesia in the UK.
  - *Pros*: highly lipid soluble, potent with long duration of action. Provides effective analgesia at low concentrations in combination with opioids.
  - *Cons*: dose-dependent motor block, cardiotoxicity due to affinity for cardiac Na$^+$ channels causing resistant life-threatening arrhythmias.

Levobupivacaine
- S-enantiomer of bupivacaine, which is gaining popularity over the racemic mixture.
  - *Pros*: clinically equipotent to bupivacaine for labour analgesia but with less arrhythmogenicity, thus better if large dose boluses required, e.g. extension of epidural block for CS.
  - *Cons*: currently more expensive than racemic bupivacaine.

Ropivacaine
- S-enantiomer of propivacaine.
  - *Pros*: less cardiotoxic than racemic bupivacaine.
  - *Cons*: gained popularity due to its apparent differential blockade of sensory fibres but not motor fibres. Studies have however shown that this is due to a significantly reduced potency (40% less potent).
  - Common solutions are between 0.1 and 0.2%. The incidence of motor block is the same at equipotent doses of racemic bupivacaine.

Lidocaine
- Short-acting amide LA.
  - *Pros*: rapid onset of action is useful to extend a pre-existing epidural block for CS.
  - *Cons*: high degree of motor block and tachyphylaxis precludes its use for labour analgesia in current modern obstetric practice. Lidocaine may be neurotoxic in high doses.

Opioids

- Opioids may act spinally or supraspinally depending on the dose, lipophilicity, and frequency of administration, i.e. bolus dosage or continuous infusion.
- Epidural opioids cross the dura and diffuse through the CSF to reach their site of action in the substantia gelatinosa of the dorsal horn of the spinal cord.
- A proportion of the administered epidural/intrathecal dose will be absorbed into the blood to exert a systemic effect.
- There is some evidence to suggest that epidural fentanyl causes segmental analgesia when given as a bolus and non-segmental systemic analgesia when given as a continuous infusion.

Morphine

- Typically used to provide longer lasting analgesia after caesarean section rather than during labour.
  - *Pros*: long lasting due to poor lipophilicity.
  - *Cons*: slow onset of action and high incidence of side effects—respiratory depression may appear up to 12h after epidural administration.

Fentanyl

- Most widely used opioid for labour analgesia in the UK.
  - *Pros*: highly lipophilic with rapid penetration of spinal cord leading to fast onset of analgesia and reduces LA requirements.
  - *Cons*: short duration of action. Nausea, vomiting, pruritus (most commonly), and respiratory depression may occur with high doses.

Diamorphine

- Intermediate lipophilicity, mostly used to provide analgesia post caesarean section.
  - *Pros*: more rapid onset of analgesia than morphine and less risk of late respiratory depression.
  - *Cons*: shorter duration of analgesic effect than morphine.

Other opioids

- Pethidine is avoided as it has an LA effect causing unpredictable sympathetic and motor block. Nausea is also very common.
- Epidural sufentanil (~5 times as potent as epidural fentanyl) is used widely in the USA but has no product licence in the UK.
- Tramadol is thought to produce less respiratory depression associated with opioids due to its selective μ1-agonism and it prolongs duration of analgesia when used in conjunction with 0.25% bupivacaine.

Other drugs

For doses see Table 11.1, p. 313. A number of other drugs, typically used in combination with LAs and/or opioids, have been or are being investigated.

Clonidine

- An α_2 agonist which acts at receptors in the dorsal horn of the spinal cord causing analgesia with no motor block.
- Descending noradrenergic pathways are subsequently activated with release of inhibitory neurotransmitters.
- Problems limiting its widespread use include hypotension and sedation.

Adrenaline

- α_1 adrenergic agonism causes vasoconstriction, which decreases systemic absorption of LA and thus prolongs its effects.
- Traditionally used as part of a test dose to determine intravascular injection—manifest as a tachycardia.
- Adrenaline can also provide analgesia via α_2 adrenergic agonism. This is associated with a dense motor block.

Neostigmine

- An anticholinesterase, which produces dose-dependent analgesia by inhibiting the breakdown of acetylcholine.
- Acetylcholine is involved in spinal modulation of pain processing, predominantly by stimulating cholinergic neurons of the muscarinic type.
- It has been used to counteract the haemodynamic depression produced by epidural clonidine, though nausea and vomiting are common side effects.
- Neostigmine is also poorly lipid soluble, so onset is delayed.

Ketamine

- An NMDA antagonist, which blocks glutamate-mediated excitatory transmission of nociceptive impulses.
- Other effects include opioid agonism and sodium channel interactions.
- The S (+) enantiomer prolongs caudal epidural block in children by up to 4 times.
- It has the added benefit of lack of respiratory depression.

Further reading

Murphy JD et al. Bupivicaine versus bupivicaine plus fentanyl for epidural analgesia: effect on maternal satisfaction. *BMJ* 1991; 302: 564–567.

Capogna G et al. Determination of the minimum local analgesic concentration (MLAC) of epidural ropivicaine in labour. *British Journal of Anaesthesia* 1998; 80: 148.

Ginosar Y et al. The site of action of epidural fentanyl in humans. The difference between infusion and bolus administration. *Anesthesia and Analgesia* 2003; 97: 1428–1438.

Zhang N, Xu MJ. Effects of epidural neostigmine and clonidine in labor analgesia: a systematic review and meta-analysis. *Journal of Obstetric and Gynaecological Research*. 2015; 41: 214–212.

Ngan Kee WD et al. Synergistic interaction between fentanyl and bupivacaine given intrathecally for labor analgesia. *Anesthesiology* 2014; 120: 1126–1136.

The test dose

The purpose of the test dose is to exclude or confirm intravascular or intra-thecal placement which is most common after initial catheter placement. However, every time a dose is injected into the epidural space it should be considered a test dose, as the epidural catheter may migrate intrathecally, subdurally, intravenously, or completely out of the epidural space.

The ideal test dose should allow the anaesthetist to rapidly detect abnormal catheter placement before endangering the patient because of drug toxicity.

An ideal drug/mixture of drugs would

- Equally detect intravascular and intrathecal injection.
- Have 100% specificity with 100% positive and negative predictive values.
- Allow detection of abnormal placement immediately (IV) or within 5min (intrathecal).
- The fact that there are huge variations in the choices obstetric anaesthetists make, confirms there is not an ideal solution.

Detection of accidental intravascular injection

Symptoms of local anaesthetic toxicity
Circumoral tingling, numbness, tinnitus.
Light-headedness, confusion, agitation, and tremor.
Loss of consciousness.
Convulsions.
Arrhythmia.
Cardiovascular collapse.

- After careful aspiration of the epidural catheter, the LA solution should be injected.
- The earliest signs of intravascular injection (circumoral tingling and tinnitus) should warn the anaesthetist to stop injecting.
- The addition of 15 micrograms adrenaline has been popular and is still advocated by some. This small amount of adrenaline will cause a transient increase in maternal heart rate after intravascular injection.
- It is highly sensitive but only 65% specific (the mother's heart rate commonly varies with the pain of contractions).
- The increase in heart rate is difficult to detect unless ECG monitoring is used.

Detection of accidental intrathecal placement

5 signs of accidental intrathecal injection
Very rapid analgesia.
Excessive sensory block.
Early motor block (hip flexion).
Early sacral block (ankle plantarflexion).
Hypotension.
  NB: *hypotension may be absent, so the block must be formally tested after the test dose to evaluate the other modalities.*

- The ideal test dose would be easily detected within 5min without excessive spread of the block and severe hypotension.
- The general principle is to use a dose of LA that could be used for a CS if given intrathecally.
- There is wide variation in practice.
  - 10–15mg bupivacaine can safely be given as a 0.1% or 0.5% solution.
  - 60mg lidocaine (3mL lidocaine 2%).
  - 10mL of 0.1% bupivacaine with fentanyl 2 micrograms/ml.
- There is not a test dose that is completely reliable at 5min and it may be safer to assess the block formally at 10min after injection.
- There is an increasing move away from small volume high concentration solutions to large volume low concentration solutions.
- The advantage of the latter is that the test dose will:
  - Significantly contribute to early analgesia.
  - Reduce the overall LA dose required to establish analgesia.
  - Reduce the early development of motor block.

Management of a suspected positive test dose

- Stop injecting.
- Re-aspirate.
- The initial aspiration test may have been negative but is now positive.
- If aspiration is still negative, the epidural catheter may still be incorrectly positioned.
- If intravascular injection is suspected, pull the catheter back 0.5–1cm and re-aspirate. If uncertainty remains, it is safer to remove the catheter completely and start again.
- If the mother develops signs of intrathecal placement.
  - Place her in the full lateral position to reduce the risk of hypotension.
  - Evaluate the block carefully with particular attention to sacral anaesthesia.
  - Give IV fluids and vasopressors as required.
- If intrathecal placement is confirmed, label the epidural catheter as SPINAL and use as a spinal catheter (see Management of dural puncture, Chapter 7 p. 212).

Further reading

Camorcia M. Testing the epidural catheter. Current Opinion Anaesthesiology 2009; 22: 336–340.
Paech M. The epinephrine test dose in obstetrics. Anesthesia and Analgesia1999; 89: 1590–1591.
Gardner IC, Kinsella SM. Obstetric epidural test doses: a survey of UK practice. International Journal of Obstetric Anesthesia 2005; 14: 96–103.
Colonna-Romano P, Nagaraj L. Tests to evaluate intravenous placement of epidural catheters in laboring women: a prospective clinical study. Anesthesia and Analgesia 1998; 86: 985–988.
Norris MC et al. Does epinephrine improve the diagnostic accuracy of aspiration during labor epidural analgesia? Anesthesia and Analgesia 1999; 88: 1073–1076.
Daoud Z et al. Evaluation of S1 motor block to determine a safe, reliable test dose for epidural analgesia. British Journal of Anaesthesia 2002; 89: 442–445.

Pain scoring

- A pain score trend can provide valuable information for the clinician regarding:
  - Effectiveness of analgesia.
  - Escalation of pain due to a new stimulus, e.g. uterine rupture.
  - Change in the nature of pain, e.g. sacral pressure with descent of the fetal head.
- The most easily applied score is the verbal numerical pain score, where the woman is asked to give a number from 0 to 100 to indicate the severity of the pain—0 being no pain and 100 being the worst pain ever.
- Aim to reduce the pain score to <30 with epidural analgesia.

Practical pain scoring

- Ask the woman to score her pain prior to analgesia.
- Determine the nature and site of the pain:
  - Tightening, crescendo pain of uterine contractions.
  - Sacral and rectal pressure from a descending fetal head or malpresentation.
  - Atypical pain—epigastric or pubic symphysis diastasis.
- Different stimuli may require different management.
- During establishment of the block, score the pain every 10min after top-ups until the pain score is <30.
- Do a pain score 10–15min after each top-up in labour or hourly with an epidural infusion.
- The most obvious sign is a comfortable, smiling woman—observe the woman through contractions and ask her how each felt.

Pain scores >30

- Establish the epidural in divided doses with up to 30mg bupivacaine with an opioid. If pain scores have never been less than 30 within 40min after initial epidural placement, consider replacing the epidural at this stage, **as the epidural will never be satisfactory**.
- If the epidural has worked well but the mother is now in pain.
  - Check the position of the epidural catheter—it may have come out of the space.
  - Ensure that the woman is getting regular intermittent bolus top-ups—severe pain should not be allowed to return prior to administering further top-ups.
  - If she is using a PCEA, make sure that she is pressing the button as required.
- If the pain score suddenly increases after being stable with effective established analgesia, determine the nature of the pain.
  - Sacral pain may be managed with a stronger LA top-up (bupivacaine 0.25% with fentanyl) in the sitting position.
  - Sudden onset severe pain may be indicative of another pathology, e.g. liver capsule haematoma if pre-eclampsia present or uterine rupture, which may warrant further investigations.
- Resite a poorly functioning epidural early.

Assessing the block

- The ideal epidural block for labour should cover the T10–S5 nerve roots with minimal motor block of the lower limbs. It can generally be called a 'light' block with evidence of a sensory block to cold sensation and a sympathetic block that usually accompanies this (warm dry feet).
- A dense sensory block (unable to feel a pinch or pinprick) is usually associated with quite a dense motor block. This type of block is typical if 0.25% bupivacaine is used and should be avoided if possible.
- Sensory, motor, and sympathetic blockade, as well as maternal satisfaction, should be assessed and documented:
  - 10min after the first dose.
  - 15–20min after the initial incremental doses to establish a block.
  - Prior to and 10min after any top-up dose for breakthrough pain, unilateral block, or missed segment.
  - If there is sudden maternal hypotension, fetal distress, or any other abnormal maternal signs or symptoms.
  - Prior to top-up for CS.

Sensory block

- It is important to establish that the woman can articulate and appreciate the differences between, touch/pressure, sharp/dull, wetness, cold ,and ice cold. Show her the 'normal sensation' by applying the stimulus to normal skin.
- Ensure that the block is assessed bilaterally about 5cm either side of the midline as indicated by the umbilicus.
- Ice or ethyl chloride are used to determine the level at which temperature sensation is altered, compared with a standard skin dermatome chart.
- A neurological pin test for pinprick sensation with both sharp and dull sensation elicited.
- Light touch can be assessed using cotton wool, touching with a finger or a Von Frey hair.
- Loss of sensation to temperature usually occurs two dermatomes higher than that to pinprick.
- Loss of sensation to pinprick usually occurs two dermatomes higher than that to light touch.
- If S1 (largest sacral nerve root) is blocked, i.e. the soles of the feet, it is unnecessary to test the perineum formally during labour. The S2 dermatome runs up the back of the leg and is also easy to test.
- In labour, it is usual to test and document the block relative to cold sensation.

Sympathetic block

- Epidural blockade can be indicated by vasomotor changes in the lower limbs.
- A sympathetic block of the feet does not develop until there is a well-defined sensory block to T10 (umbilicus).
- The soles of the feet should look pink, well perfused, and feel warm and dry. Drying of the feet is an important part of sympathetic block assessment and can only be accurately determined by examining the soles.

- Differences in foot temperature are indicative of an asymmetrical or unilateral block. Regardless of whether testing to ice demonstrates a difference, the quality of the block is unlikely to be as good on the cooler side and the mother is likely to get breakthrough pain on that side.
- Maternal hypotension is rare due to the low dose mixtures commonly used.
- Severe hypotension may occur following accidental intrathecal injection or high/subdural spread.
- Bradycardias may be seen if the cardioaccelerator fibres (T1–T4) are blocked or if there is decreased atrial pressure from reduced VR due to aorto-caval compression.

Motor block

- Motor block is minimal if low dose mixes of LA and opioid are used. There is usually some weakness or heaviness of the legs if higher concentrations of bupivacaine are used.
- Motor block can be assessed according to the traditional Bromage Scale (Table 9.1) or the modification of Breen et al. (Table 9.2).
- Epidurals act more rapidly on hip flexion and more slowly on ankle dorsiflexion. This differentiation is termed 'sacralization of the epidural block'.

Table 9.1 Bromage Scale

Grade	Criteria	Degree of motor block
I	Free movement of feet and legs	Nil (0%)
II	Just able to flex knees with free movement of feet	Partial (33%)
III	Unable to flex knees but with free movement of feet	Almost complete (66%)
IV	Unable to move legs or feet	Complete (100%)

Reprinted from Bromage PR. *Epidural Analgesia*. Philadelphia: WB Saunders; 144. Copyright 1978, with permission from Elsevier.

Table 9.2 Modified Bromage Scale as used by Breen et al.

Score	Criteria
1	Complete block (unable to move feet)
2	Almost complete block (able to move feet only)
3	Partial block (just able to move knees)
4	Detectable weakness of hip flexion while supine (full flexion of knees)
5	No detectable weakness of hip flexion while supine
6	Able to perform partial knee bend-whilst standing

Reproduced from Breen TW et al., Epidural anesthesia for labor in an ambulatory patient. *Anesthesia & Analgesia*, 77: 919–24. Copyright International Anesthesia Research Society 1993, with permission from Wolters Kluwer.

Maternal satisfaction

- A comfortable woman who feels in control and can still move freely (either standing or moving herself on the bed) indicates a successful epidural.
- Assess and document pain scores aiming to reduce the score below 30/100 (3/10).
- If she is still requiring Entonox®, the epidural block may be inadequate and needs to be reassessed and further top-ups given.
- Remember that the nature and/or intensity of the pain may change as labour advances, especially with the addition of uterine stimulants.

Further reading

Griffin RP, Reynolds F. The association between foot temperature and asymmetrical epidural blockade. *International Journal of Obstetric Anesthesia*; 1994; 3: 132–136.

Breen TW et al. Epidural anesthesia for labour in an ambulatory patient. *Anesthesia and Analgesia* 1993; 77: 919–924.

Administering analgesia

- Low dose solutions, e.g. 0.0625–0.1% bupivacaine and 2 micrograms/mL fentanyl mixture, have been found to produce effective epidural analgesia during labour.
- Other popular solutions are 0.1–0.2% ropivacaine with fentanyl or sufentanil.
- Following the administration of a titrated bolus dose of LA and opioid solution to establish a sensory block to T10, the method of administering the epidural solution to maintain analgesia throughout labour varies widely between units.

Intermittent top-ups

- Intermittent 'top-ups' can be administered either by the anaesthetist or by a midwife whenever the mother requests further pain relief or as part of a scheduled dosing regimen.
- The top-up given varies depending on local protocols and can be 0.25% bupivacaine to <0.1% bupivacaine with an opioid.

Pros
- Analgesia is titrated to the mother's requirements.
- Higher doses reduce the number of administrations.
- Low incidence of motor block with 'low dose regimes', i.e. ≤0.1% bupivacaine.
- Fewer unilateral blocks and missed segments.

Cons
- Considered labour-intensive.
- Essential that an ongoing training programme for midwives is in place.
- Top-ups may be withheld by the midwife in the second stage because of the mistaken view that the mother is more likely to have a normal delivery.

Continuous epidural infusions

- A continuous background infusion of low dose mixture (≤0.1% bupivacaine with an opioid) is administered into the epidural space via an electronic pump.

Pros
- Popular in many hospitals because of their overall efficacy.
- Fewer top-ups required overall, therefore there is a perceived reduction in workload for both midwives and the anaesthetist.
- When working well, will provide analgesia for many hours with stable haemodynamic effects.

Cons
- Purchase and maintenance costs of epidural pumps.
- Ongoing pump training for all staff is required.
- Total amount of drug administered during labour is higher compared with low dose, intermittent top-ups because analgesia is not titrated exactly to requirements and additional top-ups will be required in 70–80% of epidurals.
- If all 'seems' well, there may be a tendency not to check the block and mother's BP.

Patient-controlled epidural analgesia

- Patient controlled 'top-ups' of low dose mixture are administered into the epidural space via an electronic pump.
- Many differing dosing regimens have been reported, both with and without a continuous background infusion.
- Suggested dosing regimens with 0.1–0.125% bupivacaine and 2–3 micrograms fentanyl = 4–6ml bolus, lockout time 10–20min, background infusion 0–6ml/h.

Pros

- Safe, effective method of labour analgesia.
- Offers the mother greater control and autonomy, which is known to improve overall satisfaction.

Cons

- No significant advantage over 'top-up' regimens or infusions alone.
- Purchase and maintenance costs of pumps and ongoing pump training of all staff need to be considered.
- The mother may administer a top-up without supervision and BP monitoring.

Low dose/mobile epidurals

- A so-called 'mobile epidural' can be started in the intrathecal OR epidural space.
- Epidural analgesia does not prevent the mother from getting out of bed, walking around or sitting in a chair.
- Similarly, continuous CTG monitoring is not an indication to remain in bed for the duration of labour.
- If the mother wishes to stand, sit out, or ambulate after an epidural has been sited, the following checks should be performed 20min after completion of the epidural:
  - Ensure adequate pain relief.
  - Ensure strong, sustained ability to straight leg raise.
  - Ask mother to place feet on the floor. If her feet feel like 'cotton wool', this usually means it is NOT safe to walk.
  - Standing and first steps should be attempted initially with the anaesthetist and midwife in attendance until the mother is confident that her legs will support her weight.
  - The mother should do a deep knee bend, i.e. femur to ~45° to the vertical, under supervision.
- Continue to monitor the BP every 30min, unless required more frequently after top-ups.
- Maintain epidural analgesia with intermittent 'top-ups' of low dose solution with the mother on the bed or sitting in the chair.
- The usual checks should be performed after each 'top-up'.

Further reading

Sng BL, Sia ATH. Maintenance of epidural labour analgesia: The old, the new and the future. Best Practice & Research Clinical Anaesthesiolgy 2017; 31(1): 15–22.

Torvaldsen S et al. Discontinuation of epidural analgesia late in labour for reducing the adverse delivery outcomes associated with epidural analgesia (Review). Cochrane Database of Systematic Reviews 2004; 18: CD004457.

Peach MJ. Patient-controlled epidural analgesia in obstetrics. International Journal of Obstetric Anesthesia 1996; 5: 115–125.

Bernard JM et al. Ropivacaine and fentanyl concentrations in patient-controlled epidural analgesia during labor: a volume-range study. Anesthesia and Analgesia 2003; 97: 1800–1807.

Collis RE et al. Comparison of midwife top-ups, continuous infusion and patient-controlled epidural analgesia for maintaining mobility after a low-dose combined spinal–epidural. British Journal of Anaesthesia 1999; 82: 233–236.

Price C et al. Regional analgesia in early active labour: combined spinal epidural vs. epidural. Anaesthesia 1998; 53: 951–955.

COMET study group UK. Effect of low-dose mobile versus traditional epidural techniques on mode of delivery: a randomised controlled trial. Lancet 2001; 358: 19–23.

Haydon ML et al. Obstetric outcomes and maternal satisfaction in nulliparous women using patient-controlled epidural analgesia. American Journal of Obstetrics and Gynecology 2011; 205: 271.

Epidurals that don't work

- There is a well-recognized failure rate with epidural blockade, even in experienced hands.
- Failure rates range from 8 to 23%, reducing to 2% at re-siting.
- Failure is much higher amongst obstetric patients than surgical patients. It is therefore important to understand why epidurals fail and what can be done to remedy the situation.
- It is also important to inform the mother about the failure rate before she consents to the procedure.

Reasons why the epidural fails

- The catheter is not in the epidural space.
- The catheter has never been in the epidural space. Possible locations include the subcutaneous tissues, interspinous ligament, and paravertebral space.
- The catheter was once in the epidural space, but has migrated out. This includes 'transforaminal escape'.
- The catheter has gone beyond the epidural space into the subdural space.
- There is inadequate spread of the drug.
- Not enough volume of drug.
- Presence of anatomical barriers within the epidural space.
- Blocked epidural catheter.
- Abnormal spinal anatomy, e.g. scoliosis.

Catheter not in the epidural space

False loss of resistance

- If the catheter is not in the epidural space, the initial placement technique was incorrect.
- False loss of resistance is a common problem.
- The operator experiences a loss of resistance dorsal to the ligamentum flavum whilst still in the interspinous ligament.
- There are lacunae or cavities in the interspinous ligament that when entered can give the impression of a loss of resistance.

Indicators of a false loss of resistance

- Loss of resistance is more superficial than expected.
- The catheter is difficult to thread.
- There is no fall in meniscus level down the epidural catheter after flushing.

How to decide between true and false loss of resistance

- This comes with experience.
- Ultimately, loss of resistance must be considered to be true, as the consequence of ignoring it is an accidental dural tap, which is far worse than re-siting a failed epidural.
- Before starting the procedure, have an idea where you may expect to encounter loss of resistance.
- The average depth to the epidural space at L3/4 level is 5cm via the midline approach, with a range from 2.5 to 10cm.
- If the mother is obese, the epidural space is unlikely to be superficial. False loss of resistance is common as the needle may have to advance to 6 or 7cm before the interspinous ligament is found.

- If the catheter does not thread easily and then there is no fall of the saline meniscus due to the negative pressure within the epidural space, have a high index of suspicion that the catheter is not in the right place.
- If satisfactory analgesia is not achieved after 3×10mL epidural bolus doses, consider re-siting the epidural early.

Paravertebral block

- The epidural space is continuous with the paravertebral space laterally.
- If the needle placement is too lateral from the midline, the paravertebral space may be entered.
- A loss of resistance will be experienced and the catheter may thread easily.
- The block will be obviously unilateral and inadequate.
- A marked unilateral sympathetic block with little associated analgesia is highly suggestive.
- The only option is re-siting.

Subdural block

- The subdural space occurs between the dura and arachnoid mater.
- It is possible for the catheter to enter the epidural space, then breach the dura but not go as far as the arachnoid and subarachnoid space, which would result in CSF release and a recognized dural tap.
- If this occurs, the catheter would be sitting in the subdural space.
- A subdural block, which is a rare occurrence, characteristically results in a patchy but unexpectedly high sensory block.
- There is usually a fairly weak motor block although this is variable.
- Perineal analgesia is usually poor.
- Once recognized, the only option is to resite the catheter.

Transforaminal escape

- Collier demonstrated this phenomenon by performing epidurograms after delivery in women who have had unsatisfactory epidural analgesia (See Figs 9.1 and 9.2).
- A major cause of inadequate epidural analgesia was found to be due to escape of the catheter through the intervertebral foramina.
- The block characteristics are of a limited unilateral block, usually L1/3 dermatomes.
- After 4cm of catheter has been inserted, the catheter tends to curl up. It is therefore recommended that only 2–4cm of catheter is inserted into the epidural space.
- Interestingly, partial withdrawal of a long catheter only improves the block in 50% of women. It is thought that the catheter opens up a path through the intervertebral foramina which all subsequent epidural doses will track.
- Transforaminal escape is more common in obstetric patients and epidural venous distention is thought to be a possible causative factor.

Catheter migration with maternal repositioning

- The distance to the epidural space is greatest when lateral, and less when sitting.
- When maternal position is changed from sitting to lateral, the catheter may withdraw.
- If the catheter is taped down with the mother flexed, it will move out as she straightens.
- The key point is to allow the mother to reposition before the catheter is fixed to the skin.

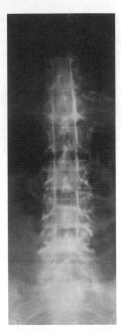

Fig. 9.1 A normal epidurogram. An even spread of contrast in the epidural space with a typical 'Christmas tree' appearance and good root spill of contrast.

Reprinted from *International Journal of Obstetric Anesthesia*, 5, Collier CB, Why obstetric epidurals fail: a study of epidurograms, 19–31. Copyright (1996), with permission from the Obstetric Anaesthetists' Association and Elsevier.

Inadequate spread of the drug within the epidural space

This assumes the catheter is in the correct space.

Not enough drug volume
- Characteristically the block is bilateral but inadequate, because it is usually too low. An upper sensory block to T10 is required.
- It can also be inadequate due to failure to block the perineum sufficiently. A lower sensory block to S3–S5 is required.
- In both cases, the management is to inject more volume of low dose local anaesthetic/opioid mixture.
- Re-siting the epidural one or two spaces above the failed catheter often improve LA spread.

Anatomical barriers within the epidural space
- Contrast X-ray studies indicate the existence of an anatomical barrier in some epidural spaces.
- A dorsomedian connective tissue band has been directly visualized with an epiduroscope.
- Midline pedicles and epidural fat pads have also been described.

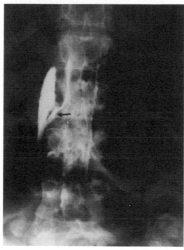

Fig. 9.2 An abnormal epidurogram. The epidural catheter emerges through the L2 intervertebral foramen (arrow). Contrast shows marked psoas and predominantly unilateral epidural spread.

Reprinted from *International Journal of Obstetric Anesthesia*, 5, Collier CB, Why obstetric epidurals fail: a study of epidurograms, 19–31. Copyright (1996), with permission from the Obstetric Anaesthetists' Association and Elsevier.

- The characteristic block is a unilateral block that occurs in ~3% of all epidurals.
- A true missed segment, which is a rare finding, can also be explained by this mechanism.
- The barrier can usually be successfully overcome by increasing the volume in the epidural space.
- Partial catheter withdrawal may also help.
- Resite higher as physical barriers are more common in the lower lumbar region.

Spinal deformity
- Scoliosis is one example where unusual distribution of the epidural solution results in an inadequate block.
- Similar difficulties may result after spinal surgery, when scar tissue reduces the spread of epidural solution.

Blocked catheter
- A patent catheter at the point of insertion can become blocked with fibrin or blood clots, resulting in poor distribution of the drug.

Further reading

Collier CB. Why obstetric epidurals fail: a study of epidurograms. *International Journal of Obstetric Anesthesia* 1996; **5**: 19–31.

Rescuing the failing epidural

The key to success is to know why the epidural is failing. A decision can then be made to spend time adjusting the catheter, increase the dose, or consider re-siting the epidural immediately. Even after re-siting, 2% of mothers will still not achieve adequate epidural analgesia.

Epidurals can be divided into 3 groups:

- Those that initially worked well.
- Those that have been partially effective.
- Those that have never worked.

Epidurals that have initially worked well

- These are worth spending some time sorting out because, initially, the catheter was in the epidural space.
- The question is 'what has changed?'
- Has the catheter moved inward or outward? Check the position at the skin.
- Check the block—is it bilateral or unilateral?
- Is it too low or not low enough?
- Have the woman's requirements changed as her labour progresses?
- If the catheter has migrated inward then withdraw it to its original site.
- If it has come out, resite the epidural, making sure that it is fixed securely after the mother has repositioned herself.
- After checking the sensory level of the block, usually to ice-cold, the height and depth of the block on both sides should be recorded and compared with previous sensory levels recorded for that epidural.
- If the block is bilateral but not extensive enough, inject more volume into the epidural space. A low concentration bolus, e.g. 10mL bupivacaine 0.1% + fentanyl 2 micrograms/ml should improve the situation.
- It is safe to give a second top-up if a recent top-up has been given, provided that the height of the block is known. Re-assess in 10–15min and consider a further 10mL bolus of low concentration mixture to improve the situation further.
- If the block height is still inadequate, re-position the woman in the full lateral position to encourage the spread of the drug in a cephalad direction and inject a similar volume of low concentration mixture.
- Never lie the mother supine to encourage cephalad spread as this will lead to profound aorto-caval compression.
- If the block is unilateral, check the length of catheter present in the space; 3–4cm is the ideal length.
- After ensuring the appropriate length of catheter is present, more volume should be injected.
- Most midline anatomical barriers can be overcome, but up to 30ml of low concentration mixture may be required to ensure bilateral spread.
- It is logical to assist the spread using gravity by positioning the mother to lie on the unblocked side.
- Give the low concentration mixture bolus in two divided doses over a period of 30min.

- If some contralateral analgesia has developed, it is worth persisting with this epidural and administering further incremental doses.
- As labour advances, the woman may experience increasing perineal pain due to descent of the presenting part.
- As before, volume is the first step to improve the spread of the block. However, if a satisfactory sensory block can be demonstrated and further analgesia is required, a higher concentration of LA can be advantageous, e.g. 5–10ml 0.125–0.25% bupivacaine, with the addition of 50 micrograms fentanyl.

Epidurals that have been partially effective

There are two common reasons for partially effective epidurals:

- Transforaminal escape of the catheter.
- Presence of a midline barrier.

Transforaminal escape

- Transforaminal escape of the catheter is characterized by a unilateral block in the lumbar region, limited to a few segments.
- The catheter needs to be withdrawn to encourage it back into the epidural space. Then proceed with further bolus doses as above.
- Success is limited to 50%, as further drug tends to escape down the preformed track.
- If no improvement is seen, the epidural catheter should be resited.
- The paramedian approach may be considered beneficial as it has been shown to encourage a straight course of the catheter. However, the most important factor is to introduce only 3–4cm of catheter into the space in the first instance.

Unilateral block

- Where a true unilateral block persists despite an appropriate length of catheter in the space, a midline barrier is thought to exist.
- Increased volume of solution can improve the spread in about 50% of cases.
- If this is unsuccessful, the epidural catheter should be resited.
- Consider using a different approach and a higher intervertebral space.
- If the analgesia has been patchy and unilateral, resite higher.

A missed segment

- This is a rare phenomenon, and closer examination of the block usually reveals a unilateral block or block that is less dense on one side (a cold or cooler foot is frequently noted on the side of pain).
- For a true missed segment to occur, there must be a demonstrable block above and below the segment with no analgesia.
- The same rules apply for improving the analgesia:
  - Increase the volume of low concentration solution.
  - Adjust the woman's position.
  - Administer additional epidural opioids, e.g. fentanyl 50 micrograms.
  - Try a bolus of higher concentration bupivacaine, e.g. 10mL of 0.125–0.25%.
- Offer to resite the epidural catheter.

Epidurals that have never worked

- The aim is to recognize these early and promptly offer to resite the epidural, rather than to persist with many ineffective top-ups.
- The woman should be warned that even after resiting, 2% of patients still do not achieve effective epidural analgesia.

Checklist for managing the failing epidural
- Check catheter position and length.
- Establish sensory block height and intensity.

If bilateral block present:
- Give increased volume 1–2 bolus doses of 10ml 0.1% bupivacaine with fentanyl 2–3 micrograms/ml.
- Consider changing woman's position to improve the spread.
- If spread is adequate but breakthrough pain persists, consider 10ml bolus of 0.125% or 0.25% bupivacaine.
- Consider additional epidural fentanyl 50 micrograms.

If unilateral block present:
- Withdraw catheter until 3–4cm remains in the epidural space.
- Position the woman on her unblocked side.
- Give up to 30ml bupivacaine 0.1% in divided doses.
- Reassess early for evidence of improvement.
- Offer to resite if no improvement.

No block:
- Give one bolus dose of 15ml 0.1% bupivacaine.
- Re-assess after 10min.
- If no block, resite the epidural catheter.

A block that has been persistently unilateral and remains only partially effective after a couple of extra top-ups and re-positioning will never be fully effective.

If it is not resited, many additional top-ups will be required and it will never be suitable to top-up for a caesarean delivery.

Explain this to the mother and encourage her to have the epidural resited.

Assessing a labour epidural for anaesthesia

- Using an *in situ* epidural for an operative delivery is a useful technique and provides good surgical anaesthesia in many cases.
- However, not all epidurals that provide analgesia for labour will provide adequate anaesthesia for surgery.
- There are several pitfalls involved with augmenting (topping up) epidurals for surgery.
- Careful assessment of the epidural is needed before the decision is made to use it as a method of anaesthesia.
- Changing to either a spinal or a general anaesthetic after a failed epidural top-up can be difficult.
- Therefore, it is important to use the most appropriate method of anaesthesia in the first instance.

Benefits

- No further invasive procedures required.
- Potentially time-saving.
- The block can be extended incrementally if rapid reduction of afterload is undesirable.

Potential pitfalls

- Can take longer to achieve an adequate block for surgical anaesthesia.
- Increased incidence of a patchy or less dense block.
- Later conversion to a spinal anaesthetic may result in a high block.
- Increased requirement for supplementary analgesia intraoperatively:
  - Studies have quoted an 84% success rate for epidural augmentation using 2% lidocaine with adrenaline.
  - 14% supplementation rate with IV analgesia.
  - 2.6% conversion rate to GA.
  - 80% of conversions to GA are due to insufficient cephalic spread of the block.

Questions to be answered when considering an epidural for surgery

How urgent is the delivery?
- Most blocks will be adequate in 15min, but some may require 30min.

How effective has it been for labour analgesia?
- Very effective: augmentation should be straightforward.
- Partially effective: may present difficulties.
- Not effective at all: should not be considered for augmentation of epidural anaesthesia at all.

Signs of an effective epidural

- A comfortable woman, not requiring additional analgesia.
- A recent low dose top-up that has been fully effective.
- A demonstrable sensory block to ice-cold temperature.
- Bilateral warm, dry feet.

- An appropriate administration of LA solution for the duration and progress of labour.
- Epidural that has not moved.
- If all of the above are present, it would be appropriate to use the epidural for the operative delivery.

What to do with the partially effective epidural?

- It has been shown that the strongest factor that was associated with a failed top-up for CS was the need for rescue top-ups above the usual protocol, examples would be:
  - Continuous infusion needing any additional top-ups.
  - Intermittent top-ups of 10mL bupivacaine 0.1% with fentanyl more frequent than hourly.
- Other associations were young maternal age, increased BMI, and increased gestation.
- A combination of the above factors may put the epidural in a high risk category and the epidural should be reviewed carefully during labour and before augmentation.
- Partially effective epidurals that could be considered for augmentation:
  - Block too low because of insufficient LA administered.
  - Perineal pain or deep pressure—often a denser block is required.
  - Unilateral block as a result of excessive catheter in the epidural space. Withdraw the catheter to 3–4cm in the space prior to augmentation.
- If the block is only partially effective and the reason is not obvious, it is safer to abandon the epidural and opt for another technique—usually a spinal if time allows.
- The worst scenario is removing the epidural catheter and not being able to establish spinal anaesthesia.
- The decision regarding the dose of spinal to inject after augmentation of the epidural has failed can be difficult.
- For suggested doses, volume, timing, and location of epidural augmentation and spinal anaesthesia after failed augmentation, see Chapter 11, pp. 306–308.

Instrumental deliveries

The same rules apply for instrumental deliveries as for CSs.

- If the epidural is inadequate for an abdominal delivery, do not be tempted to use it for an instrumental delivery.
- A failed instrumental delivery often turns into an urgent and very difficult CS, with minimal time to extend the block.
- Ensure the sensory block is adequate at the beginning of the procedure.

Further reading

Guasch E et al. Failed epidural for labor: what now? *Minerva Anestesiologica.*. 2017;83:1207–1213.

Kula AO et al.. Increasing body mass index predicts increasing difficulty, failure rate, and time to discovery of failure of epidural anesthesia in laboring patients. Journal of Clinical of Anesthiology 2017; 37: 154–158.

Bauer ME et al. Risk factors for failed conversion of labor epidural analgesia to cesarean delivery anesthesia: a systematic review and meta-analysis of observational trials. International Journal of Obstetric Anesthiology 2012; 21:294–309.

Tortosa JC et al. Effcacy of augmentation of epidural analgaesia for caesarean section. *British Journal of Anaesthesia* 2003; 91: 532–535.

Combined spinal–epidural analgesia in labour

- The CSE technique has gained popularity in the obstetric setting as it provides flexible analgesic options for a wide range of labour scenarios.
- A local anaesthetic and opioid mixture or opioid alone can be delivered directly into the CSF, leading to rapid onset of superior quality analgesia with minimal or absent motor blockade.
- No difference has been demonstrated when compared with simple epidural analgesia in duration of labour or mode of delivery.
- The technique of CSE is described in Chapter 7 p. 220. The two separate injection technique is especially useful if the mother is distressed or not co-operative. Once analgesia has been achieved the epidural can be inserted more safely.
- The deliberate puncture of the dura without intrathecal injection prior to siting an epidural catheter has been described. The advantage appears to be more reliable epidural analgesia

Pros

- Rapid onset analgesia.
- Early sacral analgesia.
- High maternal satisfaction.
- Less motor block (with low dose regimes)—some units allow and encourage ambulation.
- Reduced total local anaesthetic dose with intrathecal administration of opioid.
- Supplemental analgesia supplied by epidural catheter.

Cons

- More technically challenging with a higher incidence of failure, in particular the spinal component, probably secondary to tenting of the dura or deviation of the spinal needle in the epidural space.
- Untested epidural catheter *in situ*.
- Possible increased chance of headache from deliberate dural puncture.
- Increased incidence of opioid-mediated pruritis, especially when not given with LA.
- Case reports of meningitis exist, but these are associated with multiple punctures.
- Possible association with fetal bradycardia.
- Increased equipment costs.

Suggested intrathecal doses

- The spread of the intrathecal block and analgesia is better with plain rather than 'heavy' bupivacaine.
- Some authorities add adrenaline 2.5 micrograms to the intrathecal solution to prolong analgesia, but the effect is quite small and introduces mixing and dilution errors.

Early labour <4cm
Sufentanil 5–10 micrograms alone.

Fentanyl 25 micrograms alone.
Bupivacaine 1.5mg with 1.5 micrograms sufentanil.
Bupivacaine 1.5mg with fentanyl 6 micrograms.

Any stage of labour
Bupivacaine 2.5–5mg with fentanyl 6–25 micrograms.
Ropivacaine 2.5mg with fentanyl 6–25 micrograms.
Levobupivacaine 2.5mg with fentanyl 6–25 micrograms.
The fentanyl can be changed to sufentanil 5–10 micrograms in any of the above.

Late labour
Bupivacaine 2.5–5mg bupivacaine with fentanyl 25 micrograms.
Bupivacaine 5mg alone.

> There is no difference between CSE and epidural techniques with respect to:
> - The incidence of instrumental delivery, maternal mobility, PDPHs, CS rates, or admission of babies to the neonatal unit.
> - It is not possible to draw any meaningful conclusions regarding rare complications such as nerve injury and meningitis; however, studies are ongoing.

Further reading

Chau A et al. Dural puncture epidural technique. Improves labor analgesia quality with fewer side effects compared with epidural and combined spinal epidural techniques: a randomized clinical trial. *Anesthesia and Analgesia* 2017; 124: 560–569.
Groden J et al. Catheter failure rates and time course with epidural versus combined spinal-epidural analgesia in labor. *International Journal of Obstetric Anesthia* 2016; 26: 4–7.
Heesen M et al. Meta-analysis of the success of block following combined spinal-epidural vs epidural analgesia during labour. *Anaesthesia* 2014; 69: 64–67.
Hughes D et al. Combined spinal–epidural versus epidural analgesia in labour. *Cochrane Database of Systematic Reviews* 2003; 4:CD003401.

Regional analgesia for early labour

- Cervical dilatation of ≤4cm is considered early labour and pain is mainly visceral as uterine activity increases.
- Traditionally epidurals were avoided in early labour, as it was thought that they prolonged the duration of the first and second stages.
- Blame was partially attributed to dilution of circulating prostaglandins by fluid preloading. Nowadays this is considered unnecessary due to the low concentrations of epidural drug solutions used.
- Studies have shown that the duration of the first phase of labour appears unchanged with epidural analgesia, but the second stage of labour is likely to be prolonged.

Requests for an early epidural often accompany:
- Long latent phase.
- Dysfunctional contractions.
- Occipito-posterior position of the baby.
- Large baby.
- Atypical, rapidly escalating pain may be indicative of dysfunctional uterine contractions, abnormal fetal presentation, or other intrauterine/intrabdominal problems, and an obstetric opinion should be sought.

Indications

Maternal request
- It is unacceptable not to offer epidural analgesia to a woman because she is <4cm dilated, as long as she is considered to be in the active phase of labour or there is an obstetric commitment to deliver.

Augmentation of labour
- Contractions may appear suddenly and with force following the start of an oxytocin infusion to augment labour.

Pre-eclampsia
- To optimize BP control.

Obstetric request
- To facilitate obstetric examination or fetal scalp electrode monitoring.

Cardiac disease
- To minimize the effects of circulating catecholamines and aid in haemodynamic stability.

Morbid obesity
- To pre-empt and avoid significant GA risks.

Techniques

- A standard low dose epidural technique is appropriate for analgesia in early labour.
- If rapid pain control is necessary, a CSE technique can be used.
- Low dose CSE is also beneficial if ambulation is allowed.
- It is essential to check the adequacy of an epidural placed early on in labour as there is a greater risk of it becoming displaced.
- Epidural top-ups may be required more frequently as labour progresses or with increasing oxytocin infusion rates.

Further reading

Ohel G et al. Early versus late initiation of epidural analgesia in labor: does it increase the risk of cesarean section? A randomized trial. *American Journal of Obstetrics and Gynecology* 2006; 194: 600–605.

Wong CA et al. The risk of cesarean delivery with neuraxial analgesia given early versus late in labor. *New England Journal of Medicine* 2005; 352: 655–665.

Panni MK et al. Local anesthetic requirements are greater in dystocia than in normal labor. *Anesthesiology* 2003; 98: 957–963.

Regional analgesia for late labour

Late labour is considered to be at cervical dilatation of ≥7cm, and has been considered by some to be a contraindication to regional analgesia and should be discouraged. For some women, careful assessment and midwifery support is all that is required, but each situation must be considered on its own merit.

Indications

- An increasing number of women are labouring in midwifery-led units. Some will be transferred to medical obstetric units in late first stage or second stage of labour because of extreme maternal distress or failure to progress in the later part of their labour.
- These women need careful obstetric assessment and many will require regional analgesia for examination and augmentation despite the late stage of the labour. They should never be denied analgesia because the second stage of the labour has been reached.
- Some woman in the second stage of labour will not push because of fear and pain; regional analgesia can be beneficial.
- Some women become exhausted and an instrumental delivery becomes the likely outcome. Regional analgesia can then be used for instrumental delivery.

Techniques

Epidural

- A low dose epidural can be used, but sacral pain can be difficult to treat with the low dose solutions and good analgesia difficult to obtain — 10mL bupivacaine 0.25% with fentanyl 50 micrograms can be helpful.
- The benefit of primarily siting an epidural is that the epidural is tested in case of instrumental or caesarean delivery.

Combined spinal–epidural

- Can provide ideal, rapid analgesia in late labour, e.g. bupivacaine 2.5–5mg and fentanyl 25 micrograms, or bupivacaine 5mg alone.
- Analgesia will be shorter lived than when a CSE is used in early labour; however 30–40min of complete pain relief is usual.
- Although a proportion of women will deliver on the spinal component alone, a request for late analgesia often indicates a problem with the labour, and a request to convert analgesia to anaesthesia for instrumental or caesarean delivery is likely.
- The epidural component will remain untested for some time and may then not be reliable when required. Early testing of the epidural component of the CSE should be considered in these circumstances.

Further reading

Booth JM et al. Combined spinal epidural technique for labor analgesia does not delay recognition of epidural catheter failures: A single-center retrospective cohort survival analysis. *Anesthesiology* 2016; 125: 516–524.

Anaesthesia for Caesarean section: Basic principles

Rachel Collis

Urgency, timing and classification

The purpose of classifying the urgency of CSs is to balance the safe management of the mother with the appropriate timing of fetal delivery. The 4-point classification of urgency has been adopted in the UK (See Table 10.1). Although initially proposed as a post-delivery audit tool, it is widely used to classify and communicate the clinical urgency of every CS prior to transfer to theatre.

Categorization of urgent CS

- The traditionally accepted time of 30min from decision to delivery for category 1 CS and its effect on fetal outcome has shortcomings, which have been highlighted by the NICE guidelines.
- The delivery of the fetus within a 30min interval may not be rapid enough. For a true emergency category 1 CS, e.g. due to maternal haemorrhage or sustained fetal bradycardia, the fetus may require delivery much earlier than this.
- A 'continuum of urgency' applies to CS, rather than discrete categories. This had led to the development of traffic-light colour scale where green merges into amber and amber into red.
- GA will usually be the preferred anaesthetic technique for a true category 1; however, maternal problems such as an anticipated difficult airway or morbid obesity must be taken into consideration when deciding the anaesthetic technique and discussed pre-emptively with the obstetric and midwifery team.
- Inappropriate haste to comply with arbitrary time constraints may unduly compromise the mother's safety.
- Good communication between midwives, obstetricians, and anaesthetists is essential.
- Intrauterine fetal resuscitation, if appropriate, needs to be considered during this period, as this may improve the fetal condition such that a category 1 CS may be regraded to a category 2, therefore allowing time for a regional technique.
- The fetal condition should always be reassessed on arrival in theatre and changes in urgency clearly identified and communicated. There can be a reduction or increase in urgency.
- CTG should always be recommenced once in theatre and someone who is able to interpret the CTG should attend the mother whilst anaesthesia is performed.

Table 10.1 Classification of urgency of caesarean section

Grade	Definition (at time of decision to operate)
Category 1	Immediate threat to life of woman or fetus (usually within 30 minutes: red)
Category 2	Maternal or fetal compromise, not immediately life threatening (usually within 60 minutes: red–amber)
Category 3	Needs early delivery but no maternal or fetal compromise (amber–green)
Category 4	At a time to suit the woman and staff (green)

Adapted from Care of women undergoing emergency caesarean section. Guideline Obs 103. NHS.

Intrauterine fetal resuscitation

The anaesthetist should actively take part in both maternal and fetal resuscitation once the decision for CS has been made.

Immediate management should include

- Turn off oxytocin.
- Position the mother in full left lateral, right lateral, or knee–elbow position (if FHR persistently abnormal or cord compression).
- Administer 15L/min oxygen via a Hudson mask with a reservoir bag.
- Give fluid bolus, e.g. 1000mL Hartmann's solution (caution in pre-eclampsia).
- Treat hypotension with an IV vasopressor, e.g. ephedrine or phenylephrine.
- Consider tocolysis (especially if fetal distress is associated with prostaglandin or oxytocin administration)—discuss with obstetrician and consider terbutaline 250mcg subcutaneously or glyceryl trinitrate (GTN) sublingual spray.

Further reading

Lucas DN et al. Urgency of Caesarean section: a new classification. *Journal of the Royal Society of Medicine* 2000; 93: 346–350.

Classification of Urgency of Caesarean section: A continuum of Risk. Good Practice No. 11. April 2010 https://www.rcog.org.uk/en/guidelines-research-services/.../good-practice-11/

Thurlow JAI, Kinsella SM. Intrauterine resuscitation: active management of fetal distress. *International Journal of Obstetric Anesthia* 2002; 11:105–116.

Information and consent

Antenatal information

- All pregnant women can expect full involvement in decisions regarding their maternity care, and have an increasing demand and access to information regarding obstetric anaesthesia.
- The antenatal period should be used to provide women with access to written information, such as that provided by the OAA (labourpains.com).
- Anaesthetists should ideally be involved in antenatal education on pain relief.
- An antenatal anaesthetic assessment clinic should be available for women who require specific discussions regarding anaesthetic risks, e.g. morbid obesity, cardiac disease, known anaesthetic problems, airway problems, and any women with particular concerns who wish to see an anaesthetist.
- A system should be in place for midwives and obstetricians to refer these women for early anaesthetic review.
- Appropriate literature and interpreters should be available for women who don't speak English.

Preoperative information

Elective caesarean section

- Local guidelines should be followed in the preparation of women for an elective LSCS. The following example reflects typical practice.
- The woman is seen 1–3 days prior to surgery for preoperative clerking, midwifery assessment, and confirmation of surgical consent.
- Investigations are sent as appropriate; usually blood tests for a full blood count and group and save, or cross-match as required.
- Antacid prophylaxis is prescribed, i.e. omeprazole 20–40 mg +/− metoclopramide 10mg orally to be taken the night before and on the morning of surgery.
- The anaesthetist should complete a thorough preoperative assessment looking for problems related to a regional technique or GA. This includes examining the patient, paying particular attention to the airway, back, and auscultation for significant heart murmurs. This is a good time to reinforce the information on timing of antacid prophylaxis and starvation requirements.
- Further information on the planned anaesthetic technique should be discussed.

Regional technique

Information on what to expect when the regional technique is being performed should include:

- Positioning and monitoring, e.g. sitting or lying.
- IV access.
- The aseptic technique, e.g. very cold spray.
- LA to numb the skin of the back.
- Paraesthesia may occur momentarily during insertion of the epidural or spinal.

- Failure of insertion may occur, requiring repeated attempts or a GA.
- When the spinal anaesthetic is inserted, the patient will feel a warm bottom and legs, with tingling, leading to complete motor block of the legs.
- Nausea and vomiting is common in the first 10–15min and will be treated.
- The BP will be closely monitored during this time.
- Numbness will spread up to the chest and will be tested before surgery is allowed to proceed.
- The table is tilted to the left side.
- The drape will obscure any vision of the surgery for mother and partner, and may be lowered at delivery if the parents want to see their baby being born and subject to clinical conditions at the time. (Not all hospitals may allow this).
- The mother will feel pulling and tugging during the procedure and occasionally this may become uncomfortable. Extra analgesia can be given through the drip if necessary. In around 2% of cases a GA is necessary.
- At the end of the operation, we may insert suppositories to aid postoperative analgesia.
- A urinary catheter may be left in until bladder function returns.
- Motor function of the legs will return within 4–6h.
- Postoperative analgesia will include regular paracetamol and NSAIDs (assuming no contraindications).

Side effects explained should include the common and the serious
- Failure, including conversion to GA.
- Pruritus.
- PDPH (use local audit figures, national figures are about 1%).
- Neurological complications, transient in about 1 in 1000 and permanent in about 1 in 10,000 cases.
- Reassurance that having a spinal or epidural does not give you a 'bad back', although local bruising may occur causing local tenderness for a few days.
- The presence of the partner during the whole procedure if requested should be allowed and encouraged.
- You should enquire whether the mother (and partner) has any questions before concluding the preoperative visit.
- Documentation of this consultation should be written in the case notes. A preprinted sticky label or pre-assessment form will aid in mentioning all the relevant risks, signed to confirm that they have been discussed. This is very important because it is very often a different team conducting the anaesthetic the following day and having to discuss all the risks again will cause delay of the operating list.

General anaesthesia
Many of the general points mentioned above also apply to GA, with the exception that the partner is usually not present during induction or the operation, but will be allowed to see the baby as soon as is practicable.

- The conduct of the anaesthetic should describe the need for monitoring, IV access, preoxygenation, and cricoid pressure.

- Specific informed consent could include mentioning the risks of:
  - Awareness.
  - Regurgitation and aspiration.
  - Sore throat.
  - Muscle aches and pains.
- Specific consent should be sought for the administration of analgesia by suppository during GA and information about transversus-abdominus plane (TAP) blocks given.
- It is preferable to use IV opioids, e.g. morphine, via a PCA device for the first 24h following a CS under GA, combined with regular paracetamol and diclofenac, unless contraindicated.

Emergency caesarean section
- Labour is a difficult time to obtain informed consent. Mothers are often in severe pain, may be exhausted, under the influence of drugs such as opioids or Entonox®, or feeling extremely anxious. However, this does not alter the principles or amount of information necessary to obtain informed consent for obstetric anaesthesia.
- Research has shown that despite the influence of pain or drugs, women like to be informed and are capable of recalling the risks and benefits of regional anaesthesia. Using simple and clear information cards (e.g. giving short notes on the advantages and risks of epidural analgesia) improves recall of information and patient satisfaction.
- If time is of the essence, the consent process should occur at the same time as the woman is prepared for theatre. In an extreme emergency, consent can be verbal and a description in the notes of the conversation made afterwards.
- The volume of information may be less but the principle of informed consent still applies, and the material risks, i.e. common and serious risks, still need to be mentioned.
- Pain under regional anaesthesia is a common cause of litigation, and this needs to be mentioned prior to it occurring, with the reassurance that if it occurs, it will be dealt with swiftly, including a GA if necessary.

Further reading

Jackson GN et al. What mothers know, and want to know, about the complications of general anaesthesia. *Acta Anaesthesiologica Scandinavic* 2012; 56: 585–588.

Broaddus BM, Chandrasekhar S. Informed consent in obstetric anesthesia. *Anesthesia and Analgesia.* 2011; 112(4):912–915.

Black JD, Cyna AM. Issues of consent for regional analgesia in labour: a survey of obstetric anaesthetists. *Anaesthics and Intensive Care* 2006; 34: 254–260.

Yentis SM et al. AAGBI: Consent for anaesthesia 2017: Association of Anaesthetists of Great Britain and Ireland. *Anaesthesia* 2017;72:93–105.

Transversus Abdominus Plane Block: Anaesthesia tutorial of the week 239. 5th September 2011. Paul Townsley, James French. www.aagbi.org/sites/default/files/239%20Transversus%20 Abdominus%20Plane%20Block.pdf

Enhanced recovery for caesarean section

There is considerable evidence that a well woman who has a term singleton elective caesarean delivery (usually for breech or previous caesarean delivery) is well enough to leave hospital the following day.

- The woman and partner should be told about the possibility of early discharge well before her caesarean.
- A regional technique should be strongly encouraged.
- The woman and her partner need to be motivated towards early discharge.
- She needs to have a good level of support at home so she can rest and look after her baby whilst household duties and looking after siblings are delegated to others.
- The baby needs to be feeding well and not require additional observations or treatments.
- Units that have instigated first day discharge have increased rates typically from 2% to 50% with the majority of the other women who have had a straight forward caesarean section going home on day 2.

Key requirements for first day discharge

- There should be minimal interruption of perioperative oral intake. Women are encouraged to drink water on the morning of her caesarean. Many units now provide an isotonic sport's drink (non-carbonated) and the women are allowed to sip the drink until the time of the operation.
- Morning operating lists facilitate minimal starvation times and the best chance of day 1 discharge.
- Immediately after the operation, women are encouraged to drink water or isotonic sports drinks and eat as soon as possible after this.
- Nausea and vomiting should be treated as soon as possible. There is not a universal policy about prophylactic anti-emetics but ondansetron is the usual first line therapy.
- Post-operative pain should be treated by a single dose of a long-acting intrathecal opiates followed by regular paracetamol and non-steroidal anti-inflammatories (when not contraindicated).
- Breakthrough pain should be treated with oral opioids, a small supply of which may be required at home.
- Early mobilization is key and should be encouraged within 12h of surgery or when the neuraxial block had worn off.
- Catheters can be removed when the mother is mobilizing or the following morning, but careful bladder management is important because of the risk of urinary retention with early catheter removal.

Other considerations
- Most units do not monitor the patient's temperature in theatre or use active warming as the majority of caesarean last under 45 minutes and active measures tend to be uncomfortable for the mother.
- Delayed cord clamping to the neonate is beneficial. In term infants, delayed umbilical cord clamping increases haemoglobin levels at birth and improves iron stores in the first several months of life.
- Early skin to skin contact with the mother in theatre encourages maternal bonding, helps regulate neonatal temperature, and improves early breast feeding attempts.

Further reading

Corso E et al. Enhanced recovery after elective caesarean: a rapid review of clinical protocols, and an umbrella review of systematic reviews. *BMC Pregnancy Childbirth* 2017; 17: 91. Review

Aluri S, Wrench IJ. Enhanced recovery from obstetric surgery: a U.K. survey of practice. *International Journal of Obstetric Anesthesia* 2014 May;23(2):157–156

Wrench IJ et al. Introduction of enhanced recovery for elective caesarean section enabling next day discharge: a tertiary centre experience. *International Journal of Obstetric Anesthesia* 2015; 24: 124–130.

Antacid prophylaxis

- Regurgitation and inhalation of gastric contents can cause pneumonitis, particularly if the fluid is acidic; this can cause severe morbidity and occasionally death.
- This condition is referred to as chemical pneumonitis or Mendelson's syndrome.
- Although chemical pneumonitis is a serious condition, most deaths in Mendelson's study were associated with aspiration of solid matter.
- Gastro-oesophageal regurgitation can occur during GA if the stomach is not empty, as anaesthetic drugs relax the lower oesophageal sphincter tone.

> Pregnant women are thought to be at increased risk of regurgitation because:
> - The pregnancy hormones progesterone and relaxin cause relaxation of the smooth muscle of the stomach.
> - There is reduced barrier pressure and increased intra-abdominal pressure in pregnancy.
> - Pain, anxiety, and the use of opioids during labour increase the risk by further delaying gastric emptying.

Incidence

Since Mendelson first described the acid aspiration syndrome in 1946, the incidence has dramatically reduced. There were 66 cases in the 1946 CEMACH report.

The reasons for this dramatic reduction are multifactorial
- An increase in the use of regional anaesthesia for CS.
- Better provision of antacid prophylaxis.
- Availability of experienced obstetric anaesthetists and their assistants.
- The identification and treatment of those women at higher risk of aspiration, e.g. women receiving opioids in labour, pre-eclampsia, multiple pregnancies, previous CS, obesity, diabetes.

Methods of reducing the risk of aspiration

Based on animal work, the important factors thought to increase the chance of chemical pneumonitis are:
- Gastric pH <2.5.
- Gastric volume >25mL.

The methods employed to reduce the risk of aspiration include:
- Starvation of mothers for at least 6h before a planned CS to reduce the volume of gastric contents.
- Limits on oral intake during labour (especially solid food).
- Antacid prophylaxis: the administration of the following drugs to reduce the volume and/or acidity of the stomach contents.

Antacids

These are alkaline substances, which reduce or neutralize the acidity of the stomach contents.

Magnesium trisilicate
- First antacid to be widely used in labour but rarely used nowadays.
- It effectively reduces gastric pH.
- Slow to mix with stomach contents.
- Particulate nature is potentially hazardous and causes a pneumonitis.

Sodium citrate
- Most widely used antacid.
- Given as 30mL of 0.3M solution.
- Effective quickly (10min from laboratory studies).
- Short acting; effectiveness is unpredictable at 60min (during extubation)
- Does not seem to increase gastric volume.
- Unpalatable.
- Short shelf-life.

H_2 antagonists
- H_2 receptor antagonists, e.g. ranitidine, inhibit the secretion of acid into the stomach, which reduces the volume and acidity of the stomach contents.
- This action is not immediate and H_2 receptor antagonists are often used in combination with antacids at induction of emergency anaesthesia.
- Oral administration of ranitidine 150mg is effective in 60min.
- IV administration of ranitidine is effective in 30min and should be given at induction of emergency anaesthesia if the mother has not previously received the drug to cover extubation (when the effect of sodium citrate is unreliable).
- Adverse effects of the drugs may include dizziness, fatigue, rashes, headaches, and GIT disturbances.

Dopamine antagonists, e.g. metoclopramide
- Has been used widely and safely in pregnancy.
- 10mg metoclopramide orally or slow IV.
- These drugs inhibit vomiting and accelerate gastric emptying.
- May increase lower oesophageal tone.
- Most effective when used in conjunction with ranitidine or omeprazole.
- Adverse effects include drowsiness, restlessness, diarrhoea, and arrhythmias.

Proton pump inhibitors, e.g. omeprazole
- These drugs block the production of gastric acid by interfering with the proton pump mechanism in the gastric parietal cells.
- Omeprazole is the only proton pump inhibitor that has been widely investigated in obstetric practice.
- An oral dose of 20–40mg is effective in 60min.
- An IV dose of 40mg is effective in 30min.
- No clear advantage over ranitidine.
- Adverse effects include rashes and GIT disturbances.

There is limited evidence to support the routine administration of acid prophylaxis drugs in normal labour to prevent gastric aspiration and its consequences.

Aspiration prophylaxis protocol

Varies between individual obstetric units.

Typical aspiration prophylaxis for CS

Elective caesarean section

- 12h preop, omeprazole 20–40 mg orally.
- 2h preop, omeprazole 20–40 mg orally +/– metoclopramide 10mg orally immediately preop.
- Some units also add 0.3M sodium citrate 30mL orally. However, as it is only effective for 20min following ingestion, many units will only treat with sodium citrate if a GA is required.

Emergency CS under GA

- Omeprazole 20–40mg orally if time allows.
- Immediately preoperatively, 0.3M sodium citrate 30mL.
- Intraoperatively omeprazole 40mg and metoclopramide 10mg both IV.
- At the end of CS the stomach may be emptied with an orogastric tube, which should be removed before extubation.
- Typical aspiration prophylaxis for at risk mothers in active labour– omeprazole 20–40mg 12 hourly orally, e.g. epidural analgesia for labour.

Further reading

Calthorpe N, Lewis M. Acid aspiration prophylaxis in labour: a survey of UK obstetric units. *International Journal of Obstetric Anesthesia* 2005; 14: 300–304.

Paranjothy S1 et al. Interventions at caesarean section for reducing the risk of aspiration pneumonitis. *Cochrane Database Systematic Reviews* 20142:CD004943.

Monitoring mother and fetus

To ensure patient safety, monitoring for CS should be started prior to induction or insertion of regional technique and continued into recovery for both general and regional anaesthesia.
- Monitoring equipment should be checked before each new patient.
- Capnography is essential as deaths still occurred following undetected oesophageal intubation.
- Unexpected monitor readings should not be dismissed.

The AAGBI have published guidelines on standards of monitoring that must be used whenever a patient is anaesthetized. These include:
- Presence of an appropriately experienced anaesthetist and a trained anaesthetic assistant during the whole of the procedure.
- Accurate record keeping.
- Monitoring of the anaesthetic equipment, e.g. appropriate alarm settings, oxygen, and volatile agent analyser.

Maternal monitoring

Clinical observation
- A drop in BP in a patient undergoing a CS under regional anaesthesia may be heralded by pallor, yawning, anxiety, and a complaint of nausea.
- Frequent verbal interaction with the patient is essential and one of the most reliable methods of monitoring the mother.

Minimal monitoring requires:
- Pulse oximeter.
- Non-invasive blood pressure monitor.
- ECG.
- Capnography.
- Inspired oxygen and volatile agent analyser.
- Neuromuscular monitoring (available).
- Temperature monitor (available).
- Blood loss should be measured in every patient and additional monitoring applied dependent on patient and obstetric factors:
  - Urinary output measurements—continue monitoring closely in the postoperative period following major haemorrhage (blood loss >1500mL) and PET.
  - Invasive monitoring e.g. arterial line and CVP should be available for the very high risk mother, major PPH, and severe preeclampsia.

Fetal monitoring

- For an elective caesarean with a well-grown well baby a short period of intermittent fetal monitoring is acceptable just prior to the anaesthetic and whilst the spinal anaesthetic is beginning to work.
- In all emergency situations, monitoring of the fetal heart should be performed from prior to induction of anaesthesia to the beginning of surgery. In an emergency, induction and placement of fetal monitoring may need to happen at the same time.

- Monitoring can be intermittent, i.e. with a Doppler ultrasound, or continuous monitoring with a CTG.
- In an emergency situation, good communication is essential to facilitate adequate fetal monitoring and safe conduct of anaesthesia.
- Continuous monitoring should ideally be applied throughout the conduct of anaesthesia, including any regional techniques in any emergency or labour setting.
- Someone qualified to interpret the CTG should be present throughout.

Further reading

Hartle A et al. Checking anaesthetic equipment 2012: Association of Anaesthetists of Great Britain and Ireland (AAGBI). *Anaesthesia* 2012; 67: 660–668.

Checketts MR et al. Association of Anaesthetists of Great Britain and Ireland. Recommendations for standards of monitoring during anaesthesia and recovery 2015. *Anaesthesia* 2016; 71:85–93.

Aorto-caval compression

Introduction

- Gideon Ahltorp in 1931 first noted that signs and symptoms of cardiac insufficiency (nausea, dyspnoea, pallor, unconsciousness, and weak pulses) only occurred when the gravid uterus lay on the posterior abdominal wall. These symptoms disappeared when the lateral position was adopted or the uterus lifted upwards.
- In 1953, Howard described the concept of supine hypotensive syndrome in late pregnancy. He found that 11.2% of pregnant women developed hypotension, a decrease in systolic arterial pressure of >30mmHg, when assuming the supine position after some minutes.
- Aorto-caval compression is caused by partial occlusion of the IVC and to a lesser extent the aorta by the gravid uterus.
- Occlusion of the IVC significantly reduces the VR and CO. Despite a reduction in the CO, the BP is often maintained by means of arterial vasoconstriction.
- Occlusion of the aorta increases afterload and consequently reduces CO.
- A baroreceptor-mediated vagal bradycardia secondary to increase in systemic arterial pressure following aortic compression may cause a bradycardia and contribute to hypotension.
- Intense bradycardia <20bpm, often associated with a very low CO and maternal collapse, is thought to be caused by a severe fall in VR to the right atrium (Bezold–Jarisch reflex).
- Supine hypotension can occur as early as 20 weeks, and becomes more severe in the third trimester as the uterus increases in size.
- Hypotension occurs especially in women with poor azygos venous system collaterals.

Other contributory factors

- Polyhydramnios.
- Abnormal presentation of the fetus (breech, transverse lie).
- Multiple pregnancy.
- Maternal obesity.
- Uterine myomata.

Supine hypotension is less severe after membrane rupture, engagement of the fetal head, and descent of the head through the pelvis, and is unlikely to take place after delivery. It is most common in a term elective CS.

Lesser degrees of aorto-caval compression, insufficient to cause maternal symptoms, may nevertheless reduce placental perfusion and cause fetal compromise.

Physiological considerations

The degree of hypotension depends on the density and the extent of the preganglionic sympathetic blockade. Sympathetic block up to T5 will result in:

- Dilatation of the resistance vessels and consequently reduction in systemic vascular resistance.
- Dilatation of the capacitance vessels leading to venous pooling and reduction in VR.

- Reduction in endogenous catecholamine secretion from the adrenal medulla due to splanchnic nerve block.
- Sympathetic block above T5, in addition to vasodilatation, causes a fall in BP due to bradycardia and reduction in myocardial contractility.
- The combination of aorto-caval compression, the greater sensitivity to local anaesthetics, and the predominance of the sympathetic nervous system during pregnancy contributes significantly to the increased risk of hypotension associated with spinal or epidural anaesthesia.

Definition and incidence

- Hypotension is commonly defined as a drop of systolic BP below 100mmHg or a fall of >20% of baseline.
- The incidence of hypotension following spinal or epidural anaesthesia can be as high as 80% without prophylactic measures and is more likely if spinal anaesthesia is used.
- If untreated, it can lead to unpleasant maternal symptoms—nausea, vomiting, dizziness, and distress, and serious fetal complications— bradycardia and acidosis secondary to placental hypoperfusion.
- The induction of anaesthesia, either general or regional, with the associated arterial vasodilatation will block the main compensatory mechanism and as a result, some hypotension will inevitably occur.
- The aggressive treatment of hypotension to maintain baseline BP has been shown to be beneficial to the fetus.

Further reading

Lee SW et al. Haemodynamic effects from aortocaval compression at different angles of lateral tilt in non-labouring term pregnant women. Br J Anaesth. 2012 Dec;109(6):950–956

Lee SW et al. Management of hypotension in obstetric spinal anaesthesia. *British Journal of Anaesthesia* 2009; 103:457–458.

Ngan Kee WD, Lee A. Multivariate analysis of factors associated with umbilical arterial pH and standard base excess after caesarean section under spinal anaesthesia. *Anaesthesia* 2003; 58: 125–130.

Reynolds F, Seed PT. Anaesthesia for caesarean section and neonatal acid–base status: a meta-analysis (Review). *Anaesthesia* 2005; 60: 636–653.

Maternal position

The effects of aorto-caval compression can be minimized or relieved by:

Full lateral position to either side

- Most effective.
- Impractical to perform CS in this position, but keep woman in the full lateral if severe hypotension persists, until BP is restored to normal limits.
- High risk pregnancy (e.g. multiple pregnancy) consider inducing block in lateral position.

Tilt operating 15° to left

- A 15° left lateral tilt was proposed by Crawford in the 1970s and has become accepted by many to be the ideal position in which to place a mother prior to and during CS. There are no scientific data to validate this tilt as optimal, but it is a reasonable compromise between lying supine and tilting so far that it is dangerous to the mother. See Fig 10.1.
- Most obstetric anaesthetists underestimate the degree of tilt required, unless a tilt-measuring device is used. If the mother is actually placed in 15° left lateral tilt, most obstetricians complain that the tilt is too severe to operate.
- Only partially relieves caval compression.
- May be inadequate in high risk patients.
- Increasing the tilt, i.e. to ≥20° may improve hypotension but make the mother's position unsafe.

Wedge under right buttock

- Uterine displacement is easily achieved.
- Twists the mother's spine, which can cause discomfort.

Manual displacement of uterus to left

- Effective.
- Useful temporary measure.
- Need an additional assistant.

Whichever measure is taken, visual displacement of the uterus must occur.

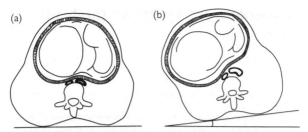

Fig. 10.1 Aorto-caval compression. (a) In the supine position, blood flow through the vena cava and aorta is significantly reduced, causing maternal and fetal compromise. The efficacy of left lateral displacement was demonstrated in 1972. The full left or right lateral position completely relieves aorto-caval compression. (b) Elevating the mother's hip 10–15cm completely relieves aorto-caval compression in 58% of term parturients.

Further reading

Krywko DM1, Bhimji SS2. Aortocaval Compression Syndrome. StatPearls [Internet]. Treasure Island (FL): StatPearls Publishing; 2017

Paech MJ. Should we take a different angle in managing pregnant women at delivery? Attempting to avoid the 'supine hypotensive syndrome'. *Anaesthia and Intensive Care* 2008; 36:775–777.

Holmes F. The supine hypotensive syndrome. *Anaesthesia*. 1995; 50: 972–977.

Intravenous pre-hydration (preload)

Crystalloids

- In the late 1960s Wollman and Marx demonstrated that hypotension can be eliminated by a crystalloid bolus before spinal anaesthesia. This remarkable success was unfortunately not reproduceable.
- Rout et al. found that even a large crystalloid bolus (20mL/kg) only reduces the incidence of hypotension to 55% compared with 71% when no crystalloid bolus was used.
- Many subsequent studies have confirmed the ineffectiveness of this measure and it is now widely accepted that a formal crystalloid preload is not essential prior to spinal anaesthesia.
- The poor efficacy of crystalloids is mainly due to their very short intravascular half-life. Therefore, if given, this should be whilst spinal anaesthesia is instituted (co-load).
- Large crystalloid preload causes haemodilution and the release of atrial natriuretic peptide, a vasodilator, leading to persistent hypotension.
- In pregnancy, low colloid oncotic pressure can be decreased further by a large preload, potentially leading to pulmonary oedema.

Colloids

- Are now rarely given except to treat severe hypovolemia.
- They are more effective in the prevention of hypotension.
- The greater efficacy of colloids is the result of their slower redistribution from the intravascular space, leading to a more sustained increase in the CVP.
- This benefit must be weighed against:
  - Increased cost.
  - Allergic reactions.
  - Pruritis.
  - Interference with blood cross-matching and clotting.
  - Possible renal impairment.

Lower limb wrapping

- There is evidence to suggest that wrapping of the legs with tight elasticated bandages prior to spinal anaesthesia significantly reduces the incidence of hypotension.
- Raising the legs can be an effective and rapid method of treating hypotension.
- Neither method is commonly employed in the UK.

Further reading

Hammond NE et al. Fluid-TRIPS and Fluidos Investigators; George Institute for Global Health, The ANZICS Clinical Trials Group, BRICNet, and the REVA research Network. Patterns of intra-venous fluid resuscitation use in adult intensive care patients between 2007 and 2014: An inter-national cross-sectional study. *PLoS One* 2017;; 12(5): e0176292.

Mercier FJ et al. Maternal hypotension during spinal anesthesia for caesarean delivery. *Minerva Anestesiologia* 2013; 79: 62–73.

Rocke DA, Rout CC. Volume preloading, spinal hypotension and caesarean section. *British Journal of Anaesthesia* 1995; 75: 257–279.

Tawfik MM et al. Comparison between colloid preload and crystalloid co-load in cesarean section under spinal anesthesia: a randomized controlled trial. *International Journal of Obstetric Anesthesia* 2014; 23: 317–323.

Rout CC et al. Leg elevation and wrapping in the prevention of hypotension following spinal anaesthesia for elective caesarean section. *Anaesthesia* 1993; 48: 304–308.

Hasanin A et al. Leg elevation decreases the incidence of post-spinal hypotension in cesarean section: a randomized controlled trial. BMC *Anesthesiology* 2017; ;17:60.

Vasopressors

Ephedrine

- Is a non-specific adrenergic agonist mainly increases BP by augmenting CO through its actions on β-receptors.
- A smaller contribution by increasing the SVR via α_1 receptor stimulation also exists.
- Ephedrine, therefore, has minimal or no vasoconstrictive effect on uteroplacental circulation, a feature that has made this drug very popular and the first line vasoconstrictor for most anaesthetists for decades.
- A survey of UK practice in 1999 showed that >95% of obstetric anaesthetists used ephedrine alone to maintain BP during spinal anaesthesia for CS. More than 60% of respondents used it prophylactically and nearly half added it to the bag of IV fluid.
- Commonly and safely given as 3–6mg IV bolus.
- Although now used less frequently than phenylephrine, it remains a safe drug and should always be available.

Advantages

- Easy to dilute and use.
- Can be given PO, IM, or IV.
- Has a very good safety record.
- Can be safely given if the mother's HR <60.

Disadvantages

- It increases HR and contractility, therefore increasing myocardial oxygen demands. This is of particular importance in women with heart disease.
- Slow onset of action and relatively long duration of action make accurate titration difficult.
- Risk of ectopics and tachyarrhythmias.
- Tachyphylaxis rapidly occurs due to depleted stores of presynaptic noradrenaline, and will become clinically ineffective.
- Its use has been linked to a fall in umbilical arterial pH. This is most probably due to its direct effect on fetal metabolism. Ephedrine crosses the placenta, and stimulation of β-receptors in the fetus increases oxygen consumption and lactate production. This has led to it predominantly becoming a second line drug.

Phenylephrine

- Based on animal studies, this pure α agonist was found to cause uteroplacental hypoperfusion because of vasoconstriction, and therefore its use in obstetrics was thought to be contraindicated.
- Clinical trials in humans using smaller doses have failed to show any evidence of adverse fetal or neonatal effects, but it is important to remember these risks, should there be an accidental over-dose.
- Phenylephrine raises BP by increasing the SVR through its direct effect on the α-1 receptor.
- From its mechanism of action, it seems logical to use phenylephrine, rather than ephedrine, to correct hypotension associated with vasodilatation arising from sympathetic block.
- It is recommended that it is given as a continuous infusion and adjusted to maintain the mothers BP to not less than 20% below her starting BP.

- Although infusions have been shown to be more efficacious in preventing episodes of hypotension, the risk of drug toxicity may be higher as the total dose of drug given by infusion will be greater and there is more potential for human or equipment error.

Suggested dose regimens
- IV 100 micrograms/ml (10mg in 100ml normal saline): run at 30–60ml/h (high dose infusion).
- IV 12.5 micrograms/ml (prepared solution): start infusion at 80–100ml/h (low dose infusion).
- IV bolus 12.5–50 micrograms as required.

Advantages
- Maternal BP is easily maintained, with a positive effect on uteroplacental perfusion.
- Its rapid onset of action and short duration make it easy to titrate when compared with ephedrine.

Disadvantages
- A reflex bradycardia is common and an anticholinergic should always be available.
- Phenylephrine is supplied commercially in different concentrations (10mg/mL, 1mg/10mL, 250 micrograms/mL, and 12.5 micrograms/mL) and extreme care is required when using this drug to ensure the correct dilution.

Other vasopressors
- The risk of bradycardia can be reduced when ephedrine is used in addition to phenylephrine. To date there is little evidence of benefit when the two drugs are combined.
- Studies that showed an increased incidence of nausea and vomiting with combination therapy, but an optimal combination ratio was not used and it is therefore difficult to reach a conclusion.
- Metaraminol, a mixed α- and β-receptor agonist, has also been used in doses of 0.25–0.5mg increments.
- Small doses of noradrenaline 10 micrograms have been used safely.
- More experimental work has been carried out on phenylephrine in obstetric practice, and its use has therefore been popularized although data suggesting that it is superior to metaraminol and noradrenaline is lacking.
- Pre-eclamptic patients may be very sensitive to these agents, and additional care should be taken to avoid adverse effects in this group of women.
- In overdose they will cause severe maternal hypertension and acute heart failure.

Recent advances
The combination of a high dose phenylephrine infusion (100 micrograms/min) and rapid crystalloid co-hydration immediately after spinal injection is the first technique to date that was found to be effective in preventing hypotension during spinal anaesthesia for elective caesarean delivery.
- This resulted in a positive outcome for the fetus.
- Studies to date have been conducted in the elective well fetus.
- Some caution must be exercised at present before extrapolation of these results to the emergency distressed fetus.

Summary

- Hypotension associated with neuroaxial blocks for caesarean delivery is common and should be minimized to avoid unpleasant maternal side effects and serious fetal consequences, i.e. fetal acidosis.
- Many methods for its prevention have been investigated and no single technique has proven to eliminate it.
- Crystalloid preload is ineffective.
- Rapid crystalloid administration during spinal anaesthesia (co-load) may be advantageous.
- Colloids are more effective than crystalloids in preventing hypotension at the expense of cost and risk of adverse reactions.
- Phenylephrine has many favourable characteristics over ephedrine and is now considered as the drug of choice when treating hypotension following spinal or epidural anaesthesia in the obstetric patient.

Further reading

Mohta M et al. Randomized double-blind comparison of ephedrine and phenylephrine for management of post-spinal hypotension in potential fetal compromise. *International Journal of Obstetric Anesthia* 2016; 27: 32–40.

Ngan Kee WD. A random-allocation graded dose-response study of norepinephrine and phenylephrine for treating hypotension during spinal anesthesia for cesarean delivery. *Anesthesiology* 2017; 127: 934–994.

Kinsella SM et al. International consensus statement on the management of hypotension with vasopressors during caesarean section under spinal anaesthesia. *Anaesthesia* 2018; 73: 71–92.

Arora P et al. Fluid administration before Caesarean delivery: Does type and timing matter? *Journal of Clinical and Diagnostic Research* 2015; 9: UC01–4.

Chooi C et al. Techniques for preventing hypotension during spinal anaesthesia for caesarean section. *Cochrane Database Systematic Reviews* 2017; 8:CD002251.

Anaesthesia for Caesarean section: Regional anaesthesia

Sarah Harries and Rachel Collis

Introduction

Regional anaesthesia is the technique of choice for caesarean delivery, provided no contraindications exist. The relationship between the increased use of regional anaesthetic techniques for caesarean delivery and decreased maternal mortality is well recognized, with epidemiological studies indicating regional anaesthesia to be 16 times safer than GA. The three commonly practised techniques—epidural, spinal, and combined spinal–epidural (CSE)—all offer significant advantages for both the mother and neonate.

Advantages

- The mother remains awake and is very much part of the delivery of her baby.
- Early maternal–baby contact, e.g. 'skin to skin' contact, encourages bonding and improves success at breastfeeding.
- The birthing partner is permitted into the operating theatre during surgery, providing emotional support for the mother.
- Reduced operative bleeding.
- Enhanced postoperative analgesia through the use of intrathecal or epidural opioids.
- Early mobilization.
- Reduced incidence of post-operative nausea and vomiting.
- Reduced incidence of postoperative deep vein thrombosis (DVT).
- The direct sedative effects of GA drugs on the neonate are avoided, i.e. delayed onset of respiration, thermoregulation and feeding.
- Eliminates the complications of GA, i.e. difficult or failed intubation, awareness, and pulmonary aspiration.

Disadvantages

- Hypotension is associated with all regional techniques and can confer significant harm to mother and neonate if not promptly treated.
- Intraoperative nausea and vomiting.
- High blocks or total spinal blocks.
- Failed block requiring conversion to GA.
- Intraoperative pain leading to dissatisfaction and complaint.
- PDPH—approximate incidence 1%.
- Neurological complications reported rarely.
- Infection-related complications again reported rarely.
- The time required to perform a regional technique or top-up an existing epidural may prohibit its use in certain situations, e.g. delivery required in <15 min.

- Whenever the anaesthetist is faced with a mother reluctant to accept a regional technique for caesarean delivery, the specific risks and benefits of general vs regional anaesthesia should be clearly emphasized, provided there are no contraindications to the proposed technique.
- The mother must not be frightened into accepting a regional technique on the grounds that GA is dangerous, as there must be a clear back-up plan for failed regional anaesthesia.

Preparation for theatre

Whatever regional technique is considered appropriate for surgery, the following should be checked and prepared prior to transfer to theatre:

- A careful history should be taken and a thorough examination performed, including examination of the lower back and an airway assessment.
- A recent full blood count (FBC) should be checked and routine group and blood screen sent to the blood bank to check for the presence of transfusion antibodies. It is acceptable not to wait for an FBC for a category 1 or 2 CS, but an antenatal FBC should be known.
- Routine cross-matching of blood is not necessary unless significant haemorrhage is anticipated, e.g. grade 4 placenta previa or accreta, in which case blood must be available in theatre or in the delivery suite fridge at the start of surgery. Electronic issue of blood is now available in many units, reducing the need for unnecessary routine cross-matching of blood, e.g. multiple previous CSs.
- Review the latest ultrasound report to confirm placental position.
- Antacid prophylaxis should be administered preoperatively, either by the oral route or IV according to unit policy.
- A clear explanation of the planned anaesthetic technique should be given, including the associated risks, and verbal consent obtained for the technique and any other procedures, e.g. IV insertion, monitoring, catheterization, and rectal medication.

Document the complications that were discussed, including:

- Risk of intraoperative discomfort, e.g. pulling, tugging, and pressure during surgery.
- PDPH ~1% for all techniques, dependent on experience of anaesthetist.
- Failed block, including conversion to GA—between 1 and 5% of regional techniques for CS are inadequate for the duration of surgery.
- Nausea and vomiting.
- Shivering.
- Itching.
- Neurological complications.
- Infection-related complications.
- Check the anaesthetic machine and all emergency drugs.
- Prepare all anaesthetic drugs prior to regional technique, e.g. vasopressors, vagolytics, oxytocin, antibiotics.
- Check IV cannula is patent and attach IV infusion.
- Apply minimal monitoring: ECG, pulse oximeter, and record the baseline BP.
- The WHO Checklist is mandated prior to all surgical procedures.

See Chapter 7 for further information on the techniques of insertion and contraindications.

Assessment of the block

There has been considerable discussion and debate regarding the most reliable method of assessing both the density and height of the block required to perform a painless CS under regional anaesthesia. At present, there is no single, universally accepted best or most predictable method of testing a block prior to the start of surgery. The fundamental block required for CS is no different if a spinal or epidural is used. The difference is that in most cases the block from a spinal anaesthetic is high, dense, and easy to assess. The block from an epidural is frequently more difficult to assess, requiring careful and subtle evaluation.

The ideal block for painless caesarean section

There are three elements to testing a regional block:
- Sensory block.
- Motor block.
- Sympathetic block.

Each should be independently tested and the results documented. See Fig 11.1 for the sensory dermatome map.

Sensory
  Dabbing cotton wool or Von Frey hair—above T8
  Sensation of ice cube pressure—above T6
  Sensation of cold—above T4
  Sensation of icy cold—T2
  Pinching of skin over abdomen felt as gentle pressure only

Motor
  Complete lumbar–sacral motor block (spinal)
  Absent straight leg raise and reduced plantar-flexion (epidural)

Sympathetic
  Hot dry soles of the feet
  Equal temperature of both feet

It is best practice to measure and document temperature and light touch testing. The method of testing light touch should be recorded, as some methods give lower results than others. The sensory testing should always be done in conjunction with motor and sympathetic block testing.

Sensory block testing

The following modalities of sensation are commonly assessed:
- Temperature sensation using:
  - Ice cube, differentiating between wet, cold and ice-cold sensation.
  - Ethyl chloride spray, differentiating between wet and dripping, cold and ice-cold.
- Pain with pinprick or a 'pinch' over the site of incision.

- Light touch sensation using:
  - Cotton wool.
  - Von Frey hairs.
  - Blunt pinprick e.g. 'Neurotip'.
  - Patient's own finger.
  - Ethyl chloride spray or ice cube, differentiating between the sensation of touch rather than cold.

Practical aspects of testing

- There is considerable scope for inter-assessor variability when testing a sensory block.
- The extent of the upper limit of the block will be different when tested by the different modalities and possibly different if alternative methods of testing any particular modality are used, e.g. continuous vs intermittent application of ice or cotton wool. Learn to use one method of testing.
- The sensation of ice-cold is normally blocked 1–2 dermatomes higher than pain, which in turn is blocked 1–2 dermatomes higher than light touch.
- Many anaesthetists only test the lower limit when using epidural anaesthesia, in the belief that during spinal anaesthesia, LA injected into the CSF at the lumbar level will inevitably block transmission along the sacral nerve roots passing through that area.
- The lower limit of the block should always be tested for all regional techniques.

Top tips for testing

- Check the block at relatively fixed time intervals, thus gaining experience of what to expect at those intervals.
- Wait for evidence of motor block before testing the sensory block for the first time.
- If the block is denser on one side than the other (noted by more motor block), start the sensory testing on that side. The mother will then appreciate if there are differences and this will help you determine subtle changes.
- Perform the first check early enough to allow positional changes or top-ups prior to fixing of intrathecal LA.
- Be prepared to repeat testing if the picture is initially vague.
- Always check the block bilaterally ~5cm from the midline. If too lateral an approach is taken, the anaesthetized dermatomes can be overestimated.
- Compare sensation with adjacent, rather than distant areas of skin.
- Continue testing past the initial level of change to seek possible further change at a higher level. This is most commonly noted when testing with an ice cube. The mother will first note cool touching, followed by cold then icy cold as the ice cube is moved cephalad.

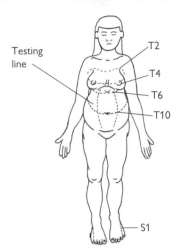

Fig. 11.1 Sensory block for caesarean section. The sensory block should be tested 5cm from the midline. S1 should be blocked to all modalities. No sensation of pinching below T10. No sensation of light touch (rubbing ice cube) below T6. No sensation of cold below T4. Sensation of icy cold at T2.

Motor block

- The dense sensory block required for CS is associated with dense motor block of the lumbar–sacral plexus.
- If the mother can straight leg raise, no matter how high the loss of sensation, the block is not suitable for a CS.
- Complete motor block of S1 plantar-flexion is characteristic of spinal anaesthesia but unusual with an epidural. Normal ankle motor function during epidural anaesthesia may indicate absent or inadequate sacral anaesthesia, which will result in pain during surgery.

Sympathetic block

- A sympathetic block of the feet does not develop until there is a well-defined sensory block to T10 at the umbilicus.
- The soles of the feet should look pink and well perfused, and feel warm and dry. Dryness of the feet is an important part of sympathetic block assessment and can only be accurately determined by examining the soles.
- Differences in foot temperature or dampness of the feet are indicative of an asymmetrical or unilateral block. Even if sensory testing does not demonstrate a difference, the quality of the block will not be as good on the cooler side.
- Observing the sympathetic block can frequently pick up the more subtle differences seen in sensory testing of epidural blocks.

Documentation

Accurately document:
- The preoperative height of block.
- The precise modalities that were used to test the block.
- The timing of testing.

- Untreated pain during CS under regional anaesthesia is currently the leading cause of complaints and litigation in the UK.
- Due to the variety of body shapes and the difference in our understanding of dermatome positions in the pregnant woman, it has been suggested that the most reproducible way of documenting the height of sensory block is through the use of a dermatome map on the anaesthetic chart.

Further reading

Russell I. Assessing the block for caesarean section. *International Journal of Obstetric Anesthesia* 2001; 10: 83–85.

Yentis SM. Height of confusion: assessing regional blocks before caesarean section. *International Journal of Obstetric Anesthesia* 2006; 15: 2–6.

Epidural anaesthesia

- In the past, epidural anaesthesia was considered to be the technique of choice for CS in mothers with cardiovascular instability, e.g. cardiac disease or severe pre-eclampsia, therefore avoiding the sudden haemodynamic changes associated with spinal anaesthesia. The CSE technique has largely replaced the need for *de novo* epidural anaesthesia in this group.
- The most common indication for epidural anaesthesia for CS is the extension of the sensory block by 'topping-up' an existing epidural that has been sited for labour analgesia. A more concentrated and greater volume of solution is required to produce the dense sensory block necessary for operative delivery.
- Epidural top-up can theoretically be used in any classification of CS (categories 1–4), although it is may be more difficult in a category 1 CS where there is immediate threat to the life of the woman or fetus, e.g. massive obstetric haemorrhage or prolonged fetal bradycardia.
- If epidural analgesia has not been effective during labour despite administration of adequate doses of LA, it is unlikely that the 'top-up' will provide adequate anaesthesia for CS. In such a case, resiting the epidural catheter may be considered, although more commonly a spinal can be inserted instead. If the clinical situation does not permit this, GA should be administered.

Advantages

- No additional procedures required. It is an extension of existing analgesia in terms of its spread and density of neural blockade.
- Greater cardiovascular stability than with spinal anaesthesia is advantageous in situations where regional blockade needs to be established gradually, e.g. parturients with severe cardiac disease.
- It can be topped-up intraoperatively to rescue an inadequate block or if surgery is prolonged.
- An epidural catheter can remain *in situ* postoperatively and be used to provide a longer duration of analgesia than is provided by a single dose of intrathecal opioid or utilized if further examination or surgery under anaesthesia is required.

Disadvantages

- Slower onset of action.
- Larger doses of LA and opioid are required.
- Less dense, patchy block than with spinal anaesthesia with a greater incidence of intraoperative pain.
- Prolonged motor and sensory block post delivery (sometimes for 8–12h).
- Risk of catheter migration to intrathecal, intravenous or subdural space.

See Chapter 7 for further details on the technique of insertion for epidural anaesthesia and the contraindications.

Checks prior to 'top-up'

The following checks should be performed on the epidural catheter in addition to the checklist already described when preparing the mother for theatre:

- Confirm that the IV line remains patent or resite prior to top-up.
- From the notes, confirm the depth of the epidural space measured at the time of catheter insertion and examine the back to ensure the depth of catheter is unchanged or that the catheter has not inadvertently fallen out or migrated further inwards.
- Exclude that any fluid or blood has accumulated at the site of insertion.
- Review the effectiveness of the epidural during labour. If recent 'top-ups' have been ineffective, re-assess the level of sensory block. If a block is asymmetrical, poor, or absent, it may be best to abandon the epidural and insert a spinal anaesthetic instead.
- Before topping-up with additional high dose local anaesthetic, assess the sensory level and motor density of block.

Place of top-up

- An epidural 'top-up' should be administered with full monitoring and preferably in the operating theatre.
- To expedite the onset of the block, an epidural top-up is sometimes administered in the delivery room.

If this is done:

- Early involvement of the anaesthetist in such situations is always beneficial.
- The anaesthetist must confirm that a means of measuring the BP and appropriate IV vasopressors are readily available to treat any hypotension.
- The anaesthetist must stay with the mother at all times to monitor her vital signs.
- CTG monitoring of the fetus must continue.
- Transfer the mother to the operating theatre in the full lateral position, as it is the safest position for her and her baby. Place her on the side of the cooler foot.

Single top-up or divided doses

- Almost all epidurals will require at least 20mL of a high concentration LA solution to produce an adequate block for CS.
- Almost all studies evaluating various solutions for CS have used either a 2mL (test dose) followed by 18mL bolus, or a single 20mL bolus.
- The most reliable and rapid method of topping up an epidural is to give a single large volume.
- A single top-up is not detrimental to the baby.
- If divided doses are given, the time to achieve an adequate block can double.
- Pre-top-up block assessment does not adequately distinguish between epidurals that will top-up easily or not.

- The total LA dose may also increase if the top-up is given in divided doses.
- Occasionally, a single 20mL bolus will produce a sensory block that produces some numbness of the lower cervical dermatones but, apart from reassuring the mother, this should require no further action.
- Some anaesthetists exercise caution, especially if top-ups are started in the delivery room, by dividing the top-ups into 10 or 5mL boluses.
- Divided doses may be safer if haemodynamic stability is important or if there is plenty of time.

Choice of drugs

Local anaesthetics
- An epidural 'top-up' should increase both the extent and density of the block that has provided analgesia for labour to a degree that is adequate for performing CS, without causing any maternal or fetal compromise.
- There are a number of possible LA solutions that may be used to 'top-up' an epidural to provide surgical anaesthesia, provided the epidural has been functioning well in labour.

The following are examples of effective local anaesthetics commonly used:
- 0.5% bupivacaine 20–25mL.
- 0.5% levobupivacaine 20–35mL.
- 2% lidocaine (often with additional 1:200,000 adrenaline + bicarbonate) 15–20mL.
- 50/50 mixture of 0.5% bupivacaine and 2% lidocaine 15–25mL.
- 0.5% ropivacaine 15–25mL.
- 0.75% ropivacaine 15–20mL.

- Bupivacaine 0.5% 20mL is generally accepted as an appropriate epidural top-up and has been found to be consistently effective when administered with opioid, e.g. 50–100 micrograms fentanyl.
- Levobupivacaine may be used in the same or an increased dose, up to 35mL of 0.5%, and may add an extra element of safety by virtue of its less cardiotoxic side effect profile.
- Studies have shown that the onset of anaesthesia is quicker with 2% lidocaine when used as the sole LA agent or in combination with 0.5% bupivacaine. There is some evidence that lidocaine-containing solutions may be less reliable, and if used on its own will not last as long. If 2% lidocaine is used, adrenaline should be added to reduce the systemic absorption of LA and improve the density of the block.
- If after 20mL of a high concentration solution there is adequate spread but inadequate density of the block, a further 5 or 10mL of the same LA solution can be given.

Opioids

- The addition of lipophilic opioids, e.g. 50–100 micrograms fentanyl or 20–50 micrograms sufentanil to the LA solution has consistently been shown to increase the quality of the sensory block and improve intraoperative analgesia.
- The site of action of all spinal opioids is the dorsal horn of the spinal cord via spinal opioid receptors. Opioids administered via the epidural route undergo systemic absorption and may cause unwanted side effects, i.e. nausea and vomiting, itching, sedation, and respiratory depression.
- Longer acting opioids, e.g. diamorphine 2.5–5mg or morphine 3–5mg may be given via the epidural catheter following delivery of the baby for postoperative analgesia. They may cause the same unwanted side effects, including late-onset respiratory depression, and the mother should be monitored postoperatively.

Adjuvant drugs

- *2mL of 8.4% preservative-free sodium bicarbonate* to 2% lidocaine epidural top-up solution has been shown to increase the speed of onset of epidural anaesthesia. The non-ionized fraction of the LA drug is increased, which in theory crosses the perineural sheath with greater efficiency. In practice, this advantage is not considered to be of any clinical significance.
- *0.1mL of 1:1000 adrenaline* to a 2% lidocaine mixture reduces the systemic absorption of lidocaine, therefore intensifies and prolongs the neural blockade. It has a direct anti-nociceptor effect by acting as an α_2 agonist within the spinal cord.
- *Clonidine* is a pure α_2 adrenergic agonist, which is thought to produce analgesia by an action within the dorsal horn of the spinal cord. It is administered as an epidural bolus of 75–100 micrograms. Clonidine has the advantage of causing less nausea and vomiting, pruritus or respiratory depression than opioids, but is associated with hypotension and sedation. It has been evaluated mostly for its postoperative analgesic effect.
- *Neostigmine* has been studied in doses of 30–300 micrograms. It produces dose-related nausea and sedation, and has a modest analgesic value.

Management of the failed block

Prior to surgery

- If the block remains inadequate before the start of surgery, a further incremental dose of LA should be administered, e.g. 5–10mL bupivacaine 0.5% or levobupivacaine 0.5%, if time allows and the patient positioned on the inadequate side.
- If there is no further extension of the block, most anaesthetists would advocate abandoning any further epidural top-ups and insertion of a reduced dose spinal anaesthetic, e.g. 1–1.5mL hyperbaric bupivacaine 0.5% in the left lateral 'Oxford' position.

The mother should then be placed on her back with a left lateral tilt, with two pillows placed well under the thoracic curvature to prevent a high block.

- If there is insufficient time to perform a spinal, a GA is the only option.

During surgery

- An inadequate block may become apparent after surgery has commenced, e.g. during peritoneal incision, exteriorization of the uterus, or swabbing of paracolic gutters. If pain becomes apparent, the mother and partner must be reassured that it will be dealt with. Pain or discomfort should be communicated to the surgeon.
- It is important to differentiate at every stage between pain and the sensation of pressure/tugging, which can cause considerable discomfort. Verbal contact and support from the anaesthetic team are essential during a CS under regional anaesthesia.
- Symptoms of pain during a CS should never be dismissed. Appropriate action should always be taken, and any management offered or refused always documented.
- If pain is apparent during peritoneal incision, i.e. before delivery of the baby, attempts can be made to improve the block with a further top-up of LA +/– opioid. The surgeon should be asked to stop surgery and wait until the patient is comfortable. Entonox® and/or a short-acting supplementary opioid, e.g. 0.5–1mg alfentanil, should be offered until the 'top-up' is effective.
- If the supplemental epidural top-up is ineffective or the urgency of delivery is such that surgery cannot stop at this stage, conversion to GA is usually the only option.
- If pain becomes apparent after delivery of the baby, surgery should be stopped and similarly a supplemental epidural 'top-up' given and the administration of Entonox® offered, and/or a short-acting supplementary opioid, e.g. 0.5–1mg alfentanil until the 'top-up' is effective. IV ketamine in 10mg increments is an additional option. If this is ineffective, GA should be offered.
- If approaching the end of surgery, local infiltration of LA at the incision site can be offered.
- Fundamentally, it is the anaesthetists' responsibility to take control of the situation and take the appropriate course of action if the mother is experiencing pain during surgery. A GA should be performed if there is any doubt.
- All patients should be reviewed in the post-delivery period. Specific information about the proposed reasons for the inadequate block should be clearly explained.

Further reading

Lucas DN et al. Extending low dose epidural analgesia for emergency caesarean section. A comparison of three solutions. *Anaesthesia* 1999; 54: 1173–1177.

Bauer ME et al. Risk factors for failed conversion of labour epidural analgesia to Caesarean delivery anaesthesia: a systematic review and meta-analysis of observational trials. *International Journal of Obstetric Anesthesia* 2012; 21: 294–309.

Allam J et al. Epidural lidocaine-bicarbonate-adrenaline vs levobupivacaine for emergency Caesarean section: a randomized controlled trial. *Anaesthesia* 2008; 63: 243–249.

Spinal anaesthesia

Spinal anaesthesia produces a reliable dense block, which has a much faster onset and provides better quality anaesthesia than an epidural technique. It is considered the first choice technique for the majority of UK anaesthetists when performing an elective or urgent CS. The role of spinal anaesthesia in a category 1 CS depends on the experience of the anaesthetist and also the obstetrician making the decision for CS. There are very few situations where the degree of urgency does not allow time for a spinal anaesthetic to be performed. If a working epidural is *in situ*, this should be topped-up for the CS to proceed. However, if the epidural has functioned poorly during labour, it should be removed and a spinal performed if time allows.

Advantages
- Rapid onset of anaesthesia.
- Dense sensory and motor block.
- Predictable extent of sensory block.
- Easy to perform in a pressurized situation, with a clear end-point.
- The addition of long-acting opioids will improve postoperative analgesia and facilitate early mobilization.
- The incidence of thromboembolic disease is reduced.

Disadvantages
- Rapid onset of sympathetic blockade, with associated hypotension, nausea, and vomiting.
- Lack of flexibility of duration with single-shot technique.
- An unexpected high block may lead to compromised respiration.
- Untreated hypotension with unrelieved aorto-caval compression can precipitate severe fetal hypoxia and acidosis.
- Maternal bradycardia due to the combination of sympathetic blockade and reduced VR initiates the Bezold–Jarish reflex.

See Chapter 7 for further details on the technique of insertion, contraindications and management of hypotension.

Choice of drugs

Local anaesthetics
- 0.5% hyperbaric bupivacaine is the only drug licensed for intrathecal use in the UK. A dose of 12.5mg has been shown to produce a reliable sensory block for surgery; however, lower doses (8–10mg) are frequently used and considered sufficient, especially when combined with an epidural technique, and may be associated with less hypotension.
- The use of 0.5% hyperbaric lidocaine has been abandoned, since reports of prolonged neurological deficits are associated with intrathecal injection.
- Plain bupivacaine has been extensively investigated and can produce a reliable block, which some say is less susceptible to the positioning of the mother.

- The final block is more dependent on the mass of drug rather than the volume of injectate, i.e.10mg bupivacaine can be given as 2mL of 0.5% solution or 10mL of 0.1% solution with equal effect.
- 0.5% levobupivacaine and 0.5–0.75% ropivacaine also produce satisfactory blocks, but are not available as hyperbaric solutions at the present time.

The required volume of LA injectate is dependent on a number of additional factors which should be considered:

- Height of the woman—although the evidence for this is limited. It may be appropriate to increase or decrease the dose a little at the extremes of stature or use a CSE.
- Decreased uterine size—prematurity, a growth restricted fetus, or severe oligohydramnios is associated with a smaller uterus. Therefore, with less vena cava compression, the cephalad spread of LA is reduced. Either increase the dose or use a CSE technique.
- Increased uterine size—multiple pregnancies and polyhydramnios lead to a contracted intrathecal space, causing a more rapid onset and extent of block due to increased cephalad spread.

Opioids

- The addition of lipophilic opioids, e.g. 10–25 micrograms fentanyl, 2.5–10 micrograms sufentanil, or 250 micrograms diamorphine, to the LA has consistently been shown to both increase the quality of the sensory block and to improve intraoperative analgesia. Intrathecal diamorphine will provide postoperative analgesia for up to 12h.
- Morphine is much slower in onset (45–60min) and does not provide good intraoperative analgesia, but is effective for the management of post-operative pain.
- The site of action of all spinal opioids is the dorsal horn of the spinal cord via spinal opioid receptors. Opioids administered via the spinal route undergo a degree of systemic absorption and may cause unwanted side effects, i.e. nausea and vomiting, itching, sedation, and respiratory depression.
- Short-acting opioids, e.g. fentanyl or sufentanil, contribute little to postoperative analgesia. Therefore, the addition of a long-acting opioid, e.g. morphine 100 micrograms, is recommended to provide optimal postoperative analgesia, provided appropriate staff and facilities are available for monitoring of vital signs every 2h for the first 24h postoperatively, as there is a small risk of developing late-onset (>12h) respiratory depression following intrathecal morphine.
- Intrathecal diamorphine has been shown to be associated with less nausea, vomiting, and itching than intrathecal morphine. However, the duration of action of diamorphine is less, i.e. 12h following surgery, compared with up to 24h after intrathecal morphine.

Adjuvant drugs
- Intrathecal clonidine is an α_2 adrenergic agonist, which produces analgesia within the dorsal horn of the spinal cord through the release of nitric oxide. Clonidine 75 micrograms added to hyperbaric bupivacaine and fentanyl has been shown to improve intraoperative and postoperative analgesia. Side effects include a prolonged motor block, hypotension, bradycardia, and sedation.
- Intrathecal midazolam 1mg has analgesic properties; however, when combined with intrathecal diamorphine, the effect is no different from that of diamorphine alone.
- Intrathecal neostigmine produces analgesia by inhibiting the breakdown of acetylcholine. Doses from 10 to 100 micrograms have been used and have been shown to improve postoperative pain for up to 24h. However, there is a high incidence of dose-related nausea and vomiting, which has limited its clinical use.

See Table 11.1 for the suggested dose and duration of action of drugs added to enhance spinal anaesthesia.

Assessment and manipulation of the block

- Perform the first check early enough, i.e. within a few minutes of positioning the mother in left tilt, to allow positional changes prior to fixing of intrathecal LA if the block is potentially inadequate.
- The extent of the sensory block should be mapped with great care, including assessment of the lower limit of the block. Bilateral motor block is expected with spinal anaesthesia.
- Although the block is usually bilateral, occasionally it is unequal and postural manipulation, especially if 'heavy' bupivacaine is used, is useful.
- The mother can be tilted or turned on to the inadequate side to improve the block.
- If the upper level of the block is inadequate, tilting the table slightly head down or flexing the hips are both effective measures.
- A sensory block to ice-cold from above T4 to S5 and to light touch to T5 should ensure a pain-free CS.
- The mother should be fully prepared for the sensation she may feel during surgery, and warned of the possibility of intraoperative discomfort or pain, and how this will be dealt with.

Table 11.1 Comparison of drug doses for epidural vs intrathecal use

Drug	Epidural route	Intrathecal route	Duration of action	Notes
Fentanyl	50–100 micrograms	15–25 micrograms	2–3h	Increased dosage produces increasing side effects, e.g. nausea, vomiting, pruritus
Morphine	3–5mg	100–200 micrograms	19–24h	Increased dosage produces increasing side effects Observe for late-onset (>12h) respiratory depression
Diamorphine	2.5–5mg	250–375 micrograms	12–20h	Associated with less unwanted side effects compared with morphine, but pruritus occurs in >80%
Sufentanil	20–50 micrograms	2.5–10 micrograms	2–4h	Increased dosage produces increasing side effects, e.g. nausea, vomiting, pruritus Not used in the UK
Clonidine	150–600 micrograms, an infusion 40 micrograms/h is required to provide lasting postoperative analgesia	75 micrograms	2–4h following an intrathecal dose with bupivacaine and fentanyl	Prolonged motor block, hypotension, bradycardia and sedation are unwanted side effects
Neostigmine	–	10–50 micrograms	10–24h	High incidence of nausea and vomiting, limiting its use

Management of the failed block

Prior to surgery

If the block is inadequate for surgery to proceed within the expected time frame, i.e. up to 15min, there are a number of possible management options:

- Change to mother's position—positioning head down or in the lateral position with the unblocked area dependent may improve a sensory block that is not quite at the limits required.
- Repeat the spinal—if there is no evidence of a sensory or motor block or the upper limit of the block is below T12, repeating the spinal is recommended. If no or minimal block is apparent, the same dose should be repeated. If there is evidence of a degree of sensory block, e.g. up to T12, a reduced dose of LA (1–1.5mL of 0.5% heavy bupivacaine) should be considered to avoid a high block. The mother should be carefully repositioned with two pillows under the thoracic curve to avoid a high block (see Figs 11.2 and 11.3).
- Insertion of an epidural—if the upper limit of the sensory block is between T12 and T4 dermatomes, insertion of an epidural catheter and augmentation of the block with incremental top-ups is recommended if time allows. 5mL of 0.5% bupivacaine or 0.5% levobupivacaine should be given and the block re-assessed every 5min until the required sensory block is reached.
- GA—if the urgency of surgery does not allow further time to improve the regional anaesthetic, a GA should be performed. The mother and fetus should be risk assessed in consultation with the obstetrician again in theatre, as the decision to convert to a GA in the morbidly obese or severely pre-eclamptic patient carries significant airway risks.

During surgery

- An inadequate block may become apparent after surgery has commenced, e.g. during peritoneal incision, exteriorization of the uterus, or swabbing of paracolic gutters. If pain becomes apparent, the mother and partner must be reassured that it will be dealt with. Pain or discomfort should be communicated to the surgeon.
- If pain is apparent during peritoneal incision, i.e. before delivery of the baby, conversion to GA is usually the only option. The surgeon should be asked to stop surgery, whilst the GA drugs and equipment are prepared. Entonox® and a short-acting supplementary opioid, e.g. 0.5–1mg alfentanil should be offered until induction of GA.
- If pain becomes apparent after delivery of the baby, surgery should be stopped and similarly Entonox® offered, and a short-acting supplementary opioid, e.g. 0.5–1mg alfentanil given. IV ketamine in 10mg increments is an additional option. If this is ineffective, GA should be offered.
- If approaching the end of surgery, local infiltration of LA at the incision site should be performed.
- It is important to differentiate at every stage between pain and the sensation of pressure/tugging, which can cause considerable discomfort. Verbal contact and support from the anaesthetic team are essential during a CS under regional anaesthesia.

- Symptoms of pain during a CS should never be dismissed. Appropriate action should always be taken, and any management offered or refused always documented.
- It is the anaesthetists' responsibility to take control of the situation and take the appropriate course of action if the mother is experiencing pain during surgery. A GA should be performed if there is any doubt.
- All patients should be reviewed in the post-delivery period. Specific information about the proposed reasons for the inadequate block should be clearly explained.

Continuous spinal anaesthesia

- This is not currently popular in the UK, although there are case reports which have described its successful use in some parturients, e.g with complex cardiac problems or severe scoliosis.
- It allows controlled and gradual development of a dense regional block while maintaining haemodynamic stability.

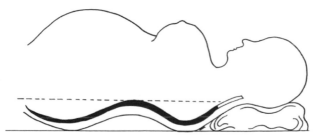

Fig. 11.2 During spinal anaesthesia, a pillow placed under the head and neck will tend to allow the intrathecal solution to travel to T2.

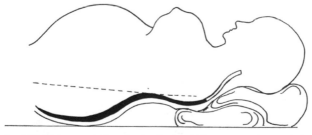

Fig. 11.3 With a second pillow placed under the mid thoracic curve, the spread of intrathecal solutions can be more easily controlled. This will prevent excessive spread of intrathecal injection, especially if performed after a failed epidural top-up.

- Small incremental doses, i.e. 0.25mL of plain 0.5% or 0.25% bupivacaine, are titrated against the required height of the sensory block and maternal BP.

Further reading

Onishi E et al. Optimal intrathecal hyperbaric bupivacaine dose with opioids for Caesarean delivery: a prospective double-blind randomized trial. *International Journal of Obstetric Anesthesia* 2017; 31: 68–73.

Husiani SW, Russell IF. Intrathecal diamorphine compared with morphine for postoperative analgesia after caesarean section under spinal anaesthesia. *British Journal of Anaesthesia* 1998; 81: 135–139.

Cowan CM et al. Comparison of intrathecal fentanyl and diamorphine in addition to bupivacaine for caesarean section under spinal anaesthesia. *British Journal of Anaesthesia* 2002; 89: 452–458.

Russell IF. At Caesarean section under regional anaesthesia, it is essential to test sensory block with light touch before allowing surgery to start. *International Journal of Obstetric Anesthesia* 2006; 15: 294–297.

Kinsella SM et al. International consensus statement on the management of hypotension with vasopressors during Caesarean section under spinal anaesthsia. *Anaesthesia* 2018; 73: 71–92.

Crespo S et al. Intrathecal clonidine as an adjuvant for neuroaxial anaesthesia during caesarean delivery: a systematic review and meta-analysis of randomized trails. *International Journal of Obstetric Anesthesia* 2017; 32, 64–76.

Combined spinal–epidural (CSE)

The CSE technique is the technique of choice for anaesthesia for CS in an increasing number of clinical situations, in both the elective and emergency setting. It combines the speed of onset and reliability of a spinal anaesthetic with the flexibility to extend the sensory block by supplementation with slow boluses of LA via the epidural catheter. It allows a reduced dose of intrathecal LA to be injected when necessary, therefore minimizing many of the side effects frequently seen with a single-shot spinal technique.

Indications for CSE

The indications broadly fall into the following categories:

Minimizing hypotension
- When cardiovascular stability is paramount (e.g. valvular heart disease, complex congenital heart disease, and severe pre-eclampsia, a low dose of intrathecal LA (1.5mL hyperbaric 0.5% bupivacaine) may be administered and the sensory block supplemented by incremental epidural top-ups, which are titrated against the BP. The CSE technique has significantly reduced the need to administer GA to mothers with severe cardiac disease.
- Increased uterine size (e.g. multiple pregnancies and polyhydramnios) are associated with increased aorto-caval compression and excessive cephalad spread of intrathecal LA, both contributing to increased hypotension and uterine hypoperfusion. A reduced spinal dose minimizes the associated symptoms and complications.

Unpredictability of block height
- When it is difficult to estimate the ideal intrathecal dose for the desired block height (e.g. short or tall stature), a CSE is beneficial.
- Prematurity or a severely growth restricted fetus is associated with less cephalad spread of LA and a less predictable sensory block; the presence of the epidural catheter to extend the block, if necessary, is useful.

Prolonged surgery
- If prolonged or technically difficult surgery is anticipated, the block may be extended via the epidural (e.g. placenta previa, previous CS, presence of adhesions from previous abdominal surgery, or surgical access difficult due to morbid obesity).
- If additional surgery is planned at the same time (e.g. oophrectomy).

GA contraindicated
- When a GA is strongly contraindicated (e.g. malignant hyperpyrexia, suxamethonium apnoea, or cases of previous failed intubation or anticipated difficult airway), a spinal may be administered and epidural top-ups given to extend the block. The presence of the epidural catheter should minimize the need to convert to GA.

Postoperative analgesia
- When epidural analgesia is considered beneficial in the postoperative period (e.g. chronic pain conditions, allergy to opioids, history of opioid abuse).

Advantages
- Rapid onset of anaesthesia.
- Good quality sensory block.
- Flexible and titratable to prevent rapid changes of BP.
- Allows rapid extension of the regional block.
- Reduces need for conversion to GA.
- Epidural may be used for postoperative analgesia.

Disadvantages
- More difficult technique to learn and perform.
- Higher rate of failure of spinal component.
- Rapid decrease in BP is still possible.
- Untested epidural catheter, therefore it cannot be totally relied upon to function as you would expect.
- Complications of both spinal and epidural techniques ever present.
- Possibility of increased infection rate.
- Possibility of conus damage.

See Chapter 7 for further details on the technique of insertion, contraindications and management of hypotension.

Choice of drugs

Local anaesthetics
- The dose of intrathecal LA administered will depend on the indication for CSE anaesthesia.
- 'Back-up' in the event of inadequate spinal anaesthesia or anticipated prolonged or difficult surgery:
  - A standard dose of 10–12.5mg bupivacaine can be administered.
  - Care should be taken when flushing the epidural catheter with saline solution after insertion, as small volumes (2–3mL) of injectate can cause significant cephalad spread of LA and a high block will become quickly apparent.
- Minimize hypotension:
  - An intrathecal dose of 5–7.5mg bupivacaine can reduce the speed of onset and extent of the block.
  - It has been shown that reduced doses can produce the required sensory block for pain-free surgery, with less associated hypotension.
  - Extending the sensory block can be achieved by injecting 5–10mL of saline through the Tuohy needle before catheter insertion.
  - The epidural catheter can also be flushed with 5mL of saline to extend the block.
  - The sensory block produced by these small doses is adequate in ~50% of cases, depending on the exact dose used and opioids added.
  - The main drawback is the reduced surgical anaesthesia time of <1h following a reduced intrathecal dose.

- The anaesthetist must be familiar with testing the intrathecal block and topping-up the epidural component before and during surgery before attempting a low dose technique.
- If additional supplementation of the sensory block is required, slow incremental top-ups should be given via the epidural catheter i.e. 3–5mL bupivacaine 0.5%, and the block re-assessed every 5min.

Opioids
- The addition of an intrathecal opioid, e.g. fentanyl 15–25 micrograms or sufentanil 2.5–10 micrograms, will enhance the quality of the sensory block and improve intraoperative analgesia, and must always be given if <10mg of bupivacaine is used.
- Long-acting opioids provide optimal postoperative analgesia and are strongly recommended, provided appropriate staff and facilities are available for monitoring of vital signs every 2h for the first 24h postoperatively.

Assessment of the block
- The extent of the sensory block should be mapped with great care, including assessment of the lower limit of the block. Bilateral motor block is expected from the spinal component.
- Re-assess the level of the block after each supplementary epidural bolus.
- The mother should be fully prepared for the sensation she may feel during surgery and warned of the possibility of intraoperative discomfort or pain, and how this will be dealt with.

Management of the failed block
Prior to surgery
- If there is no apparent sensory or motor block from the spinal component of the CSE, the two options are either to repeat the spinal using the same dose or to start topping-up the epidural *de novo* using slow incremental boluses of 5–10mL bupivacaine 0.5% or levobupivacaine 0.5%. If there were any difficulties siting the epidural catheter, it may be advisable to choose to repeat the entire CSE technique.
- If there is a degree of sensory block, further incremental dose of local anaesthetic should be administered via the epidural catheter, e.g. 5–10mL bupivacaine 0.5% or levobupivacaine 0.5%, titrated against the BP and the patient positioned appropriately.
- If the block remains inadequate, the CSE or just the epidural may be re-sited and further slow incremental epidural top-ups administered.
- Depending on the urgency of the clinical situation, a GA may be necessary. The obstetrician should be made aware if there are any unexpected difficulties or delays in performing the regional technique.

During surgery

- Remember that the epidural catheter may be untested until this stage.
- An inadequate block may become apparent after surgery has commenced, e.g. during peritoneal incision, exteriorization of the uterus, or swabbing of paracolic gutters. At whatever stage of surgery pain becomes apparent, reassurance of the mother and partner that it will be dealt with is paramount, and any pain or discomfort should be communicated to the surgeon.
- If pain is apparent during peritoneal incision, i.e. before delivery of the baby, attempts can be made to improve the block with a further top-up of LA ± opioid. The surgeon should be asked to stop surgery and wait until the patient is comfortable and the administration of Entonox® offered, and/or a short-acting supplementary opioid, e.g. 0.5–1mg alfentanil, until the 'top-up' is effective.
- If the supplemental epidural top-up is ineffective or the urgency of delivery is such that surgery cannot stop at this stage, conversion to GA is usually the only option.
- If pain becomes apparent after delivery of the baby, surgery should be stopped and similarly a supplemental epidural 'top-up' given and the administration of Entonox® offered, and/or a short-acting supplementary opioid, e.g. 0.5–1mg alfentanil, until the 'top-up' is effective. IV ketamine in 10mg increments is an additional option. If this is ineffective, GA should be offered.
- If approaching the end of surgery, local infiltration of LA at the incision site should be offered.
- It is important to differentiate at every stage between pain and the sensation of pressure/tugging which can cause considerable discomfort. Verbal contact and support from the anaesthetic team are essential during a CS under regional anaesthesia. Give the mother an indication of the stage of surgery and an estimate of how long surgery will last.
- Symptoms of pain during a CS should never be dismissed. Appropriate action should always be taken, and any management offered or refused documented.
- All patients should be reviewed in the post-delivery period. Specific information about the proposed reasons for the inadequate block should be clearly explained.

Further reading

Van de Velde M et al. Combined spinal–epidural anesthesia for cesarean delivery: dose-dependent effects of hyperbaric bupivacaine on maternal hemodynamics. *Anesthesia and Analgesia* 2006; 103: 187–190.

Choi DH et al. Combined low-dose spinal–epidural anesthesia versus single-shot spinal anesthesia for elective cesarean delivery. *International Journal of Obstetric Anesthesia* 2006; 15: 13–17.

Beale N et al. Effect of epidural volume extension on dose requirement of intrathecal hyperbaric bupivacaine at caesarean section. *British Journal of Anaesthesia* 2005; 95: 500–503.

Hamlyn EL et al. Low-dose sequential combined spinal–epidural: an anaesthetic technique for caesarean section in patients with significant cardiac disease. *International Journal of Obstetric Anesthesia* 2005; 14: 355–361.

James KS et al. Combined spinal–extradural anaesthesia for preterm and term caesarean section: is there a difference in local anaesthetic requirements? *British Journal of Anaesthesia* 1997; 78: 498–501.

Common complications

The following complications are frequently seen when performing any regional technique for CS.

Hypotension

A fall is the systolic and diastolic BP is frequently seen within minutes of administering the regional technique, due to aorto-caval compression being unmasked by sudden autonomic blockade. The autonomic system normally mitigates the haemodynamic effects of aorto-caval compression. Bradycardia <60/min is often associated with the sudden hypotension.

Manifestations
• Nausea and vomiting.
• Light-headedness.
• Pallor.

Management
• Increase left uterine displacement by ensuring a tilt of 20° or place in full left lateral position.
• Prompt treatment with vasopressors ± a vagolytic, e.g. glycopyrronium bromide 200–400 micrograms. The discussion of choice and administration of vasopressors is detailed in Chapter 10, pp. 294–296.
• Increase IV fluid infusion.
• Expedite surgical delivery if there is concern for fetal well-being.

Respiratory difficulty

It is not uncommon for mothers to complain of difficulty taking a deep breath or chest tightness as the block extends cephalad. This perceived difficulty in taking an adequate breath or cough is due to paralysis of the lower intercostal muscles, which contributes to forced expiration and the increased abdominal size, limiting diaphragmatic movement in the supine position. This always improves after delivery when diaphragmatic splinting is relieved.

Management
• Reassure mother and partner.
• Re-assess the upper limit of the block by assessing motor function in the hands.
• Place a pillow or wedge under the shoulders to the mid thorax. This improves diaphragmatic breathing.
• Monitor pulse oximetry and administer oxygen by face mask if SpO_2 <95%.

Headache
• The sudden onset of headache at the time of spinal insertion or immediately after lying down is thought to be due to air entering the intrathecal space and rising cranially. Reassurance should be offered.
• Headache in the days following a regional technique should always be investigated further.

- The PDPH rate associated with spinal anaesthesia when using atraumatic needles is less than 1%. Features of the headache include:
  - Frontal pain, usually bilateral and posture-related.
  - Neck stiffness, again posture-related.
  - Nausea and vomiting.
  - Tinnitus.
  - Visual disturbance or photophobia.
- The headache that follows spinal dural puncture is often not as severe as that associated with an accidental dural puncture with a Tuohy needle. However, the symptoms should not be dismissed and all management options discussed, as detailed in Chapter 15.
- Other causes of headache post delivery should also be excluded, e.g. dehydration, pre-eclampsia.
- Headache following an inadvertent dural puncture at the time of epidural or CSE insertion is frequently severe. Approximately 60–70% will require an epidural blood patch. See Chapter 15, pp. 420–424, for details of management.

Anaesthesia for Caesarean section: General anaesthesia

Stephen Morris and Rhidian Jones

Lessons from National Audits

The number of obstetric general anaesthetics (GA) has fallen as the use of regional anaesthesia has increased. The Hospital Episode Statistics for England and Wales for 2013 found only 8% of obstetric procedures were done under GA. This, coupled with the reduced training time available for trainees and reduced numbers of intubations in all areas of practice, has led to concerns about the ability of trainees to manage obstetric GA and intubation safely.

CEMACE 2006–2008

Airway related deaths in obstetrics have decreased substantially since the middle of last century, when 32 deaths occurred between 1967 and 1969.

Of the 7 deaths directly related to anaesthesia in the CEMACE report (2006–2008), 3 deaths were linked to GA. Unfortunately 2 of these were of similar causes to the previous triennial audit:

- Inability to recognize oesophageal intubation.
- Gastric aspiration on extubation.

The report emphasized the importance of rehearsing failed intubation drills, situational awareness, and ensuring adequate ventilation. It also advised that a wide bore orogastric tube should be used to relieve pressure and contents in a patient with a potentially full stomach and to extubate the trachea fully awake. The report also questioned the possibility that both cases could have been done under regional anaesthesia, especially as one case had an epidural already sited. The decision, and reasoning, for a GA should be clearly documented in the patient's notes.

NAP4 2009

Further lessons in airway management have been learnt as a result of NAP4 (National Audit Project 4), which recorded all airway complications during 2009. Four GA failed intubation obstetric cases were reported, two of which were rescued with supraglottic airway devices and one with a surgical airway. Recommendations arising from the report suggested obstetric anaesthetists should:

- Be familiar with failed intubations strategies.
- Be skilled with supraglottic airway devices for rescuing the airway.
- Have a fibreoptic scope available within the maternity suite.
- Ensure recovery staff are familiar with complications associated with caesarean section under GA.

MBRRACE-UK 2009–2012

In the MBRRACE UK report of 2014 (covering 2009–2012) there were 2 airway-related deaths, both as a result of postoperative hypoventilation. The emphasis has changed from deaths to 'Lessons for Anaesthesia' and reinforced the need for drills in the management of perioperative airway crises including severe bronchospasm and mechanical obstruction as well as difficult/oesophageal intubation.

Indications for general anaesthesia

Despite the identification of problems with GA, there will always be the need to give a GA quickly but safely to the pregnant woman; indeed it may be lifesaving. Historically, some indications that were regarded as absolute may now be regarded as relative, particularly as the use of continuous spinal catheters and CSE anaesthesia have removed the need for GA in some cases. A clinical decision based on the risks and benefits of GA must be made for each patient.

- Category 1 CS, where there is immediate threat to the life of the mother or the baby and there is absolutely no time for a regional technique.
- Failure of regional anaesthesia. Either inability to establish a block or failure to provide adequate intra-operative anaesthesia.
- Maternal refusal of regional technique, despite an adequate explanation of the options having been given by an experienced anaesthetist.
- Regional technique contraindicated.

Contraindications to regional anaesthesia

Absolute

- Uncorrected hypovolaemia/ongoing haemorrhage.
- Localized infection.
- Allergy to local anaesthetic drugs.
- Present or potential raised intracranial pressure.

Relative

- Inadequate haemostasis pathological/pharmacological.
- Platelet count <70×10^3/L.
- Fixed cardiac output states, sympathetic-dependent pathology, e.g. severe aortic stenosis.
- Structural abnormalities of the lumbar spine/cord, e.g. spina bifida.
- Some spinal operations such as insertion of rods for scoliosis correction.

Contraindications to general anaesthesia

There are very few contraindications to GA. If intubation has failed or has been very difficult in the past, the most senior anaesthetist available must be consulted about the need for further GA. If the appropriate equipment is not available, then induction of GA should not begin.

Airway assessment

The following maternal factors will increase the likelihood or consequences of airway management difficulties:

Anatomical factors

- Increased chest diameter and enlarged breasts can make laryngoscopy with a standard Macintosh handle difficult.
- Respiratory tract mucosal oedema makes airway obstruction and bleeding more likely.
- Tongue enlargement may prohibit compression with the laryngoscope.
- Maternal obesity.

Physiological factors

- Increased oxygen consumption—this is increased 15–30% above normal and is mainly due to the demands of the fetoplacental unit and the uterus. This leads to an increased rate of desaturation.
- Functional residual capacity (FRC)—this is decreased by up to 20% in the third trimester, as the diaphragm is displaced cephalad by the enlarging uterus. This reduces both the residual volume and expiratory reserve volume, such that the FRC is greatly reduced. This is more significant in the supine position and removes one of the largest stores of oxygen available to the body, making pregnant women very susceptible to hypoxia during induction of anaesthesia.

Other factors

- Left lateral tilt used to minimize aorto-caval compression may distort the laryngeal view.
- Cricoid pressure applied excessively or inexpertly may make intubation difficult by compressing the trachea or soft tissues.
- It is well recognized that there is a higher incidence of difficulty in the obstetric population. Work from the UK has shown:
  - Incidence of grade 3 view ≈ 1 in 500.
  - Incidence of grade 4 view ≈ 1 in 1800.
  - Incidence of failed intubation ≈1 in 250 (1 in >2000 in non-obstetric).
  - Incidence of severe airway problems ≈ 1 in 4000, which was illustrated in the NAP4 Audit with 1 case of 'Can't intubate, can't oxygenate'.
- Although anaesthesia-related deaths are a small proportion of the overall maternal mortality figures, GA-related deaths are usually due to lack of airway management skills and experience, and thus are potentially preventable.
- Increased use of regional techniques in the management of CS leading to a reduction in anaesthetists' experience of obstetric GA.

Maternal history

- Details of any previous difficulty must be sought. The patient may have been told of a problem. There may be a letter or medic alert bracelet, and any previous anaesthetic record available should be examined. Bear in mind that a previous successful intubation does not guarantee success this time.
- Pre-eclampsia, especially with concurrent upper respiratory tract infection (URTI) can be complicated by airway oedema and can increase the Mallampati score.
- A change in voice may indicate laryngeal oedema.
- Obstructive sleep apnoea increases the risk of difficult facemask ventilation as well as tracheal intubation.
- Obesity increases the risk of GA, and weight increase in pregnancy as well as booking BMI should be recorded.

Maternal examination

Airway assessment is a basic skill and should always be undertaken regardless of the type of anaesthesia planned, in case of a complication (e.g. total spinal) that requires tracheal intubation. It is also important to anticipate difficult mask ventilation and access to the airway from the front of the neck.

Mallampati scores have been reported to increase during pregnancy and labour, and should be assessed immediately before GA.

Markers of difficult intubation &/or ventilation

- Large breasts.
- Large tongue.
- Reduced head/neck flexion.
- Small jaw/receding mandible.
- Inability to bring lower incisors in front of the upper ones.
- Short neck.
- Short thyro-mental distance.
- Protruding maxillary incisors.
- Less than 5cm between incisors on mouth opening (3 fingers).
- Obesity >90kg booking.
- Mallampati score ≥3.
- Risk of airway oedema.
- If two or more of the above are detected, senior help should be sought and considerations given to avoiding GA. If the patient is anticipated to be difficult to manage under a GA, but refuses to have a regional anaesthetic, a senior anaesthetist with appropriate skills should be present and awake fibreoptic intubation considered.
- Scoring systems are not good at predicting the difficult airway, in part due to its rarity. However, the combination of decreased neck extension, Mallampati grade 3 or 4, and decreased mouth opening is associated with a high incidence of difficult intubation.

Communication and preparation

- Rapid effective communication of the likelihood of a GA CS allows time for an airway assessment to be made and an appropriate management plan to be instituted.
- If difficulties with intubation are considered likely, senior/additional help should be sought as early as possible, and the whole multi-disciplinary team should be aware of the potential problems which can be verbalized during the WHO checklist.
- Lack of abnormality of the airway assessment does not exclude an airway problem developing later.
- A GA should only be induced in the presence of a properly checked anaesthetic machine and equipment, with minimum monitoring established and with the help of a dedicated trained anaesthetic assistant.
- Even in a category 1 caesarean section it is important to remember that the mother's interests still come first, and the anaesthetist should resist pressure to induce anaesthesia if they believe intubation not to be possible.

Equipment

The intubation trolley/cart should contain the following equipment and should be available immediately in case of any difficulties with airway management:

- Face masks of various sizes.
- Oropharyngeal and nasopharyngeal airways.
- Short- and long-bladed Macintosh laryngoscopes.
- Short-handled laryngoscope.
- Video-laryngoscope.
- Bougie/tube introducer.
- Selection of tracheal tubes—6.5 to 8mm (including microlaryngeal tube).
- Proseal™ laryngeal mask airway (LMA) or I-gel™ size 3 and 4.
- A device for cricothyroidotomy and equipment for ventilation (anaesthetists working on the labour ward should be familiar with the connections).
- Scalpel size 10.

- The role of video-laryngoscopy in obstetric anaesthesia GA is becoming increasingly routine. Training in the elective GA setting is strongly recommended.
- Although fibreoptic intubation by the inexperienced has no place during a failed intubation, it should be available to the experienced practitioner who is skilled at asleep fibreoptic intubation with cricoid pressure in place.

Drugs for general anaesthesia

Induction agents

There is currently considerable debate as to which induction agent should be used for GA in obstetrics. Traditionally thiopental has been used for the rapid sequence induction, but its position is being challenged by propofol. The specific factors to be considered for each induction agent are outlined.

Thiopental

- Well known to generations of anaesthetists.
- Rapid predictable sleep with eye closing makes it the easiest drug to use when suxamethonium must be administered quickly.
- There is reliable anaesthesia for 5–7min, which allows the brain concentration of inhalational agent to come up to a sleep dose.
- Relatively cardio-stable.
- At a dose of 4mg/kg, sedation at birth of the baby is minimal.
- At higher doses (8mg/kg), fetal depression will occur.
- Rapid redistribution in the maternal and fetal circulation allows the baby to be born in a vigorous condition.

Propofol

- Very familiar to anaesthetists in non-obstetric practice.
- Lack of a clear induction end-point and an unreliable sleep dose make it a difficult drug to use for rapid sequence induction.
- At 2.5mg/kg, the baby is born in a vigorous condition. In higher doses it is associated with neonatal sedation.
- Rapid wakening is associated with propofol use, but this was not associated with increased awareness in NAP5, although the numbers were very small.
- Higher incidence of hypotension (and therefore reduced uterine perfusion).
- No requirement for pre-mixing.
- No risk of confusion with IV antibiotic syringe.
- Total IV anaesthesia has been described and is the anaesthetic of choice for patients with a history of malignant hyperthermia. At doses >6mg/kg/h it is associated with neonatal sedation. At this dose, it may lead to maternal awareness, especially if opioids have not been used.

Ketamine

- Has been described for induction of the severely haemodynamically compromised mother as it is extremely cardiovascularly stable.
- It has a slower induction time and an end-point is difficult to detect.
- It can cause hallucinations and delirium, especially in the unpremedicated mother.
- At 1mg/kg the condition of the neonate is comparable with thiopental.
- At 2mg/kg, which is probably a more appropriate dose for the mother, neonatal depression can be expected.

Benzodiazepines
- Their slow onset makes these drugs less appropriate under normal circumstances than the other agents, with increased risk of aspiration.
- Midazolam at an induction dose of 0.2mg/kg is associated with prolonged sedation in the neonate and doubling of the time to sustained respiration compared with thiopental.
- They are also associated with poor feeding, neonatal hypothermia, hypotonia, and neonatal jaundice.

Neuromuscular agents

In a similar vein to the ongoing debate regarding the ideal induction agent, the role of suxamethonium as the neuro-muscular agent of choice for rapid sequence induction is being challenged by rocuronium. The factors to consider are outlined below.

Suxamethonium
- At the present time, it remains the drug of choice in obstetric practice because it provides rapid ideal intubating conditions with spontaneous reversal of effect.
- Is given in a dose of 1–1.5mg/kg.
- Spontaneous ventilation returns in 5–8min.
- Muscle fasciculations may increase oxygen consumption and speed up desaturation.
- Time to neuromuscular reversal may be slightly prolonged in pregnancy due to the physiological dilution of plasma pseudocholinesterase.
- Suxamethonium does not cross the placenta, therefore the neonate is not affected. However there is a case description of neonatal paralysis in a pseudocholinesterase-deficient neonate born to a deficient mother.
- The neuromuscular blocking effect is not altered by magnesium sulphate ($MgSO_4$), but fasciculations are attenuated and therefore difficult to see.
- Contraindications to suxamethonium are the same as for the non-pregnant population.

Non-depolarizing neuromuscular blockers
- An intermediate acting agent is required to maintain paralysis during CS after neuromuscular recovery from suxamethonium.
- Vecuronium, atracurium, and rocuronium have been extensively investigated following the initial suxamethonium dose.
  - They do not cross the placenta.
  - Their effect is prolonged by MgSO4, and neuromuscular function must be closely observed in the mother at reversal and into the postoperative period.
- Rocuronium has been extensively described to facilitate a rapid sequence induction when suxamethonium is contraindicated.
- It can be used in a dose of 1–1.2mg/kg, with good intubating conditions within 60s.
- This dose will cause paralysis for about 45min.
- It can be rapidly reversed by sugammadex (16mg/kg), making it a viable alternative to suxamethonium for a modified rapid sequence induction.

Inhalational agents

Nitrous oxide

- Is a useful carrier gas with oxygen, reducing the minimum alveolar concentration (MAC) of volatile agents.
- It freely crosses the placenta, and concentrations will continue to increase in the neonate for 15min during maternal administration.
- Concentrations >50% may cause neonatal depression.
- The use of nitrous oxide and oxygen alone will cause light anaesthesia, increased maternal catecholamines, adverse acid-base status in the baby, and an increased risk of awareness.
- Its main advantage is that it does not cause uterine relaxation and can be used to reduce the concentration of the volatile agents required.

Volatile agents

- All cause dose- and time-dependent neonatal depression.
- Induction to delivery time should be <11min.
- All cause dose-dependent uterine relaxation and their use should be restricted to < 1 MAC end-tidal concentration when nitrous oxide is used to supplement anaesthesia.
- Agents such as sevoflurane, isoflurane, and desflurane have the advantage of low blood gas solubility, allowing rapid induction and recovery.
- Sevoflurane should ideally be available as it is the best agent should anaesthesia with spontaneous ventilation be required.

Opioids

- Are not usually given as part of a rapid sequence induction in obstetric practice, but are being considered to reduce the risk of awareness.
- They cause neonatal depression and delayed recovery of spontaneous respiration in the mother should there be a failed intubation.
- 20 micrograms per kg of alfentanil will help obtund the intubation response and can be given at induction if hypertension or tachycardia must be avoided.

Conduct of general anaesthesia

The OAA in conjunction with the Difficult Airway Society have published a number of algorithms relating to safe obstetric GA, failed tracheal intubation, and the 'can't intubate can't oxygenate' scenario. In addition there are helpful tables relating to patient management after failed tracheal intubation. These should be displayed clearly in the obstetric theatre and staff should practice scenarios regularly in drills and simulation training (Fig 12.1).

Pre-theatre preparation

History and examination

Although often a pressured situation, it is essential a brief anaesthetic history is taken following the decision that a GA is required.

• Airway assessment (as above).
• Starvation status.
• Medication history and allergies noted.
• If indicated a focused systems examination should also be performed.

Pre-medication

All mothers should receive medication to increase gastric pH and reduce gastric volume before delivery:

• Omeprazole 20–40mg 12 hourly orally in labour, if high risk.
• Ranitidine 50mg IV or omeprazole 40mg IV, if not previously given orally.
• 30mL sodium citrate 0.3M immediately prior to induction.

Fetal resuscitation

In emergencies, continue active fetal resuscitation measures:

• Stop oxytocin infusion.
• Place mother in the full left lateral position during transfer to theatre.
• Give oxygen via facemask.
• IV infusion of crystalloid.
• Hypotension should be corrected by the use of IV vasopressor.
• Consider use of tocolytic i.e. terbutaline 0.25mg SC.

Pre-induction

Setting the scene

• All personnel should be present in theatre: theatre scrub team, obstetricians, neonatologists, and anaesthetists.
• Explain to the mother what is going to happen.
• A time-out period should occur to perform the WHO checklist.
• Antibiotic prophylaxis should ideally be given before skin incision.
• For a category 1 CS, the patient should be prepped, draped, and catheterized prior to induction, and the baby should be delivered as soon after induction as possible.
• It is imperative that the anaesthetist knows the location of another anaesthetist and how to get hold of them if they experience difficulties.
• Administer high flow O2 by facemask from arrival in theatre, and apply nasal cannulae (see Pre-oxygenation).

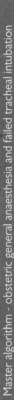

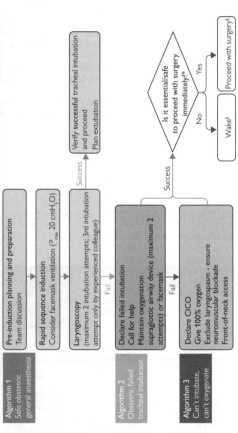

Fig. 12.1 Master algorithm—obstetric general anaesthesia and failed tracheal intubation

Positioning the mother
- Before induction of anaesthesia, the patient should first be positioned supine with a left lateral tilt on the operating table in theatre to reduce aorto-caval compression.
- Take time to optimize the position for airway management, including table height, so that repositioning is unnecessary in event of difficulty.
- The head position should be that described as 'sniffing the morning air', neck flexed, head extended, ensuring that the mouth can be maximally opened. This can only be achieved with a pillow placed away from the shoulders (neck flexion) and plumped up behind the head with the patient's chin raised (head extension),
- Braided, tied, and knotted hair on the occiput is an additional problem that prevents neck extension. Hair should be untied and spread across the pillow.
- Scarves around the head are a similar hazard, as they can hide knotted hair and should be removed. Headscarves worn for religious reasons can be loosely applied around the head.
- Encourage the patient to extend her head (raise her chin) during pre-oxygenation. This improves the overall position of the head and allows accurate inspection of the neck before application of cricoid pressure.

Optimizing laryngoscopy in the obese
- Position the head using the 'ramped' position (Figs 12.2–3) for the obese, which brings the tragus and sternum onto the same horizontal plane. This improves pre-oxygenation and the view at laryngoscopy and makes intubation easier.
- Careful choice of laryngoscope blade and handle.

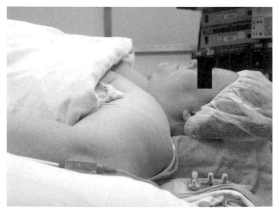

Fig. 12.2 The 'sniff' head position without ramp.

Reprinted by permission from Springer Nature: Springer Nature. *Obesity Surgery*. Laryngoscopy and morbid obesity: a comparison of the 'sniff' and 'ramped' positions, Collins JS et al., © Springer Nature and International Federation for the Surgery of Obesity and metabolic disorders, 2004.

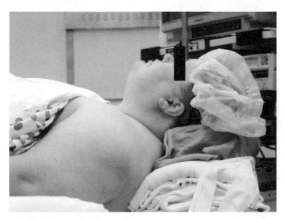

Fig. 12.3 The 'ramped' head position.

Reprinted by permission from Springer Nature: Springer Nature. *Obesity Surgery*. Laryngoscopy and morbid obesity: a comparison of the 'sniff' and 'ramped' positions, Collins JS et al., © Springer Nature and International Federation for the Surgery of Obesity and metabolic disorders, 2004.

- Use arm boards if necessary to ensure the patient's breasts are not going to interfere with laryngoscope manipulation.
- Some functions of the operating table may not work if the patient's weight is above a certain threshold, which can cause difficulty in safe positioning.

Pre-oxygenation

- There is an increase in oxygen consumption of up to 12–16% at term, compared with non-pregnant controls.
- In early labour, oxygen consumption may further increase up to a total of 30% of the non-pregnant state.
- A healthy, non-pregnant patient will tolerate up to 3min of apnoea before desaturating. A pregnant woman with her increased oxygen requirement and decreased functional residual capacity will desaturate much faster, particularly if she is obese. A realistic time may be as short as 60–90s before desaturation occurs.
- Following application of O_2 via nasal cannule at 4L/min, there are three different methods of pre-oxygenation, all using flow rates ≥ 10 litres/min:
  - Tidal volume breathing for 3min.
  - Eight deep breaths.
  - Waiting for a fractional end-tidal O_2 measurement of >0.9. This technique is probably the most accurate and now more practical with increased availability of end-tidal O_2 monitoring.
- A tight-fitting mask should be used to minimize air entrainment. The mother may be very anxious and repeatedly push the mask away from her face. She must be persuaded not to do this as pre-oxygenation must start again if she does so.
- The advantage of pre-oxygenating for 3min is that it allows the anaesthetist to make final checks before induction of anaesthesia.

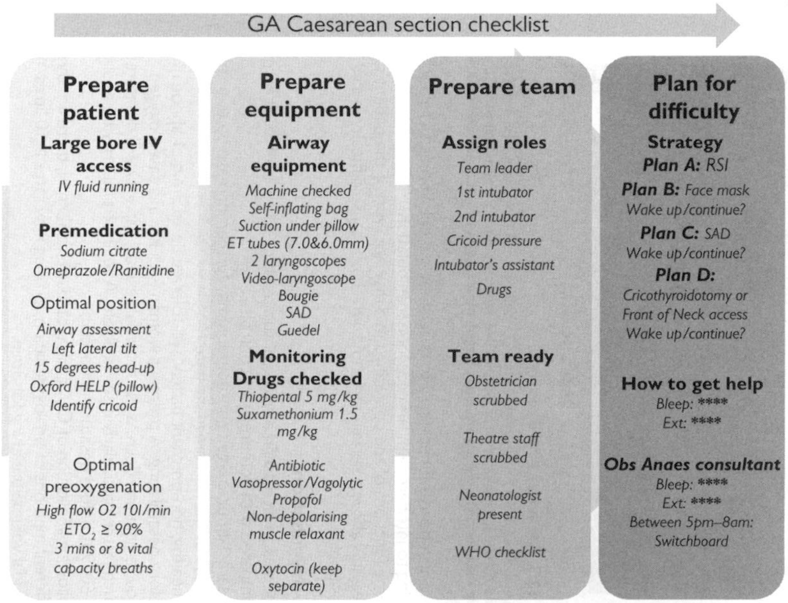

GA Caesarean section checklist

Prepare patient	Prepare equipment	Prepare team	Plan for difficulty
Large bore IV access *IV fluid running* **Premedication** *Sodium citrate* *Omeprazole/Ranitidine* *Optimal position* *Airway assessment* *Left lateral tilt* *15 degrees head-up* *Oxford HELP (pillow)* *Identify cricoid* *Optimal preoxygenation* *High flow O2 10l/min* *ETO₂ ≥ 90%* *3 mins or 8 vital capacity breaths*	**Airway equipment** *Machine checked* *Self-inflating bag* *Suction under pillow* *ET tubes (7.0&6.0mm)* *2 laryngoscopes* *Video-laryngoscope* *Bougie* *SAD* *Guedel* *Monitoring* **Drugs checked** *Thiopental 5 mg/kg* *Suxamethonium 1.5 mg/kg* *Antibiotic* *Vasopressor/Vagolytic* *Propofol* *Non-depolarising muscle relaxant* *Oxytocin (keep separate)*	**Assign roles** *Team leader* *1st intubator* *2nd intubator* *Cricoid pressure* *Intubator's assistant* *Drugs* **Team ready** *Obstetrician scrubbed* *Theatre staff scrubbed* *Neonatologist present* *WHO checklist*	**Strategy** **Plan A:** *RSI* **Plan B:** *Face mask* *Wake up/continue?* **Plan C:** *SAD* *Wake up/continue?* **Plan D:** *Cricothyroidotomy or Front of Neck access* *Wake up/continue?* **How to get help** *Bleep: **** Ext: ***** **Obs Anaes consultant** *Bleep: **** Ext: ***** Between 5pm–8am: Switchboard*

Fig. 12.4. GA Caesarean section checklist.
Reproduced with permission of Dr Lucy French, Cardiff, 2015.

Induction

Most frequently rapid sequence induction of anaesthesia is performed with the following drugs:
- Thiopental 5–7mg/kg or propofol 2.5mg/kg.
- Suxamethonium 1.5mg/kg OR rocuronium 1mg/kg if the patient has a contraindication to suxamethonium.
- If required, obtund sympathetic response to intubation with, e.g. alfentanil 20 micrograms/kg or consider a 50mg/kg bolus of MgSO4 in patients with pre-eclampsia.
- Increase the oxygen flow via the nasal cannulae as consciousness is lost and the period of apnoea begins, as this will prolong the time to desaturation.

Cricoid pressure

- Badly applied cricoid pressure has been implicated during intubation difficulties.
- Ensure cricoid pressure is applied correctly and not altered by table tilt; often best achieved if applied from the patient's left side.
- Single-handed cricoid pressure can flatten the neck on the pillow, reducing neck extension.
- Two-handed cricoid pressure can improve intubation position but reduces help to the anaesthetist, unless there is a second assistant.
- Excessive backward and poorly directed pressure can obliterate the laryngeal opening. The pressure should be no greater than 30Newtons or 3kg, which can be practiced on a weighing scales in theatre.
- Only trained and regularly updated anaesthetic assistants should apply cricoid pressure.

Intubation

- Make the first intubation attempt the best attempt.
- Adequate time must be allowed for the suxamethonium to work. In the pregnant woman, this is usually more than 30 seconds. Attempts at laryngoscopy before full relaxation may lead to dental damage and mucosal bleeding, both of which will increase the likelihood of intubation difficulties.
- Keep facemask in place until fasciculations have finished. If they are not seen (vide supra MgSO4) attempt intubation after 45 seconds.
- Depending on individual circumstances, a long-blade, short-handled laryngoscope, or videolaryngoscope may be used for the first intubation.

Second intubation attempt

- Do not have more than two attempts or use more than two devices.
- The BURP manoeuvre (Back—Upward—Right—Pressure) may improve the laryngeal view. Note: 'Right' means patient's right, which is to the assistant's left.
- Take care when using rigid intubation guides/bougies as they can cause pharyngeal, laryngeal, and tracheal trauma
- Failure to intubate must be acknowledged without delay and communicated to the rest of the theatre team.

Assessing tracheal tube position

- Capnography is the gold standard to confirm correct tracheal placement.
- Bilateral auscultation of the chest is important, particularly if laryngoscopy is >grade 2.
- The cuff should be placed below the vocal cords and inflated gradually until the air leak with manual ventilation stops and the pressure in the cuff is between 20 and 30cmH$_2$O.

Maintenance of anaesthesia

Pre-delivery

- Ventilate to normocapnia of pregnancy (4.0–4.5kPa) with 50:50 mixture of O$_2$ and N$_2$O.
- Most monitors will calculate a MAC when using a mixture of volatile and nitrous oxide. Use overpressure to rapidly titrate the volatile to a MAC of 1.0. In the absence of this function an end-tidal volatile MAC of >0.5 should be aimed for.
- MAC is reduced by 20–30% in pregnancy.
- Use a nerve stimulator to confirm the offset of suxamethonium. Then use small doses of a non-depolarizing agent to maintain neuromuscular blockade.

Post delivery

- Level the table to improve surgical access.
- Reduce O$_2$ to 30%, if maternal SpO$_2$ will allow, with 70% N$_2$O or 70% air.
- Give oxytocin 5IU IV slowly and consider a planned oxytocin infusion as uterine atony can be more problematic due to the effects of volatile anaesthesia.

Analgesia

Aims

- To allow early mobilization of the mother.
- Minimal maternal side effects.
- Minimal fetal side effects.
- Minimal secretion in breast milk.
- To allow normal maternal bonding with the newborn.
- To allow early discharge from hospital.
- Undoubtedly balanced analgesia using multimodal analgesic therapy is the ideal.

Intraoperative

- Give IV opioid analgesia:
  - Fentanyl 100 micrograms.
  - Morphine 10mg in titrated aliquots.
  - Alternatively administer morphine 4mg or diamorphine 2.5mg epidurally if catheter is *in situ* but there was no time for topping-up.
- NSAID if no contra-indication e.g. diclofenac 100mg rectally if consent obtained previously, or diclofenac 75mg IV.
- Paracetamol 1g IV.

Local anaesthetic techniques

Potential viable adjuncts or alternatives to systemic analgesia include:

- Transversus abdominus plane (TAP) blocks can be performed at the end of the operation, ideally with the aid of ultrasound. See Chapter 8 for details of insertion, p. 234.
- Quadratus lumborum blocks have also been shown to produce superior post-operative analgesia.
- Local wound infiltration by surgeons.
- Bilateral ilio-inguinal nerve blocks, sub-fascial or sub-rectus infiltrations.

Postoperative

- A morphine patient controlled analgesia (PCA) device is recommended for postoperative analgesia
- If not contraindicated, regular paracetamol and NSAIDs should be prescribed in addition to the PCA.

Failed intubation

In order to maximize safety, it is essential that every anaesthetist has a clear strategy for airway management. The use of a simple protocol is preferable in which the only requirements are the competent use of a small number of airway adjuncts (Fig 12.5).

Priorities

- Declare a failed intubation.
- Call for help.
- Oxygenate the patient.
- Optimize the patient's head position.
- Do not turn the patient into the lateral position as this will hinder ongoing airway manoeuvres.

Oxygenation—facemask

- Four-hand ventilation involves one operator holding the facemask and performing jaw thrust whilst the second squeezes the bag.
- There is an increased risk of bleeding with nasopharyngeal airways, because of the congested mucosa seen in pregnancy.
- It is important that the jaw thrust is properly applied to ensure that three primary areas of airway obstruction (tongue, soft palate, epiglottis) are bypassed, maximizing chances of ventilation.
- With the above manoeuvres, oxygenation should be possible in most cases, but cricoid pressure may need to be removed or adjusted to improve airway patency.

Oxygenation—supraglottic airway device

- There are numerous reports of the successful use of the classic LMA in 'Can't intubate, Can't oxygenate' scenarios.
- Second generation supraglottic airway devices (SAD) such as the ProSeal™ LMA and I-gel™ provide a better pharyngeal seal, and have the added benefit of a channel that acts as a conduit for gastric contents.
- It is essential to release cricoid pressure during insertion of the SAD. Once correctly placed, and if a good seal is demonstrated, reapplying cricoid pressure is unnecessary unless a first generation SAD is used.
- Inserting a SAD in a patient who is emerging from a thiopental/ suxamethonium anaesthetic may be difficult, and 50% of rescue attempts in obstetric patients in NAP4 were unsuccessful.
- If oxygenation is impossible, declare an emergency to the theatre team and call for specialist help (ENT surgeon/intensivist).

Cannula cricothyroidotomy/scalpel-bougie-tube

- It is important to decide on a rescue technique before induction of anaesthesia, as a failed intubation and ventilation situation is not the time to be making such a decision.
- The technique chosen will depend on the equipment available and the previous experience/training of the anaesthetist.

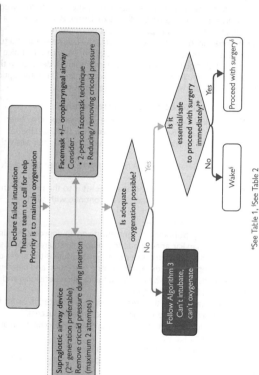

Algorithm 2 – obstetric failed tracheal intubation

Declare failed intubation
Theatre team to call for help
Priority is to maintain oxygenation

Supraglottic airway device
(2nd generation preferable)
Remove cricoid pressure during insertion
(maximum 2 attempts)

Facemask +/– oropharyngeal airway
Consider:
• 2-person facemask technique
• Reducing/removing cricoid pressure

Is adequate oxygenation possible?

No — Follow Algorithm 3
Can't intubate,
can't oxygenate

Yes — Is it essential/safe to proceed with surgery immediately?*

No — Wake§

Yes — Proceed with surgery†

*See Table 1, †See Table 2

Fig. 12.5 OAA and DAS Failed intubation algorithm 2

- NAP4 found that approximately 60% of cannula techniques failed, whereas surgical techniques were almost universally successful.
- It is essential to exclude laryngospasm, so at this stage ensure complete neuromuscular blockade.
- If large cannulae (≥ 4mm) are used, ventilation can be achieved with a standard self-inflating bag and expired CO_2 monitored.
- If jet ventilation is used, with a non-kinking cannula, keep inflation pressures to a minimum and use a 1-second inflation breath followed by a 4-second expiratory pause to allow exhalation. Barotrauma is a serious risk, and upper airway patency must be optimized.
- Some authorities advocate the use of a scalpel—bougie—tracheal tube technique rather than cannula and jet ventilation. As with the choice of all techniques that require specialized equipment, it will depend on the training of the individual. If a cannula technique is tried first, the option of a scalpel technique remains—the reverse is not true.

Does surgery need to continue immediately?

- At any point in the algorithm where maternal oxygenation has been achieved, the question arises whether to continue the anaesthetic with an unprotected airway or to risk death of the fetus and allow the mother to wake.
- Further guidance is detailed in OAA/DAS (Fig 12.1) to prompt swift decision-making
- In practice, the primary duty of the anaesthetist is to the mother, and there are only two absolute indications to continue with surgery:
  - Maternal cardiac arrest.
  - Life-threatening haemorrhage.
- A GA for a CS using spontaneous ventilation and an unprotected airway is a difficult and unfamiliar anaesthetic technique; it requires expertise, but may be the only option in these cases. Sevoflurane is the agent of choice, and be prepared for excessive uterine relaxation and bleeding. Trainee anaesthetists should be careful in taking such decisions, and senior help should be sought urgently.
- In a maternal cardiac arrest, the uterus must be evacuated in order for cardiopulmonary resuscitation to have any chance of success.
- In massive obstetric haemorrhage, bleeding is unlikely to be controlled until the placenta has separated.
- Other factors affecting the decision to continue include maternal obesity, recent solid food intake, and the lack of a regional anaesthetic alternative.
- It may be possible to convert the SAD rescue airway technique into a definitive airway by intubating with a fibrescope through the SAD or by using exchange catheters.
- If a jet ventilation technique is used, anaesthesia must be provided with an intravenous propofol infusion.
- If it is not deemed safe to continue, the patient should be awoken and other methods of anaesthesia reconsidered.

- The choice of rocuronium as the muscle relaxant for intubation in the expectation of using sugammadex in event of failure results in additional decisions to make in an already stressed environment. Airway manoeuvres (SAD insertion, cricothyroidotomy) may be easier to perform and more effective in a patient who is fully paralysed, so the timing of sugammadex administration needs to be carefully considered.

Training and assistance

- Training, using simulator-based scenarios, can be useful for practising failed intubation/ventilation. This will allow skills, knowledge of equipment, flexibility of thinking, and team-work to be taught.
- In the operating theatres, the skill of managing an airway with a mask and oropharyngeal airway needs a raised profile and should be practised on non-obstetric patients.
- Any elective obstetric GA should be used as a training opportunity to teach a rapid sequence induction, providing there are no concerns regarding the airway. Appropriate seniority should always be available for training and managing more difficult patients.
- All anaesthetists covering the maternity unit should be familiar with the airway equipment available and trained to put it together and to ventilate a manikin before they are faced with a GA on a patient.
- A skilled assistant is part of the successful management of GA and must be available at all times. It is important that assistants are also trained in and practice failed and difficult intubation drills with the team so that they clearly understand the principles of their management.

Awake fibreoptic intubation

Indications

The indications for awake fibreoptic intubation in obstetric practice are limited to:

- An elective or category 3 caesarean section where there is a history of previous failed/difficult intubation or concern that intubation will be difficult.
- After a failed intubation when the mother is woken and regional anaesthesia is still not possible.

Unless the anaesthetist is considered an expert in the technique of awake fibreoptic intubation, it is considered best practice never to attempt the technique as part of a failed intubation with the mother anaesthetized.

Options available if difficulty anticipated

- Regional anesthesia—CSE or spinal catheter—offers lowest risk of unexpectedly high block.
- Secure airway with patient awake, i.e. fibreoptic intubation would be the technique of choice.
- Avoid intubation and use alternative airway.
  - LMA has been used in 1067 selected elective cases in Korea.
  - ProSeal™ LMA has been used in cases of failed intubation in obstetrics.
- CS under local infiltration only.

Technique of awake fibreoptic intubation

Both oral and nasal routes have been successfully used and a careful pre-operative explanation is needed.

- Glycopyrronium bromide (5 micrograms per kg IM) can be given to reduce secretions.
- A topical vasoconstrictor to shrink the nasal mucosa (e.g. oxymetazoline or phenylephrine).
- Maximize airway space by sitting patient up and avoiding sedation.
- Multiple techniques have been described for anaesthetizing the airway; choose the one you are most familiar with.
- Smaller endotracheal tubes than usual should be selected, e.g. size 6mm; armoured or tapered tip (as provided with the intubating LMA) and preloaded on the fibrescope.
- GA is only induced when tube placement has been confirmed by capnography.
- Direct laryngoscopy should be performed afterwards to give an impression of the ease of conventional intubation.
- Extubation should be performed awake when protective airway reflexes have returned.
- A survey in one UK region showed that 91.4% would choose awake intubation if regional was contraindicated or had failed in a patient with a known difficult airway. However, only 6/74 choosing awake fibreoptic intubation had obstetric experience of this.
- It is important to involve colleagues experienced in fibreoptic intubation as recommended in the CEMACH 2000–2002 report.

Extubation and postoperative care

- Deaths from extubation problems in obstetric patients have been reported.
- If the patient was difficult to intubate, extreme care should be taken at extubation.
- There is debate as to whether extubation should be done in the left lateral position or the upright position.
- The sitting upright position allows free excursion of the diaphragm, which is particularly relevant in the obese patient. If the intra-abdominal pressure is high, it is still possible to regurgitate in the sitting or reclining position.
- Passage of an orogastric tube to empty the stomach prior to extubation should be performed if there is any concern about increased volume of gastric contents.
- Laryngeal competence is impaired for some hours after anaesthesia, so the patient is at risk of aspiration of gastric contents during recovery.
- Initial postoperative care should be in an environment with staff trained to the level of a general theatre recovery area.
- If there have been any intubation difficulties the mother must be fully informed of the problem. Patients should be given a letter to keep, clearly describing the problem and management; a copy should be kept in the notes and the GP informed.

Aspiration

This is rare in modern practice, but Curtis Mendleson (1913–2002) first highlighted the serious consequences of pulmonary aspiration in 1946. This leads initially to a chemical pneumonitis and atelectasis of varying degree. Later the condition can be complicated by the development of adult respiratory distress syndrome (ARDS) and/or polymicrobial pneumonia. In Mendleson's original description, deaths were caused by asphyxiation due to solid matter. The chemical pneumonitis associated with the aspiration of gastric acid, although serious, recovered without specific treatment in all cases.

Aspiration continues to be a small but important cause of anaesthetic-related maternal deaths. Failure to manage the airway appropriately and secure rapid endotracheal intubation exposes the mother to the risk of aspiration.

Relevant gastrointestinal physiology

- Gastro-oesophageal reflux is common in pregnancy.
- pH studies show increased gastric acidity.
- Increased intragastric pressure due to the pregnancy.
- Decreased lower oesophageal tone.
- In labour, there is decreased gastric emptying associated with pain and opioid drugs.

Additional risk factors

- Poor cricoid application (due to left lateral tilt).
- Failed intubation.
- Peripartum opioids, either systemic or regional.
- Obesity.
- Diabetes mellitus (gastroparesis) increasingly common in pregnancy.
- Non-fasted women—this is a controversial area as feeding in labour has been encouraged. Aspiration though, however rare, may be used as an argument against feeding in labour, especially as it is the aspiration of solid material that is most life-threatening.

Prevention

The following changes in clinical practice have significantly decreased the incidence of aspiration:
- Increased use of regional techniques.
- Antacid prophylaxis in labour and prior to operative delivery.
- Light diet and isotonic drinks only in labour.
- Improved training in obstetric anaesthesia.

Presentation

- Presents initially as tachypnoea, tachycardia and raised airway pressures, decreased O_2 saturations, and localized wheeze/crepitations.
- The extent of the symptoms and signs depends on the acidity and volume of the aspirate.
- ARDS is possible within 24–72h, presenting with increasingly high airway pressures and respiratory rate, low paO_2, and high $paCO_2$. A prolonged period of ventilation may be necessary.

Management

Acute management

- Call for help. Inform obstetricians.
- Maintain airway and give 100% O_2.
- Check endotracheal tube and cuff. Re-intubate if required.
- Suction lower airway until aspirates clear.
- Avoid excessive intermittent positive pressure ventilation (IPPV) until suctioned.
- Consider bronchodilators if there is marked bronchospasm.
- Consider bronchoscopy/lavage if clinically no improvement.
- Pass nasogastric tube and empty stomach.

Further management

- Liaise with critical care and plan for transfer.
- Evidence of high oxygen requirement may indicate that postoperative ventilatory support may be required.
- If there is evidence of atelectasis, consider physiotherapy and continuous positive airway pressure (CPAP).
- Prophylactic antibiotics are not required.
- Corticosteroids do not affect outcome.

Investigations

- Chest X-ray—early changes include diffuse infiltrative shadowing in the right lower lobe, classically with a variable degree of atelectasis, which may be profound if bronchial occlusion has occurred. The left lateral tilt used in obstetric patients can change this pattern, and infiltrates are seen more commonly on the left.
- Arterial blood gases.
- Bronchoscopy—consider if aspiration of solids is possible, severe atelectasis, or little clinical improvement.

Preventing awareness

The 5th National Audit Project of the Royal College of Anaesthetists (NAP5) looked at cases of accidental awareness under general anaesthesia (AAGA) in a 12-month period from June 2012 to May 2013.

- There were 14 cases of AAGA in obstetrics, 12 of which were at CS (category 1:5, category 2:4, category 3/4:3).
- AAGA was always associated with difficulty or delay at intubation.
- Obstetric cases made up only 0.8% of the anaesthetics given in the 12 month but 10% of the reported AAGA.
- This confirmed that the incidence of awareness is higher than in the non-obstetric population i.e. between 1:670—1:920.
- The possibility of AAGA should be mentioned in the preoperative assessment.

High incidence is probably caused by:

- AAGA was always associated with difficulty or delay at intubation.
- Anxious, unpremedicated patient, with a high cardiac output that rapidly redistributes the induction agent.
- Rapid sequence induction with muscle relaxation.
- Reduced dose of anaesthetic agents because of fear of increased sedation in the baby.
- Short interval between induction of anaesthesia and start of surgery.
- A reduced dose of inhalational agent because of fear of uterine relaxation.
- Higher incidence of difficulty with intubation resulting in delay in initiating inhalational supplementation.

Problems can be reduced by:

- Giving an adequate dose of thiopental (no less than 5mg/kg).
- Using nitrous oxide with oxygen.
- Using an over-MAC technique at the start of surgery guided by end-tidal vapour analysis.
- Using agents with low blood/gas partition coefficients such as sevoflurane, isoflurane, or desflurane.
- Using high gas flows initially to increase rapidly the brain partial pressure of volatile agent.

Role of bispectral index (BIS) monitoring

Because of rapidly changing depth of anaesthesia and a short induction to delivery time, there is little evidence to support depth of anaesthesia monitoring with bi-spectral index during general anaesthesia for CS; however, it is being currently considered by some obstetric units. Although an adequate dose and concentration of anaesthetic agents must be used, pregnancy is also associated with a reduction in MAC requirement of about 20–30%. This can be seen from the first trimester.

Further reading

Lipman S et al. The demise of general anesthesia in obstetrics revisited: prescription for a cure. *International Journal of Obstetric Anesthesia* 2005; 14: 2–4.

Mushambi MC et al Obstetric Anaesthetists' Association and Difficult Airway Society guidelines for the management of difficult and failed tracheal intubation in obstetrics. *Anaesthesia* 2015; 70:1286–1306.

Rahman K et al. Failed tracheal intubation in obstetrics: no more frequent but still managed badly. *Anaesthesia* 2005; 60: 168–171.

Han TH et al. The laryngeal mask airway is effective (and probably safe) in selected healthy parturients for elective Cesarean section: a prospective study of 1067 cases. *Canadian Journal of Anaesthesia* 2001; 48: 1117–1121.

Popat MT. Awake fibreoptic intubation skills in obstetric patients: a survey of anaesthetists in the Oxford region. *International Journal of Obstetric Anesthesia* 2000; 9: 78–82.

Collins JS et al. Laryngoscopy and morbid obesity: a comparison of the 'sniff' and 'ramped' positions. *Obesity Surgery* 2004; 14: 1171–1175.

Thurlow JA et al. Intrauterine resuscitation: active management of fetal distress. *International Journal of Obstetric Anesthesia* 2002; 11: 105–116.

Chiron B et al. Standard preoxygenation technique versus two rapid techniques in pregnant patients. *International Journal of Obstetric Anesthesia* 2004; 13: 11–14.

Hart EM, Owen H. Errors and omissions in anesthesia: a pilot study using a pilot's checklist. *Anesthesia and Analgesia* 2005; 101: 246–250.

Russell R. Failed intubation in obstetrics: a self-fulfilling prophecy? *International Journal of Obstetric Anesthesia* 2007; 16: 1–3.

Stacey M. General anaesthesia and failure to ventilate. In Dob D, Cooper G, Holdcroft A, ed. *Crises in Childbirth.* 2007.

Lucas DN, Yentis SM. Unsettled weather and the end for thiopental? Obstetric general anaesthesia after the NAP5 and MBRRACE-UK reports. *Anaesthesia* 2015; 70: 375–392.

Krohg A et al. The analgesic effect of ultrasound-guided quadratus lumborum block after caesarean delivery: a randomised clinical trial. *Anaesthesia Analgesia* 2018; 126: 559–565

Post-delivery symptom control

Gemma Keigthley and Sarah Harries

Analgesia after vaginal delivery

The severity of pain and analgesia required after delivery usually depend on the mode of delivery. Accurate pain scoring is essential when determining the strength of analgesics that may be required. A verbal rating scale (0–3) is recommended, aiming for a pain score of <2, i.e. no pain (0) or mild pain (1) on movement.

Analgesia after vaginal delivery

Normal vaginal delivery

- A normal vaginal delivery may not require any analgesics post delivery or simple analgesia such as paracetamol 1g 6 hourly and an NSAID, e.g. ibuprofen 400mg 6–8 hourly as required.

Vaginal delivery with episiotomy or perineal tear

- The pain following a difficult vaginal delivery should not be under-estimated, and often requires a regular prescription of paracetamol 1g 6 hourly and an NSAID, e.g. diclofenac 100mg PR at the time of repair, followed by diclofenac 50mg 8 hourly or ibuprofen 400mg 6–8 hourly with food.
- Moderate strength opioids, e.g. tramadol 50–100mg or codeine phosphate 30–60mg may also be needed, and should be prescribed up to 6 hourly as required. Avoid codeine in breastfeeding mothers.

Additional notes

- Always prescribe a laxative, e.g. lactulose 15mL, 12 hourly, with IV or PO opioid prescription, following an episiotomy or extensive perineal tear repair.
- All the drugs mentioned, with the exception of codeine, have been safely used in mothers who are breastfeeding, despite the manufacturer of tramadol advising to avoid its use during lactation.
- Caution must be exercised in using any NSAID in mothers with moderate to severe pre-eclampsia or a creatinine >70mmol/l, in addition to any other usual contraindications for NSAID use.

Analgesia after caesarean delivery

General recommendations

- Effective analgesia following caesarean delivery is one of the important pillars of enhanced recovery following obstetric surgery, ensuring early discharge from hospital.
- A balanced analgesia approach is highly recommended.
- Paracetamol with an NSAID and an opioid have been extensively investigated, and this combination is safe and efficacious.
- Intrathecal and epidural opioids have been extensively shown to be safe, highly acceptable to the mother, and provide excellent analgesia.
- Breastfeeding is safe when ordinary therapeutic doses are used, however, the current consensus is that codeine should not be given to breastfeeding mothers.
- NSAIDs are contraindicated in a number of situations, and care should be exercised when prescribing them. They are not contraindicated in all asthmatics; if the patient has taken them without problem previously, they may be used normally.
- A small number of studies have shown that an epidural infusion or PCEA, if an epidural catheter is *in situ*, provides excellent post-caesarean delivery if continued. If surgery is complicated or other adjuncts contraindicated, this approach may be very beneficial.
- Early mobilization is strongly recommended after delivery, and continuing epidural analgesia into the post-delivery period may impede this.

General anaesthesia

Intra-operative

- Paracetamol 1g IV and an NSAID, e.g. 100mg diclofenac PR or 75mg diluted IV after delivery of the baby, plus 10–20mg morphine in titrated IV boluses.
- Consider bilateral transversus abdominis plane (TAP) blocks or wound infiltration with 20mL 0.5% bupivacaine or levobupivacaine.
- When compared to a placebo, TAP blocks have been shown to improve post-caesarean section analgesia, however, they are inferior to intrathecal opioids.

Postoperative

- IV morphine via a PCA device.
- Paracetamol 1g 6 hourly PO/PR/IV and diclofenac 100mg 12 hourly for 2–4 doses, followed by diclofenac 50mg PO 8 hourly OR ibuprofen 400mg PO 6–8 hourly with food.
- Moderate strength opioids, e.g. tramadol 50–100mg PO/IV, codeine phosphate 30–60mg PO, or liquid morphine 5mg PO may be required for breakthrough pain or step-down analgesia after 24 hours. However codeine should not be given to breastfeeding mothers.

Spinal anaesthesia

Intra-operative
- Intrathecal morphine 100 micrograms and intrathecal fentanyl 10–20 micrograms or intrathecal diamorphine 250 micrograms before delivery.
- Paracetamol 1g PR and diclofenac 100mg PR after delivery.

Post-operative
- Paracetamol 1g 6 hourly PO/PR.
- Diclofenac 100mg PO/PR 12 hourly for 2–4 post-operative doses, followed by diclofenac 50mg 8 hourly OR ibuprofen 400mg PO 6 hourly with food.
- Moderate strength opioids, e.g. tramadol 50–100mg PO/IV, codeine phosphate 30–60mg PO or liquid morphine 5mg PO may be used for breakthrough pain. Codeine should not be given to breastfeeding mothers.

Epidural top-up

Intraoperative
- Epidural fentanyl 50–100 micrograms before delivery followed by epidural morphine 4mg or epidural diamorphine 2.5mg
- Paracetamol 1g PR and diclofenac 100mg PR after delivery.

Postoperative
- As for after spinal anaesthesia.

Combined spinal–epidural

Intraoperative
- Either as for single-shot spinal anaesthesia (see above) or intrathecal fentanyl 20 micrograms before delivery, followed by epidural morphine 4mg or epidural diamorphine 2.5mg,
- Paracetamol 1g PR and diclofenac 100mg PR after delivery.

Postoperative
- As for after spinal anaesthesia.

Additional notes
- Always prescribe a laxative, e.g. lactulose 15mL, 12 hourly, with IV or PO opioid prescription.
- All mothers receiving morphine or diamorphine via the intrathecal, epidural, or IV route should be monitored closely for the first 24 hours, i.e. pulse, BP, respiratory rate, and oxygen saturation should be measured and documented every 30min for the first 2h, followed by 2 hourly intervals up to 24 hours.
- Regular prescription of codeine and other opioids should be avoided for at least 24 hours after intrathecal morphine because of the risk of late respiratory depression.
- Caution must be exercised in using any NSAID in mothers with moderate to severe pre-eclampsia or a creatinine >70mmol/l, plus any other usual contraindications for NSAID use.

Management of nausea and vomiting

Post-delivery nausea and vomiting is multifactorial, therefore all underlying causes should be considered to prevent maternal morbidity.

Causes

- Opioids.
- Pain.
- Ergometrine.
- Antibiotics.
- Post-operative ileus.
- Postdural puncture headache (PDPH).
- Postpartum eclampsia.
- Intracranial pathology, e.g. cerebral venous thrombosis.

Treatment

Antiemetics

- Ondansetron is excreted in small amounts in the breast milk and has no clinical effects on the baby and is safe to use, despite the manufacturers advice to avoid it. Routine use of ondansetron 4mg IV intra-operatively has been shown to reduce post-operative nausea and vomiting and allow early return to normal diet. No data are available for the new generation 5-hydroxytryptamine 3 antagonists.
- Cyclizine 50mg IV 8 hourly is safe to use during lactation.
- Dexamethasone 4–8mg IV is compatible with breastfeeding in a single dose but there is no data for prolonged use.
- Metoclopramide 10mg IV is safe to use but often of limited benefit.
- Prochlorperazine 3mg via the buccal route, is a useful alternative if post-operative nausea and vomiting is difficult to control.
- If nausea and vomiting is persistent or has an atypical presentation, uncommon causes should be considered early.

Drug side effects

Opioids

Opioids in spinal and epidural blocks are commonly used, and their side effect profile is similar by both routes.

Pruritus

This is a troublesome and very common side effect, with an incidence of 83% in the postpartum mother.

The mechanism of pruritus is complex:

- A specialized subpopulation of unmyelinated chemonociceptors and dedicated spinal neurons responsible for the itch sensation have been identified.
- The central nervous system containing an 'itch centre'.
- Activation of the medullary dorsal horn with antagonism of inhibitory transmitters.
- Regulation of the serotonergic pathway.

Treatment options

- Although commonly prescribed, IV or oral chlorphenamine does not have a direct effect as the itch is not due to histamine release, but the mother may find this drug beneficial because of its sedative properties.
- A reduction in itch intensity has been described in some patients given ondansetron, and it may be worthwhile giving this drug to a mother who is also nauseous.
- Sub-anaesthetic doses of propofol may be beneficial but should not be given without full and immediate anaesthetic support.
- Naloxone will reverse the pruritus associated with opioids but may also reverse the analgesic effect. Data suggests that an IV continuous, low dose naloxone infusion has the largest body of evidence supporting its use in preventing opioid-induced pruritus; however, doses above 2micrograms/kg/h. are not recommended as they are more likely to reverse analgesia. An initial dose of 50 micrograms is recommended.
- Additional IV options in the order of decreasing efficacy:
  - Droperidol 1.25–2.5mg (higher doses are ineffective).
  - Nalbuphine 3mg.
  - Droperidol has also been used as a bolus dose in the epidural.
- Reassurance that the 'itch' is not an 'allergic' reaction is the most important strategy, as it is a relatively short-lived problem (<24h).
- Better understanding of the receptors and mechanisms of pruritus will probably lead to more effective treatment options in the future.

Delayed gastric emptying

- This is well described after all epidural opioids and is dose related.
- Mothers receiving epidural fentanyl in labour will also be at risk.

Nausea and vomiting

- Should be treated with conventional antiemetic therapy as described.

Urinary retention

- Uncommon in obstetric practice, BUT bladder emptying must be carefully monitored and enquired after following catheter removal.

Maternal respiratory depression
- Uncommon in obstetric practice at the spinal doses used.
- May be increased risk if given with systemic IV opioids.
- Respiratory rate and sedation scores should be compulsory for a period of 12–24h in a well-managed clinical area after long-acting opioids (morphine or diamorphine) in the intrathecal and epidural space.

Neonatal respiratory depression
- Major respiratory depression in the neonate is rare after conventional epidural or spinal doses in obstetric practice.
- Epidural opioids have been implicated in poor establishment of breastfeeding.

Non-steroidal anti-inflammatory drugs

Non-steroidal anti-inflammatory drugs (NSAIDs) are safe in the postnatal period and for breastfeeding mothers.

Caution in prescribing post-delivery in the following setting
- In patients where bleeding has been problematic.
- Low platelet counts <100.
- Oliguria due to hypovolaemia or renal impairment.
- Pre-eclampsia/eclampsia because of the renal component of the disease. NSAIDs can be introduced after assessment of renal function and a normal platelet count has been established.

Advice on drugs and breastfeeding

The administration of drugs to breastfeeding mothers can cause harm to the nursing infant. Drugs can inhibit lactation or cause direct harmful effects to the infant due to excretion in breast milk.

For many medications, there is insufficient evidence available to provide accurate guidance on drug safety during breastfeeding. Therefore, for this reason alone, manufacturers often advise avoiding medications that are probably quite safe.

General principles for prescribing drugs to lactating women

- Is the medication really necessary?
- Choose the safest drug available.
- Control of pain and nausea is important.
- Minimize drug exposure by administering medications just after breastfeeding or before the infant is due to have a lengthy sleep period.
- Breastfeeding is the gold standard in infant nutrition. The risks of a potentially harmful drug being excreted in milk have to be balanced with the advantages of continued breastfeeding.

Further reading

British National Formulary Appendix 5: Breastfeeding. Codeine: restricted use as analgesic in children and adolescents after European safety review, *Medicines and Healthcare products regulatory agency*, Published: 25 June 2013.

Charuluxananan S et al. Ondansetron for treatment of intrathecal morphine-induced pruritus after cesarean delivery. *Regional Anesthesia and Pain Medicine* 2000; 25: 535–539.

Yeh, HM, et al. Prophylactic intravenous ondansetron reduces the incidence of intrathecal morphine-induced pruritus in patients undergoing caesarean delivery. *Anesthesia and Analgesia* 2000; 91: 172–175.

Anaesthesia and analgesia for specific obstetric indications

Sarah Harries

Feticide

Definition

A therapeutic feticide involves the injection of potassium chloride into the fetal heart under ultrasound control when severe fetal abnormalities are present and the decision has been made to terminate the pregnancy. This is in line with recommendations from the Royal College of Obstetricians and Gynaecologists, which state that the decision to terminate a pregnancy after 21 weeks and 6 days gestation should ensure that the fetus is born dead.

Key issues

- The feticide procedure and the delivery that follows are always conducted in difficult circumstances. The mother and partner must be approached in a sensitive and understanding manner.
- The feticide may be performed in the fetal medicine unit or on the labour ward.
- If asked to administer analgesia, anxiolysis, or sedation for the procedure in whatever setting, check that the necessary monitoring and resuscitation equipment are readily available.
- Following the feticide, labour is induced with prostaglandins.
- The onset of labour may be prolonged, with an increased risk of retained products following delivery.

Management

- The anaesthetist may be requested to administer analgesia ± sedation routinely for such procedures, or only for the very anxious patient.
- Oral analgesia and sedation, e.g. tramadol 100mg or morphine 5mg, with lorazepam 2mg, are effective if administered prior to the procedure.
- IV midazolam in 1mg increments ± IV fentanyl 10–20 micrograms/IV alfentanil 100–200 micrograms increments may be safely administered during the feticide for the anxious patient, provided appropriate monitoring is applied.
- Following induction with prostaglandins, labour usually proceeds rapidly.
- Analgesia should be offered, either systemic opioids or regional techniques, in the usual way.
- If anaesthesia for retained products of conception is required, an assessment of the risks and benefits of general vs regional anaesthesia should be done. Rapid sequence induction and tracheal intubation are recommended following mid-trimester terminations.
- If an anaesthetist considers for religious or cultural reasons that they are unable to manage a women undergoing a feticide, they should communicate this to a senior anaesthetist as early as possible.

Intrauterine death

Definition

Unexpected death of the fetus after 20 weeks gestation occurs in <1% of pregnancies, and frequently no specific maternal or fetal cause can be found. It may be detected by a prolonged period of absent fetal movements and later confirmed by the absent of a fetal heart beat on ultrasound scanning.

Key issues

- Intrauterine death is a devastating event for parents, and the management of the subsequent delivery is emotionally difficult and stressful for all staff involved.
- There are major obstetric consequences:
  - Deranged clotting leading to DIC.
  - Sepsis.
  - Postpartum haemorrhage.
  - Retained products of conception.
- Tissue thromboplastin, the stimulus for disseminated intravascular coagulation (DIC), is released from the fetus 3–5 weeks following fetal death; however, it may be released from the placenta much earlier if placental separation has occurred.
- Labour is usually induced as soon as feasible after the diagnosis has been confirmed, with the aim to deliver the fetus vaginally.
- Labour may be prolonged and difficult, especially if the fetus is near term gestation, and may require assisted delivery, e.g. forceps extraction or hysterotomy.

Management

- The situation always demands sympathy and sensitivity from all staff.
- The mother should be assessed for signs of a coagulopathy or sepsis prior to discussion about the methods of analgesia available for delivery.
  - Check FBC, clotting screen, point of care viscoelastometric haemostatic assays (VHA), U&E, serial temperature, pulse rate, and BP.
  - Clotting abnormalities should be corrected with fibrinogen concentrate, FFP, or cryoprecipitate. Discussion with the haematologist is helpful for any degree of clotting dysfunction.
- Any signs of infection should be treated with broad-spectrum antibiotics, e.g. IV penicillins and metronidazole, as untreated sepsis can trigger a severe coagulopathy.
- Analgesic options for labour should be discussed early:
  - Systemic opioids, e.g. IV PCA fentanyl or morphine are often used as first-line analgesics and provide a degree of sedation for the mother. PCA remifentanil should not be used unless the mother is constantly monitored by a trained midwife.
  - Adjuvant sedatives, e.g. incremental IV midazolam 1mg are helpful to distract from the delivery process and will provide a degree of amnesia if this is the mother's wish.
  - Epidural analgesia will provide effective analgesia and allow the mother to remain more lucid and in control. Epidural analgesia is contraindicated if a coagulopathy is present or uncorrected.

Complications

- Uterine rupture should always be considered in a mother with a previous uterine scar.
- PPH is a risk especially associated with coagulopathy or retained products .
- Pre-eclampsia should be excluded.
- Hysterotomy in the presence of uncorrected coagulopathy is particularly high risk and not recommended. Correction of the underlying coagulopathy must be the first priority prior to delivery.
- Intrauterine death of one twin is a recognized complication in a monochorionic twin pregnancy. Management is usually conservative, and the pregnancy is allowed to continue with the viable remaining twin.

Breech presentation and abnormal lie

Definition

The position of the fetus at term is defined by its lie, i.e. the relationship of the longitudinal axis of the fetus to that of the mother, and the nature of the presenting part foremost in the pelvis, e.g. cephalic (head), breech (buttock), or compound.

Breech presentation

The fetus lies longitudinally with its buttocks in the lower pole of the uterus. The presenting part may be buttocks with hips flexed and knees extended (frank breech), buttocks with hips and knees flexed (complete breech), or a foot or knee presenting before the buttocks (footling breech). It occurs in 3–4% of singleton term pregnancies.

Abnormal (transverse) lie

The fetus lies across the uterine cavity, not along the longitudinal axis, with a variable presenting part. The fetus must be converted to a longitudinal lie for a vaginal delivery to be successful. It occurs in 0.3% of term pregnancies.

> **Key issues**
> - An antenatal diagnosis of a breech presentation or abnormal lie is not absolute as the fetus frequently turns in the final weeks prior to delivery. This should be confirmed with ultrasound.
> - Fetal presentation is dependent on several factors: uterine tone, the tone and pressure of surrounding structures including the maternal abdominal wall, fetal mobility, and the amount of amniotic fluid present.
> - Breech presentation and abnormal lie are both associated with grand multiparity, polyhydramnios, placenta praevia, and other obstructive lesions in the pelvis, e.g. large uterine fibroids.
> - Both breech presentation and abnormal lie are associated with an increased risk of cord prolapse and consequently fetal compromise.
> - If a mother presents to delivery suite with a malpresentation, early anaesthetic assessment of the mother is important because of the high incidence of intervention. The anaesthetic assessment should be documented and handed over to subsequent shifts of staff.
> - Effective team-work between obstetrician, anaesthetist, and midwife is essential to ensure a safe delivery and best outcome for mother and baby.

Management

Breech presentation

Several antenatal management options are possible, provided there is no evidence of an obstructing structure in the pelvis:
- Vaginal breech delivery.
- Planned CS.
- External cephalic version (ECV).

- The Term Breech Trial demonstrated that perinatal mortality, neonatal mortality, and serious neonatal morbidity are significantly lower following a planned CS compared with a planned vaginal breech delivery. As a result of this trial, many women opt for a planned CS if breech presentation persists. Consequently, obstetricians and midwives skilled at performing vaginal breech deliveries are likely to be less readily available in the future.
- Vaginal breech delivery has been shown to be associated with greater intrapartum hypoxia than a vaginal cephalic delivery, due to prolonged compression of the umbilical cord during the second stage of labour.

External cephalic version

- An ECV is performed for breech presentation at ≥37 weeks gestation, with the aim of turning the fetus to a cephalic position to facilitate a vaginal birth.
- ECV has been shown to reduce the incidence of breech presentation at term and the incidence of CS for non-cephalic births.
- Obstetricians trained and skilled in the procedure should perform it.
- Routine tocolysis to relax the uterine muscles is recommended to improve the success of ECV.
- Routine CTG recording should be undertaken before and after an ECV.
- Suggested tocolytic agents:
  - β sympathomimetic agents, e.g. inhaled salbutamol, IV infusion of ritodrine, have demonstrated increased success of ECV.
  - Nitroglycerin, e.g. sublingual GTN spray.
  - No significant difference between these different agents has been found in terms of success rate.
- Epidural anaesthesia has been shown to have a positive effect on the success rate of ECV but not to the extent where it is wholly recommended.
- A spinal injection of 2.5mg bupivacaine and 10 micrograms sufentanil has been used in the USA to provide analgesia for the procedure, which can be painful, and some mothers do not tolerate it. However, it does not improve the success and may mask the pain associated with complications, e.g. abruption. If this treatment was to be translated to UK practice, 15 micrograms fentanyl with bupivacaine would be a suitable alternative to the sufentanil.
- Significant maternal hypotension, requiring aggressive management with vasopressors, can occur with ECV under spinal block.
- Contraindications to ECV include: previous CS or uterine surgery, oligohydramnios, compromised or premature fetus, antepartum haemorrhage, pre-eclampsia, or maternal refusal.
- Risks associated with the procedure include: uterine rupture and placental abruption; thus it should only be performed where there is a dedicated obstetric team available to manage these complications.
- In the UK, it is unusual for anaesthetic teams to participate in this procedure, other than to be on 'stand-by' in the event of any complications requiring immediate delivery by CS.
- However, there are some institutions where the administration of epidural or general anaesthesia is advocated for ECV.
- Fetal scanning following the ECV will confirm the new position and fetal well-being.

Labour management
- This frequently presents when the mother presents in advanced labour with an undiagnosed breech presentation. Some mothers at this stage will opt for a vaginal birth, although an emergency caesarean is an option.
- Continuous fetal monitoring is essential throughout labour, with the facilities available to proceed to emergency CS if required.
- Adequate analgesia should be offered and maintained for the duration of labour and delivery, as the mother wishes. Perineal analgesia and anaesthesia are essential for the second stage.
- There are clear benefits to effective epidural or CSE analgesia for the delivery; however, there is a lack of definitive evidence to substantiate this.

Effective epidural analgesia:
- Prevents premature 'pushing' prior to full dilatation, which can be associated with a breech presentation. Involuntary maternal pushing can result in the small breech presenting part being pushed through a cervix which is not fully dilated. This can lead to head entrapment.
- Provides sacral analgesia for an extended episiotomy or the application of forceps to the after-coming head.
- Can be extended rapidly in the event of fetal distress and the need for an emergency CS.
- After the insertion of an epidural, usual delivery suite protocols for top-up regimes, infusions or PCEA should be followed.
- The anaesthetist should remain in close proximity to the delivery room to deal swiftly with any complications.

Caesarean section
There are many situations when a CS may be required for breech presentation; planned CS, emergency CS following a known or undiagnosed breech presenting in labour. Or Category 1 CS if fetal distress occurs during planned vaginal breech delivery.
- Regional anaesthesia confers significant benefits over GA for CS, and should be attempted provided time allows.
- If an epidural is sited for labour analgesia, it should be checked frequently to ensure an adequate sensory block is present and the block can be extended rapidly for an emergency CS, e.g. 20mL 0.5% bupivacaine or levobupivacaine + 50–100 micrograms fentanyl.
- If an emergency CS is required during the second stage of labour, extraction of the fetus may be extremely difficult. Additional uterine relaxation may be required, e.g. 50–100 micrograms IV GTN or sublingual GTN spray.
- Elective CSs are usually straightforward, although difficulties in extracting the fetus can occur.

Abnormal lie
The management options include: planned CS or stabilization of fetal head in the pelvis, followed by immediate induction of labour, usually with a controlled artificial rupture of membranes.

Caesarean section

- A planned CS is indicated if the reason for the abnormal lie is due to an obstruction in the pelvis preventing descent of the fetal head, e.g. placenta praevia.
- Hypotension may be difficult to manage as the fetus lies across the vena cava, and usual lateral tilt may not relieve the obstruction.
- Emergency CS may be indicated if during or following induction of labour, the umbilical cord prolapses into the pelvis, causing fetal distress.
- The anaesthetic technique will depend wholly on the situation and the time available. Regional anaesthesia confers significant benefits over GA for CS, and should be attempted provided time allows.

Stabilization of fetal position

- Abnormal lie is associated with grand-multiparity and polyhydramnios.
- It may be possible to turn the fetus of these women to a cephalic position and induce labour immediately, usually by controlled artificial rupture of membranes in the obstetric operating theatre.
- The major risk of this procedure is cord prolapse, precipitating the need for an immediate caesarean delivery.
- There are a number of possible management options for this procedure and will ultimately depend on applying a risk–benefit analysis for each individual situation. Discussion with the obstetrician regarding the risks of immediate delivery is essential.

Management options

- CSE anaesthesia—the spinal component should be sufficient to allow an immediate CS to be performed if necessary, whilst the epidural component could be used for labour analgesia if no complications occur.
- Spinal anaesthesia—an intrathecal dose for immediate CS and management of labour analgesia, as required, thereafter.
- Anaesthetist 'on-standby' in the operating theatre ready to administer a GA if required for immediate delivery. This option is not recommended in certain situations, e.g. the morbidly obese patient or an anticipated difficult airway.

Further reading

Hannah ME et al. on behalf of Term Breech Trial Collaborative Group. Planned Caesarean section versus planned vaginal birth for breech presentation at term: a randomized multicentre trial. *Lancet* 2000; 356: 1375–1383.

Khaw KS et al. Randomized trial of anaesthetic interventions in external cephalic version for breech presentation. *BJA* 2015; 114 (6): 944–950.

Twins and other multiple pregnancies

Definition

Multiple gestations have become a more common occurrence with the increasing success of *in vitro* fertilization (IVF). However, certain restrictions now apply which limit the number of embryos that can be implanted at any one time, which should decrease the number of extreme multiple births. The incidence of twin pregnancies is 1 in 80, triplets 1 in 8000, and quads 1 in 800,000 after natural conceptions.

Key issues

Multiple pregnancies are associated with a number of major obstetric complications, placing them at increased risk during pregnancy and delivery:

- Pre-eclampsia.
- Anaemia.
- Intrauterine growth rate (IUGR).
- Intrauterine death.
- Malpresentations.
- Premature labour.
- Prolonged labour.
- Malpresentation of second twin following delivery of first twin.
- PPH secondary to uterine atony.
- Many of the minor complaints of pregnancy, e.g. heartburn, exertional breathlessness, backache, pelvic-related pain, will be present in excess.
- Aorto-caval compression is much more severe. Mothers suffer symptoms of supine hypotension in the third trimester and particularly following sympathetic blockade during regional anaesthesia.
- The anaesthetist has a key role to play in the safe management of these mothers during their delivery.

Management

- In a twin pregnancy, if the first twin is cephalic presentation and there is no evidence of other co-existing problems, there is usually no reason why these women cannot labour, although some may not wish to do so.
- In triplet and quadruplet pregnancies, a planned CS between 34 and 36 weeks gestation is the preferred mode of delivery, before preterm labour is threatened.

Labour

- The labour may be long, and the second fetus may present abnormally, necessitating instrumental delivery, cephalic version, or immediate CS.
- The early insertion of an effective epidural is beneficial in a twin pregnancy as it allows rapid top-up for a 'trial of instrumental delivery', external or internal version of the second twin, or CS if there are problems following delivery of the first twin.

- The anaesthetist should be aware at all times of the progress of labour in twin births, and be present during the second stage of labour to respond and treat appropriately if the decision is made to transfer to theatre or for emergency CS.
- Elective epidural top-up with 10mL bupivacaine or levobupivacaine 0.5% for the delivery of the second twin will facilitate intrauterine manipulation, instrumental delivery, and rapid extension of the epidural block for CS. The mother will have successfully delivered her first twin at this stage, and this stronger top-up will not impede her effort.

Caesarean section

The usual choices for anaesthetic technique apply. Points to consider:

- Engorged epidural veins may increase the risk of a bloody tap.
- Compressed epidural and subarachnoid spaces increase the risk of a high regional block, so the dose of LA injected intrathecally should be reduced.
- Aorto-caval compression is likely to be more severe; therefore, maintain left lateral position for as long as possible following establishment of the regional block.
- Surgery for triplet or quadruplet deliveries may be prolonged. A CSE technique may be preferable by allowing modification of the spinal dose and minimizing the risk of hypotension from aorto-caval compression.

Complications

- The incidence of pre-eclampsia and preterm labour is increased, often necessitating early delivery.
- The risk of a PPH is increased following both vaginal delivery and CS, due to the large uterus and atony following delivery. Close observation, large-bore venous access, and additional oxytocic drugs, e.g. IV/IM ergometrine and a continuous oxytocin infusion are recommended.

Further reading

De Castro et al. Trial of labour in twin pregnancies: a retrospective cohort study. *BJOG* 2016; 123: 940–945.

Carvalho B et al. Vaginal twin delivery: a survey and review of location, anaesthesia coverage and interventions. *IJOA* 2008; 17: 212–216.

Vaginal delivery after CS

Definition
If a woman has undergone a transverse lower segment incision CS for a previous delivery, subsequent vaginal delivery is possible provided a risk assessment is undertaken by the responsible obstetrician and no obvious contraindications exist. It is often termed 'trial of labour' (TOL) or VBAC (vaginal birth after caesarean section).

Key issues
The alarming rise in CS rate over the last 20yrs has driven the need to reconsider vaginal delivery after a previous CS. VBAC is safe and effective in carefully selected mothers and has a success rate of 72–76%. Repeat elective CS is also safe, but does carry additional risks e.g. haemorrhage, thromboembolism, bladder damage, adhesions.

Contraindications to VBAC
- Previous classical (vertical uterine incision) CS.
- Extensive uterine surgery.
- Previous rupture.
- ≥3 CSs.

Caution is recommended prior to advising VBAC
- Twin pregnancy.
- Fetal macrosomia.
- 2 previous CSs.
- Short interdelivery time period <18 months between delivery.
- The main risk is uterine dehiscence or rupture during labour, therefore induction agents, e.g. prostaglandins and oxytocics, should be used cautiously.
- Epidural analgesia for labour is not contraindicated and may be beneficial if extension of the block is required for CS. In the past, there has been concern about epidural analgesia masking the pain of uterine rupture. Provided close observations of mother and continuous fetal monitoring is performed, early signs of uterine dehiscence will be detected.
- A low dose epidural analgesia regime as per usual labour ward protocols is recommended.

Management
- A low dose epidural is beneficial.
- Continuous CTG monitoring is mandatory.
- The mother and the epidural should be frequently assessed by the anaesthetist.
- Low dose epidural techniques do not usually mask the pain of uterine rupture, therefore breakthrough pain in a well-functioning epidural must be taken seriously.
- The epidural should be topped-up frequently, so it can be rapidly converted to a block suitable for an emergency CS.

Complications

The main complication is uterine scar rupture, which can present with:
- Severe abdominal pain, continuous in nature.
- Intrapartum bleeding.
- Maternal tachycardia, hypotension, or collapse.
- Fetal distress or demise.

Management includes immediate delivery by CS and prompt resuscitation of the mother.

Further reading

Royal College of Obstetricians and Gynaecologists. *Birth after Previous Caesarean Section. Royal College of Obstetricians and Gynaecologists Guidelines.* No. 45. October 2015.

Premature fetus

Definition

The premature fetus is defined as a delivery between 20 and 37 weeks gestation. Its incidence in the UK is ~10% of all pregnancies. Delivery of the premature fetus usually follows spontaneous onset of preterm labour or premature rupture of membranes, but may be necessary due to obstetric complications, e.g. pre-eclampsia or significant growth restriction.

Key issues

Risk factors for preterm delivery include:
• Previous preterm delivery.
• Multiple pregnancy.
• Infection, e.g. chorioamnionitis, pyelonephritis.
• Abnormal placentation, e.g. placenta praevia.
• Cervical incompetence.
• Smoking.
• Extremes of age <15 and >40yrs.
• In many cases, no apparent risk factors are found.

Delivery prior to 32 weeks gestation is associated with major morbidity and mortality for the baby. Neonates have a higher incidence of respiratory distress syndrome, acidosis, and intracranial haemorrhage.
• Once the diagnosis of preterm labour has been confirmed, the obstetrician must decide if tocolysis is appropriate to stop the labour or to allow spontaneous labour to continue.
• Tocolytic drugs include β-sympathomimetics, e.g. salbutamol or terbutaline; calcium antagonists, e.g. nifedipine, glyceryl trinitrate; and the oxytocin receptor antagonist—atosiban.
• The greatest benefit of tocolysis is to delay delivery and allow sufficient time for corticosteroid therapy to aid fetal lung maturity.
• Two doses of steroid, e.g. betamethasone, 12h apart, are beneficial if administered to the mother when the gestational age is <34 weeks. Delivery should be delayed until 24h following the first dose if possible.
• The method of delivery of the premature infant <30 weeks is controversial. Some obstetricians would advocate a CS, as labour is too great a stress for the fetus, particularly if growth-restricted.
• There is a higher incidence of operative delivery with the premature fetus; early anaesthetic assessment of the mother and optimization of any co-existing systemic disease is essential.
• If pre-eclampsia is present, request an up-to-date FBC and clotting studies if a regional technique is planned for delivery.
• A woman faced with premature delivery is often very frightened and distressed. Take time to explain the anaesthetic plan of management and answer her concerns.

Management

Labour

- If time permits, an epidural for labour analgesia can be beneficial. It will prevent the early sensation to push prior to full dilatation and a precipitous delivery of the premature baby, which can increase the risk of intracranial haemorrhage.

Caesarean section

- A 'classical' CS with a vertical incision in the uterus may be necessary if the gestational age is <28 weeks. The lower segment of the uterus has not developed at this stage.
- A regional anaesthetic technique is appropriate for either a classical or lower segment CS; however, the dose of LA required to provide an adequate block will be greater than that required for a term CS.
- As the uterus is smaller, due to the preterm fetus and reduced liquor volume, compression of the epidural and subarachnoid spaces will not be as pronounced and therefore will not assist in the cephalad spread of LA to the same degree. The usual intrathecal dose for a term CS may result in an inadequate block.
- A CSE technique has the advantage of extending the block, if the intrathecal component if found to be inadequate on assessment.
- Surgery and extraction of the fetus is often more difficult and the mother and partner are extremely anxious; therefore, an adequate block is essential.
- In the extreme preterm situation, syntocinon may not be fully effective in promoting uterine contraction as the receptors are not fully developed. Ergometrine should be considered post delivery to prevent uterine atony.
- GA is acceptable, but the mother will not see the baby after delivery 'however brief' and sometimes the baby will die before the mother has recovered sufficiently to see her baby.

Placenta praevia

Definition

Placenta praevia occurs when the placenta either completely or partially covers the internal cervical os, or is implanted at its margin. It is associated with considerable morbidity and mortality. The incidence is ~1 in 200 pregnancies, but is higher with previous uterine scars, multiparity, and increasing maternal age.

Grading of placenta praevia

I   placenta extends into the lower uterine segment but does not reach the internal cervical os.

II placenta extends into the lower uterine segment and reaches but does not cover the internal cervical os.

III placenta eccentrically covers the internal cervical os.

IV placenta covers the internal cervical os centrally.

I and II are considered minor praevia, and III and IV major praevia
   The grading can be further divided into anterior and posterior praevia. In anterior placenta praevia, the placenta is frequently incised prior to delivery of the baby which can lead to brisk initial blood-loss.

Key issues

• Placenta praevia can present with painless insidious vaginal bleeding, catastrophic obstetric haemorrhage, or be asymptomatic.

• The management of a patient with placenta praevia will depend on the grading of the praevia at abdominal ultrasound. However, many grading systems have been superseded by ultrasonic techniques relating the leading edge of the placenta to the cervical os.

• Clinical suspicion often follows antepartum bleeding, but is raised in any woman with vaginal bleeding and a high presenting part or abnormal lie, irrespective of previous imaging.

• The differential diagnosis is placental abruption, which is usually associated with abdominal pain and uterine tenderness or irritability. An ultrasound will differentiate these two diagnoses although both problems can be seen together.

Management

Initial resuscitation

• Following presentation with a vaginal bleed, an urgent ultrasound will confirm the diagnosis and the position of the praevia.

• In the event of major haemorrhage, two large-bore cannulae should be inserted and fluid resuscitation commenced.

• Blood should be sent for FBC, clotting studies and 4–6 units of cross-matched blood requested.

Vaginal delivery
- It is possible for a minor praevia, i.e. the leading edge of the placenta must be >2cm away from the os, to have a successful vaginal delivery.
- Epidural analgesia should be encouraged for labour as it may be rapidly extended if a CS is required.
- Continuous fetal monitoring in labour is essential.

Elective caesarean section
- Women with major placenta praevia who have bled are usually admitted and managed as an in-patient from the time of their first major bleed. They may have repeat episodes of bleeding, each time being managed with resuscitation, sometimes requiring blood transfusion, and close observation of mother and fetus.
- Whenever possible, elective CS is delayed until 38 weeks to minimize neonatal morbidity.
- Traditionally, regional anaesthesia has been relatively contraindicated for an elective CS for major praevias. However, an experienced anaesthetist would preferentially manage a major anterior placenta praevia with a regional technique, either a single-shot spinal or preferably a CSE technique.
- CSE has the advantage of extending the regional blockade if surgery becomes prolonged.
- A senior anaesthetist and obstetrician should be present for the CS.
- Two large-bore cannulae should be inserted prior to commencing surgery, and invasive BP monitoring is recommended for a major anterior praevia.
- Major haemorrhage during surgery should be anticipated. This is of particular concern with an anterior placenta praevia as the placenta is frequently incised prior to delivery and considerable haemorrhage can occur before it is possible to give uterotonics. Cross-matched blood should be available in theatre or in the delivery suite fridge prior to surgery.
- Resuscitation of the mother will be optimized by the use of rapid infusion devices, with the facility to warm all infusion fluids. The use of cell salvage has been previously encouraged; however, the results of the SALVO trial would question its role in future.

Emergency caesarean section
GA should be performed in any mother with:
- Uncontrolled bleeding despite resuscitation.
- Cardiovascular instability.
- Coagulopathy.
- Fetal distress.
- As above, a senior anaesthetist and obstetrician should take responsibility for surgery.
- Resuscitation should continue throughout transfer to theatre and preparation for GA.
- It is not advisable to start surgery before blood is available for rapid infusion at the time of uterine incision.

Complications

- PPH is a major risk, due to atony of the lower uterine segment and bleeding from the raw placental bed. Discuss with the obstetrician before starting surgery the plan for additional oxytocics following the first IV dose of oxytocin 5IU.
- Early use of ergometrine, continuous oxytocin infusion, misoprostol PR, and carboprost should be considered.
- The lower segment of the uterus is less responsive to uterotonics, which may be very much less effective than expected.
- If bleeding is uncontrolled following delivery, early use of a B-Lynch suture or intrauterine balloon tamponade may avoid the need for a caesarean hysterectomy.
- Uterine embolization may be considered provided the patient is cardiovascularly stable for transfer or there is sufficient time to organize assistance from interventional radiology in an emergency situation.

Further reading

Harnett MJ et al. Anesthesia for interventional radiology in parturients at risk of major hemorrhage at cesarean section delivery. *Anesthesia and Analgesia* 2006; 103: 1329–1330.

Placenta accreta

Definition

Placenta accreta occurs when a placenta praevia implants over a previous uterine scar, following either previous CS or uterine surgery. The normal cleavage plane between placenta and myometrium is lost, and following delivery it becomes impossible to separate the placenta from the uterus, resulting in potentially life-threatening haemorrhage and the need for a caesarean hysterectomy.

Classification

Dependent upon the extent of infiltration:
- **Placenta accreta**—placenta grows through the endometrium to the myometrium.
- **Placenta increta**—placenta grows into the myometrium.
- **Placenta percreta**—placenta grows through the myometrium to the uterine serosa and on into surrounding structures, e.g. bladder or broad ligament.

Data from Konijeti R., Rajfer J., and Askari A. Placenta Percreta and the Urologist. *Rev Urol.* 2009 Summer; 11(3): 173–176.

Key issues

- The incidence of placenta accreta is rising due to an increase in deliveries by CS, with an incidence of 20–30% in mothers with a placenta praevia and one previous scar, and 40–50% with a placenta praevia and two or more previous CS scars.
- Placenta increta and percreta are both rare but more severe.
- CS is the only possible mode of delivery. This should be planned in advance with a senior anaesthetist and senior obstetrician.
- Preoperative MRI or detailed ultrasound scanning should be performed in those women considered to be at high risk, as the anaesthetic technique and surgical procedure may be influenced by the degree of risk.
- Bleeding at the time of delivery can be catastrophic.

Management

Anaesthetic management
- The anaesthetic management is dictated by the likelihood of major haemorrhage, maternal preference, and the level of obstetric and anaesthetic experience of dealing with such cases.
- The risk of haemorrhage, transfusion, and hysterectomy should be discussed with the patient as part of the consent procedure, and a minimum of 6 units of blood available in theatre prior to surgery.
- The facility for rapid infusion of warmed fluids and blood is essential, and cell salvage is currently recommended.
- Invasive BP monitoring is essential.
- There is increasing evidence to support the safety of regional anaesthesia provided the patient is normovolaemic before neuroaxial techniques are employed.
- CSE would be the regional technique of choice, as the block can be extended if surgery is prolonged.

- In cases of significant haemorrhage and hypovolaemia, fluid resuscitation and conversion to GA is advised.
- Many experienced anaesthetists would still choose to perform an elective CS for a placenta accreta under GA.
- Resuscitation should follow guidance on major obstetric haemorrhage (see Chapter 18).

Surgical management
- Surgery should be performed by a senior obstetrician with skilled surgical assistance, and the equipment to proceed to a hysterectomy readily available.
- The placenta may have to be divided to facilitate delivery.
- Poor contraction of the lower uterine segment causes continued bleeding following delivery.
- A plan for the use of additional oxytocic agents should be decided prior to surgery commencing.

Haemorrhage may be controlled by:
- Bimanual compression of the uterus.
- B-Lynch suture.
- Ligation, embolization, or balloon occlusion of the internal iliac arteries.
- Temporary aortic compression, either manual with the operator's fist, arterial clamp, or with an intra-aortic occlusion balloon.
- Hysterectomy.

Interventional radiology
- Interventional radiology has an increasing role in the management of women with a diagnosed placenta accreta.
- Consideration should be given to preoperative insertion of bilateral internal iliac balloons under radiological control. If uncontrolled bleeding occurred, the balloons could be inflated to occlude the uterine blood supply; however, cases of arterial rupture, limb ischaemia and thrombosis have been described with significant morbidity.
- This has been successfully achieved in many units in the UK and usually necessitates the CS being conducted within the radiology department, which requires advanced planning.
- Uterine embolization may be performed in the emergency situation, provided the mother is cardiovascularly stable for transfer.

Complications
- Continued observation throughout the postnatal period is vital as haemorrhage may be delayed.
- Any ongoing coagulopathy should be corrected.
- Damage to the bladder, ureters, and other surrounding structures may result from surgery.

Further reading
Fitzpatrick, KE et al. The management and outcomes of placenta accreta, increta and percreta in the UK: a population-based descriptive study. *British Journal of Obstetrics and Gynaecology* 2014; 121: 62–71.

Controlled rupture of membranes

Definition

Artificial rupture of membranes (ARM) is a method commonly employed to induce labour, provided the cervix is favourable. A controlled ARM is required when the fetal head is high and not fully engaged in the pelvis. The main danger during a controlled ARM is the cord prolapsing into the birth canal in front of the presenting part and causing severe fetal distress.

Key issues

- Due to the high risk of cord prolapse, a controlled ARM should be performed in the obstetric theatre with facilities and staff fully prepared to proceed to a category 1 CS if necessary.
- Mothers suitable for controlled ARM include those with abnormal lie following stabilization of the fetal head position, polyhydramnios, or multiparity.

Management

- There are a number of possible management options for this procedure and these will ultimately depend on applying a risk–benefit analysis for each individual situation.
- Discussion with the obstetrician regarding the risks of immediate delivery is essential.
- A full explanation of the regional technique, including the possible complications, should be given to the mother and documented.
- An assessment for GA should be made.

Combined spinal–epidural anaesthesia

- A CSE technique will cover all eventual obstetric possibilities.
- The spinal component should be an intrathecal dose sufficient to allow an immediate CS to be performed, e.g. 12.5mg 0.5% heavy bupivacaine + 20 micrograms fentanyl.
- The epidural component can be used for labour analgesia if no complications occur at the time of the ARM.
- In addition, a long-acting opioid can be administered into the epidural space for postoperative analgesia if a CS is required.

Spinal anaesthesia

- Insertion of a single-shot spinal with a sufficient intrathecal dose for CS would cover the immediate concerns of a cord prolapse at the time of ARM.
- If the ARM is uneventful, labour analgesia can be offered, depending on what the mother requests when labour is established,
- This option for regional anaesthesia should be taken if the mother presents any risks for a possible CS under GA, e.g. difficult airway, obesity, malignant hyperpyrexia.

Anaesthetist 'on-standby'
- Instead of choosing to administer a regional technique, which may not be ultimately used, the anaesthetist can be 'on standby' in the operating theatre.
- Some mothers may not want a regional technique.
- If an immediate CS is required due to a prolapsed cord, a GA would be required for delivery.
- This option is not recommended in a mother with significant risks of GA, e.g. the obese patient or an anticipated difficult airway.

Complications

The major risk of this procedure is cord prolapse, precipitating immediate caesarean delivery by GA, if a regional technique has not been administered.

Fetal distress

Definition

The most important thing to appreciate when dealing with cases of 'fetal distress' is that the term covers a wide range of degrees of risk to the fetus. The diagnosis may be made on a variety of criteria, either antenatally or intrapartum, and encountered in numerous different modes of fetal assessment, e.g. CTG, fetal blood sampling, fetal ECG ST analysis (STAN).

The diagnosis of intrapartum fetal distress usually indicates that the obstetrician considers that the fetus needs early or immediate delivery, and the timing of delivery is graded according to the following categories for CS:
- Category 1: threat to life of mother or baby that requires immediate delivery (usually under 30 minutes but more urgent delivery may be required).
- Category 2: compromise to mother or baby that requires early delivery. (Usually 30–60 minutes)
- Category 3: early delivery where neither the baby nor mother is compromised (may be more than 60 minutes).
- Category 4: elective CS (no urgency).

However, there are very few precise methods of diagnosing fetal distress which strongly correlate with measures of poor fetal outcome, either biochemical or clinical.

Key issues
- Effective team-work and communication is essential. Discuss the patient with the obstetrician, midwives, and obstetric theatre team.
- Ascertain the degree of urgency immediately and ask for a review if you feel the situation has changed.
- The mother is your first priority and, as her anaesthetist, her safety is your prime concern. In difficult situations, everyone else will be focused on the baby and you may be the sole voice for the mother. Don't be afraid to speak up for her.

During transfer to theatre, every effort should be made to improve the fetal condition and provide 'intrauterine resuscitation', which includes:
- Position the mother in full left lateral to reduce aorto-caval compression.
- Administer oxygen by face mask.
- Treat hypotension with increments of vasopressor, e.g. IV ephedrine or phenylephrine.
- Stop oxytocic drug infusions.
- Consider tocolytic drugs, e.g. IV terbutaline 100–250 micrograms, IV GTN 50 micrograms, or sublingual GTN 200–400 micrograms.
- Always reassess the situation with the obstetrician after transfer to theatre. Reapply the CTG monitor—if the fetal heart is more reassuring, the options for the anaesthetic technique for delivery should be discussed again. It is common that the degree of urgency has changed and this must be clearly stated to the theatre team.

Management of delivery

- The management of 'fetal distress' depends on the stage of labour and the degree of concern. It is essential to establish immediately with the obstetrician the required 'decision to delivery' time.
- A neonatologist should be contacted as soon as the diagnosis of fetal distress is made to attend the delivery and provide emergency resuscitation of the newborn.

First stage of labour

- 'Fetal distress' during first stage almost always necessitates delivery by emergency CS.
- GA is usually required for a category 1 section when the mother's life is in danger or the 'decision to delivery' time is <15min. In extreme urgency, most anaesthetists would accept that they could achieve anaesthesia more rapidly and reliably with GA.
- It is acceptable to consider performing a 'rapid sequence spinal' for category 1 CS, when the mother's life is not in danger, although the fetus may be significantly distressed. An experienced anaesthetist may decide to have ONE attempt inserting a spinal, whilst the woman is being preoxygenated via a tight-fitting mask and the fetus monitored continuously. If the attempt is successful, the CS may proceed; however, there should be a low threshold for stopping and no time is lost before converting to a GA. There must be no compromise in standards of monitoring or sterility of technique.
- The degree of urgency following the decision for CS can change in either direction, therefore it is vital that the fetal heart is monitored continuously. In some cases, a category 1 CS is rapidly moved to theatre assuming that a GA is necessary, but as the fetal condition stabilizes, perhaps as a result of intrauterine resuscitation, it becomes apparent that there is sufficient time to perform a regional technique or no CS is necessary at all.
- Alternatively, the initial assessment may indicate sufficient time for a regional technique; however, during transfer, deterioration in the fetal condition necessitates a change of plan to a GA.

> In every situation, prompt and effective communication between anaesthetists, midwives and obstetricians is vital.
> It is important for all professionals involved to know their own roles clearly and understand the factors affecting the decision-making of other disciplines.

Second stage of labour

- Fetal distress in the second stage occurs quite frequently when the vertex is visible. This is often successfully managed with experienced midwifery care. The mother should be encouraged to push as effectively as possible to ensure rapid delivery.
- If fetal distress occurs in the second stage of labour, when the presenting part is below the ischial spines, an emergency assisted ventouse or outlet forceps delivery in the delivery room may be appropriate. This may be performed under a pudendal nerve

block—10mL of 1% lidocaine is injected just below and medial to the ischial spines bilaterally, and it should be supplemented with perineal infiltration for the episiotomy.
- If the obstetrician considers a trial of instrumental delivery to be appropriate, the woman should be transferred rapidly to the obstetric theatre with continuous fetal monitoring in place. This usually occurs when the fetal head is still in the mid-cavity of the pelvis or malpresented. Stay with the mother and, if a good working epidural is *in situ*, start topping up the epidural block immediately.
- If the decision to delivery time is <15min, the most appropriate decision is an emergency CS. It is essential that the degree of urgency for CS is discussed before deciding on a particular anaesthetic technique. Again, stay with the mother and, if a good working epidural is *in situ*, start topping up the epidural block immediately.

Further information on the anaesthetic technique is detailed in Chapters 11 and 12.

Recognition of the 'at risk' fetus

Regular communication with the midwives and obstetricians while working in the delivery suite is of paramount importance to enable you to spot the 'at risk' fetus and form an early management plan of 'what to do if ... ' in your mind. It is good practice to attend all staff handover rounds and have regular updates on new admissions and each woman's progress in labour.

'At risk' labour includes:

Maternal factors
- Slow labour, induced or augmented with syntocinon.
- Induction for >2 weeks postdates.
- Pre-eclampsia.

Fetal factors
- IUGR ('small for dates').
- Meconium staining of liquor.
- Poor biophysical profile.
- Fetal Doppler studies showing absent or reversed end-diastolic flow in the umbilical arteries.
- Fetal abnormalities.
- Twins.

> Identification of any of these conditions in early labour allows time for an early epidural block to be established in the usual way, which could then be topped-up for all but the most immediate of CS.

Further reading

Lucas D et al. Urgency of caesarean section: a new classification. *Journal of the Royal Society of Medicine* 2000; 93: 346–350.

Cord prolapse

Definition

Cord prolapse occurs when the umbilical cord lies in front of or beside the presenting part, in the presence of ruptured membranes. The incidence of cord prolapse is 0.2–0.4% with a cephalic presentation; however, this increases to 2–4% with multiple pregnancies and malpresentations.

Key issues

Cord prolapse is an obstetric emergency, as compression of the umbilical cord will severely compromise the fetal blood supply and precipitate immediate fetal distress. Delivery by category 1 CS must be performed extremely quickly, i.e. within minutes, to ensure no hypoxic damage to the fetus.

Predisposing factors include:
- High/ill-fitting presenting part.
- High parity.
- Prematurity.
- Multiple pregnancy.
- Polyhydramnios.
- High head at the time of either spontaneous or artificial membrane rupture.

Management

- Although speed is essential, the situation should not prevent a rapid preoperative assessment prior to CS.
- Reassurance and an explanation of the problem must be given to the mother and partner.
- Antacid prophylaxis—ranitidine 50mg IV/omeprazole 40mg IV and 30mL 0.3M sodium citrate PO, should be given.
- Oxygen 15L/min should be administered via a tight-fitting face mask.
- There are two suggested positions to limit the extent of pressure on the umbilical cord during transfer to theatre:
  - Knee–chest.
  - Exaggerated Simm's—left lateral.
- In addition, the presenting part must be pushed out of the pelvis with manual upward pressure by the obstetrician or midwife. This must continue until surgery is commenced.
- Alternatively, the presenting part can be pushed out of the pelvis by filling the bladder with 400–700mL of saline via a catheter, which often also inhibits uterine contractions.
- If time allows, tocolytic drugs are used to stop labour, as uterine contractions make it difficult to prevent excessive cord pressure, e.g. IV salbutamol or terbutaline 100–250 micrograms, or IV GTN 50–100 micrograms.
- If fetal blood supply remains compromised, GA is the only option and a standard technique is applied with the usual safety precautions.

- The drugs required for a GA should always be prepared in advance and refrigerated, in the event of a category 1 CS for cord prolapse.
- Regional anaesthesia may be considered by an experienced anaesthetist only if the cord is free from compression and there is no evidence of fetal compromise, which is more likely with bladder filling.
- Standard spinal anaesthesia in the lateral position is the regional technique of choice.
- Topping-up an *in situ* epidural should only be used if it is working well and the anaesthetist is very confident that anaesthesia will be satisfactory.
- Simulated drills of cord prolapse involving the delivery suite and theatre teams should be performed regularly, and any learning points from the drills addressed.

Placental abruption

Definition

Placental abruption is defined as premature separation of a normally implanted placenta. There may be a complete or partial separation and it occurs in ~1% of pregnancies.

> ### Key issues
>
> There are many associated risk factors:
> - Pre-eclampsia, eclampsia, or chronic hypertension.
> - Premature rupture of membranes.
> - Increased uterine size, e.g. multiple pregnancy, polyhydramnios.
> - Increasing parity.
> - Previous history of abruption.
> - Amniocentesis.
>
> Classical signs include: abdominal pain, haemorrhage, uterine tenderness or irritability, coagulopathy, fetal distress or demise.
> - The presence of abdominal pain often differentiates an abruption from bleeding secondary to a placenta praevia.
> - It may present with either profound revealed or concealed bleeding, requiring rapid resuscitation of the mother. Blood loss with a concealed retroplacental haemtoma is frequently underestimated.
> - Close observation of the mother is required as cardiovascular stability is often maintained until >40% of circulating blood volume is lost.
> - Coagulation abnormalities occur early following an abruption with very low platelet numbers and fibrinogen <1g/L. VHA fibrogen estimation is very helpful. Urgent correction of a coagulopathy is necessary to minimize further maternal bleeding.
> - Stabilization of the mother and immediate delivery can be life saving for the mother and fetus.
> - The perinatal mortality rate following a major placental abruption is as high as 50%.

Management

- Establish IV access with two large-bore cannulae and commence fluid resuscitation, administer oxygen by face mask, give 1 gram IV tranexamic acid and send blood for urgent FBC, nearside fibrinogen estimation or thromboelastography, and clotting studies, and cross-match 4–6 units of blood, depending on the degree of concern.
- Following VHA point of care testing results, early administration of fibrinogen concentrate, platelets, and additional clotting products can be life saving to the mother.
- Rapid assessment of the cardiovascular status of the mother and viability and gestational age of the fetus is important, as this will determine the ultimate obstetric management of delivery.

Viable fetus
- If bleeding is minimal or has stopped, the mother is haemodynamically stable, and the fetus not compromised, it may be appropriate to adopt a watch and wait policy, particularly if the gestational age is <34 weeks. The mother should be given betamethasone to aid fetal lung maturity. The mother should stay on the delivery suite for close maternal and fetal monitoring, and the decision for delivery reviewed regularly.
- If bleeding continues and/or the fetus demonstrates signs of distress, immediate delivery by CS is indicated.
- CS should not be delayed until blood results, cross-matched blood, or blood products are available, if the mother or fetus remain compromised.

Choice of anaesthetic technique
- GA is the technique of choice for the mother who is cardiovascularly compromised, or coagulopathy is present or suspected.
- Resuscitation of the mother will be optimized by the use of rapid infusion devices with the facility to warm all infusion fluids.
- Invasive BP and CVP monitoring should be considered if the mother remains cardiovascularly unstable or if there is evidence of co-existing pre-eclampsia.
- Regular VHA point of care and/or laboratory checks on platelet count and clotting studies should be performed.
- Regional anaesthesia is not contraindicated provided the mother is normovolaemic and there is no evidence of clotting abnormalities. A single-shot spinal technique would be appropriate.
- If an abruption becomes apparent during labour and the mother has a working epidural in situ, it may be safely 'topped-up' for the CS.
- Despite the urgency of the situation, it is important to complete a rapid preoperative anaesthetic assessment and not forget to administer antacid prophylaxis.

Dead fetus
- If the placental separation has caused intrauterine death, vaginal delivery is the preferred mode, provided there is no ongoing catastrophic maternal haemorrhage.
- The uterus frequently becomes irritable, and precipitous delivery is characteristic.
- Clotting abnormalities are very common.
- Following resuscitation, any coagulopathy should be corrected, and platelet and clotting studies re-checked regularly.
- Epidural analgesia is not contraindicated for labour, provided the clotting results are entirely normal and platelet count >100.

Complications
- Always exclude co-existing pre-eclampsia when faced with a placental abruption. Effective fluid management can be difficult and the mother can rapidly develop pulmonary oedema.
- The risk of uterine atony following delivery is increased, particularly if blood has extravasated into the uterine musculature, i.e Couvelaire uterus. At CS, all blood clots should be fully evacuated from the uterus

and the uterus massaged to aid contraction. Additional oxytocics may be required to maintain uterine contraction, e.g. IV/IM ergometrine, IV oxytocin infusion, or misoprostol PR.
- DIC complicates ~10% of all abruptions but is more common if fetal death has occurred. DIC causes consumption of factors I, II, V, and VIII, and platelets. Use of VHA fibrinogen estimation is very useful to guide early management of clotting abnormalities. DIC is reversed by transfusion of fibrinogen concentrate, FFP, and platelets, under the guidance of the haematologist.
- Acute renal failure may result if DIC or hypovolaemia remains uncorrected.

Instrumental vaginal delivery

Definition

An instrumental delivery facilitates successful vaginal delivery and may be performed with either a suction device (ventouse) or forceps. The type of forceps can be further subdivided into outlet (Wrigleys), non-rotational (Neville–Barnes), or rotational (Keillands) forceps.

> ### Key issues
>
> The reason for instrumental delivery should be clarified with the obstetrician at the time the decision is made, together with an assessment of the likelihood of success.
>
> Reasons include:
> * Failure to progress in the second stage of labour (usually >2h).
> * Maternal exhaustion.
> * Presence of significant cardiac disease.
> * Fetal distress.
>
> These factors guide any decisions about the most appropriate place to conduct the delivery, i.e. the delivery room or theatre, and the type of anaesthetic that will be required.
> * If there is any doubt regarding the estimation of success of an instrumental delivery, the mother should be transferred to theatre for the procedure.
> * Anything other than a simple 'lift-out' technique will require the mother to be prepared to proceed for emergency CS if the instrumental delivery is unsuccessful.

Management

Simple 'lift-out'
* This may be appropriate if the fetal head is very low and there is a very high likelihood of successful vaginal delivery.
* Perineal anaesthesia, S2–S5, is essential for any assisted vaginal delivery.
* In patients without a working epidural, the obstetrician may choose to perform a pudendal nerve block, for a simple 'lift-out' procedure with either a ventouse or outlet forceps in the delivery room. Further local anaesthetic should be infiltrated for the episiotomy.
* If the patient has a working epidural in situ, a light 'top-up' of ~10mL of 0.25% bupivacaine or levobupivacaine can be given, preferably with the mother in a sitting position to ensure a dense sacral block.
* Care should be taken to ensure that all appropriate monitoring and emergency drugs are readily available, whenever an epidural is 'topped-up' in the delivery room.

Trial of instrumental delivery

- If the obstetrician considers a 'trial of instrumental delivery' to be appropriate, the woman should be transferred to the obstetric theatre. This usually occurs when the fetal head is still in the mid-cavity of the pelvis or malpresented. If there is no fetal compromise, transfer the mother before topping-up an epidural. If there is fetal compromise, stay with the mother and, if a good working epidural is *in situ*, start topping-up the epidural block immediately.
- A trial of instrumental delivery should always be performed in the operating theatre with the equipment and staff to proceed to immediate CS.
- A GA is not usually indicated for a vaginal delivery, as the mother cannot bear down and it is likely to fail.

Prior to transfer to theatre

- A thorough preoperative assessment should be completed, followed by an explanation of the anaesthetic technique and delivery plan, including the possibility and consequences of proceeding to CS.
- FBC and a request for blood group and save should be sent to the laboratory immediately. However, it may be necessary to proceed to theatre before the results are available.
- Make it your responsibility to ensure prompt transfer to a well-prepared theatre.
- Assess the sensory and motor block if an epidural is in situ, review the timing of last top-up and consider commencing a further epidural top-up if it has worked well for labour analgesia.
- Stay with the mother and ensure regular BP measurements are performed and hypotension promptly treated.
- Review need for further antacid prophylaxis.

Anaesthetic techniques

- A dense sensory sacral block extending to T10 will be required for the instrumental delivery, with the facility to extend the sensory block rapidly to light touch to T5 if the instrumental delivery fails.
- When deciding on the anaesthetic technique, a balance must be struck between ensuring the woman is able to push as effectively as possible and providing the ideal conditions for rapid conversion to a CS.
- The anaesthetic technique will depend on whether an epidural has been sited for labour analgesia and its efficacy. If no epidural is in place, the decision between a single-shot spinal and a CSE technique is often determined by the time available.

Epidural top-up

- If an epidural is *in situ*, review how it has performed in labour and the timing of the last top-up, and assess the sensory block prior to commencing with further incremental top-ups.
- If there is a high likelihood of successful vaginal delivery and the epidural has been functioning well, 10mL of 0.5% bupivacaine or levobupivacaine + 50–100 micrograms fentanyl should be given and the

block re-assessed. Anaesthetists sometimes favour 2% lidocaine with the addition of adrenaline and bicarbonate as it may be faster acting.
- Ensure evidence of sacral anaesthesia prior to starting the instrumental extraction.
- Incremental epidural top-ups in this way will still allow effective maternal effort for pushing, without causing intercostal motor block.
- If attempted instrumental delivery is unsuccessful, a further 10–15mL of 0.5% bupivacaine or levobupivacaine +/– 50–100 micrograms of fentanyl should be given and the sensory and motor block re-assessed for CS.
- Epidural diamorphine or morphine may be administered for postoperative analgesia if a CS becomes necessary.

Spinal anaesthesia
- If a spinal is inserted, the dose MUST be sufficient for delivery to proceed to a CS.
- The woman's ability to push will be reduced by the higher intercostal motor blockade.
- The addition of a long-acting opioid, e.g. intrathecal morphine, may prove to be unnecessary if the trial is successful, but post-delivery monitoring for late respiratory depression must be the same as after a caesarean delivery.
- Alternatively, the decision to omit a long-acting opioid from the intrathecal mixture will increase postoperative pain scores if a CS is necessary, and LA nerve blocks and parenteral opioids will be required.

Combined spinal–epidural
- A CSE technique confers advantages if a *de novo* regional technique is required.
- A low dose spinal technique, e.g. 5mg bupivacaine and 10–20 micrograms fentanyl, will facilitate a pain-free instrumental delivery. However, if vaginal delivery is unsuccessful, the epidural may be topped-up incrementally with 5–10mL aliquots of 0.5% bupivacaine or levobupivacaine until an adequate sensory block for CS is achieved.

- It is essential that the anaesthetist fully understands all obstetric possibilities when proceeding with a trial of instrumental delivery.
- Failure of instrumental delivery may necessitate an immediate and often very difficult CS; the lower the fetal head, the more difficult the CS will be.
- Inadequate regional anaesthesia will require conversion to GA.

Complications

- Following a prolonged labour, difficult or failed instrumental vaginal delivery, the mother is at risk of major PPH either due to uterine atony or following trauma of the structures within the birth canal.
- An infusion of oxytocin should be continued following delivery, with close observation of the mother in the immediate postpartum period for bleeding.
- Bleeding is often underestimated, particularly if a prolonged repair of the perineum is required or the instrumental delivery fails. Weigh all swabs to assess blood loss accurately or observe for continued bleeding from the vagina during surgery.
- A difficult instrumental delivery will be painful in the postnatal period. Consider epidural diamorphine or morphine if a large episiotomy has been performed or extensive vaginal tear has occurred.
- Ensure adequate analgesia is prescribed regularly, with a laxative to prevent constipation.

Uterine inversion

Definition

Puerperal uterine inversion is the displacement of the fundus of the uterus, usually occurring during the third stage of labour, and is a serious but infrequent complication of childbirth. Although rare, it can be a life-threatening emergency due to associated blood loss and cardiovascular instability.

Key issues

The reported incidence of uterine inversion varies considerably in the literature and is quoted to be between 1 in 2000 and 1 in 40,000 births.
It may be classified as:
- Complete—the fundus passes through the cervix.
- Incomplete—the fundus remains above the cervix.
- May complicate excessive cord traction at CS.
  The contributing causal factors include:
- Fundal implantation of the placenta.
- Excessive cord traction or pulling on the placenta prior to the beginning of placental separation.
- Poor uterine tone.
- Abnormal adherence of the placenta.

The classical presentation of uterine inversion is an obviously displaced uterus during placental delivery, which is commonly associated with PPH, severe pain, and clinical shock that appears out of proportion to the blood loss.
- Shock is thought to be due, in part, to the parasympathetic response to traction on the uterine suspensory ligaments, and may be associated with profound bradycardia.
- This is an obstetric emergency and there should be no delay in instituting treatment.

Management

- Treatment of haemorrhagic shock, i.e. high flow oxygen, aggressive IV fluid resuscitation, atropine to treat any bradycardia, and replacement of the uterus must occur simultaneously.
- Any delay in replacement of the uterus will increase uterine oedema, impeding later replacement, and may exacerbate cardiovascular instability.
- Immediate GA is usually required to facilitate uterine replacement unless a spinal or recently topped-up epidural is already *in situ*.

Replacement of uterus

This may be achieved by:
- Manual replacement—the uterus is pushed back through the cervix to its normal position.

- Hydrostatic correction—the woman is placed in a steep Trendelenberg position, warm normal saline is delivered to the posterior fornix of the vagina which causes gradual stretching of the orifice, aiding correction of the inversion.
- The use of an intrauterine tamponade balloon may be placed to reduce the risk of reinversion.

If unsuccessful, tocolytic drugs can be given to increase cervical relaxation:
- β_2 receptor agonists—salbutamol 250 micrograms IV bolus.
- Magnesium sulphate—4g IV over 10min.
- GTN—50–100 micrograms IV bolus.
- The halogenated vapour of GA agents will cause uterine and cervical relaxation.

Severe cases may require laparotomy and combined abdominal–vaginal correction.

Complications

Severe PPH is the most frequent consequence of uterine inversion.

Further reading

Haeri S et al. Intrauterine tamponade balloon use in the treatment of uterine inversion. *BMJ Case Reports* 2015; pii: bcr2014206705.

EXIT procedures

Definition

Ex utero intrapartum treatment (EXIT) procedures offer the advantage of performing life-saving upper airway surgery on a newborn baby at the time of CS, before the umbilical cord is severed and therefore maintaining uteroplacental gas exchange until an airway can be secured.

> ### Key issues
>
> The range of indications for EXIT procedures include:
> - Congenital high airway obstruction syndrome.
> - Reversal of tracheal balloon occlusion when managing severe congenital diaphragmatic hernia.
> - Giant fetal neck masses.
> - Lung or mediastinal tumours.
> - Transfer from EXIT to ECMO (extracorporeal membrane oxygenation).
>
> The advantage of EXIT procedures is that they allow for intubation and ventilation at birth.
> - If intubation is not possible, fetal tracheostomy can be performed, or any lung or neck masses causing anatomical distortion can be resected on placental support.
> - The mother usually requires GA for the CS, with increased volatile concentration (2–3 MAC) to facilitate prolonged uterine relaxation.
> - Uterine relaxation and placental circulation have been maintained for as long as 2–3h to enable secure airway management prior to delivery of the fetus.

Management

The key aims of management are:
- Partial delivery of the fetus.
- Prolonged uterine relaxation.
- Preservation of the uteroplacental circulation.
- Delayed uteroplacental separation.

Procedure
- Preoperative indometacin 50mg rectally is given prophylactically as a tocolytic, and routine antacid prophylaxis.
- A lumbar epidural catheter may be sited for intraoperative and postoperative pain relief.
- Rapid sequence induction of anaesthesia is performed, with left lateral tilt.
- High doses (2–3 MAC) of inhalational agents are used to maintain uterine relaxation.
- IV GTN or terbutaline may also be administered to reduce uterine tone.
- Maternal BP must be maintained in order to continue perfusion through the placenta.
- Administration of agents causing smooth muscle relaxation is balanced against vasopressors and fluid administration as necessary.

- Using ultrasound, the placental edges are mapped and the hysterotomy performed avoiding the placenta.
- The fetal head is exposed and intubation can be attempted.
- The indication for the EXIT procedure will determine the fetal exposure necessary; this should be kept to a minimum in order to reduce heat loss and the risk of umbilical cord compromise or premature placental detachment.
- The key to successful outcome of EXIT procedures is the co-ordination of multiple personnel from various disciplines including anaesthesia, paediatric surgery, obstetrics, radiology, neonatology, and midwifery.

Further reading

Dahlgren G et al. Four cases of the ex-utero intrapartum treatment (EXIT) procedure: anaesthetic implications. *International Journal of Obstetrics and Anesthesia* 2004; 13: 178–182.

Retained placenta

Definition

The third stage of labour involves the separation, descent, and delivery of the placenta. The retroplacental myometrium must contract, allowing the placenta to come away from its bed and be expelled. The placenta is considered retained if it fails to deliver within 60min of birth.

Key issues

Retained placenta is a common cause of PPH with an incidence of ~2% worldwide, and is a significant cause of maternal morbidity and mortality. The reasons may be broadly divided into:
- Failed separation due to poor or absent uterine contraction.
- Failed separation due to morbid adherence, e.g. to a fibroid, uterine scar or in the presence of placenta accreta.
- Successful separation but retained by a contracted uterus and closed cervical os.

Risk factors for a retained placenta include:
- Previous retained placenta.
- Snapped umbilical cord.
- Previous injury to or scarring of uterus.
- Preterm delivery.
- Induced labour.
- Multiparity.

Management

Early management
- Initial management may be conservative, e.g. bladder emptying and waiting for signs of spontaneous separation and delivery of the placenta.
- Early initiation of breastfeeding may assist placental separation.
- Active management of the third stage involves use of IM oxytocin and ergometrine mixture (Syntometrine®) or oxytocin alone, with controlled cord traction after uterine contraction.
- A second dose of Syntometrine® should be given, followed by an oxytocin infusion at 10IU/h to aid separation.
- Blood loss may be concealed, and close observation for maternal pallor, tachycardia, and hypotension must be maintained:
- Establish IV access with a large-bore cannula.
- Measure blood loss and assess cardiovascular stability.
- Check FBC ± clotting studies, and send sample for group and save or cross-match depending on blood loss.
- Alternative non-surgical therapies include umbilical venous injection of saline, plasma expanders, or prostaglandins.
- If the placenta has not been expelled after 1h of oxytocin infusion or there is significant bleeding ± haemodynamic instability, the placenta must be removed manually.

Manual removal of placenta

- Manual removal of placenta should be performed in the theatre environment, preferably under regional anaesthesia, provided no contraindications exist, e.g. uncorrected hypovolaemia, coagulopathy.
- A sensory (temperature) block to T6 is required for pain-free manual removal of placenta as the uterine fundus is often manipulated.
- Always assess the sacral component of the block before surgery starts.
- Regional anaesthesia may be established by:

Epidural top-up

- 15–20mL 0.5% bupivacaine ± short-acting opioid e.g. 50 micrograms fentanyl should be administered if there is an indwelling epidural catheter.
- Continuous monitoring of ECG and pulse oximetry, and intermittent BP should be performed.

Spinal anaesthesia

- 2.0–2.5mL heavy 0.5% bupivacaine ± short-acting opioid, e.g. 15–20 micrograms fentanyl, should be injected into the intrathecal space.
- Site the spinal with the mother in the lateral position if she is uncomfortable.
- A full CS dose of intrathecal LA should be used as the postpartum uterus does not augment the extent of cephalad spread of LA.

General anaesthesia

- GA may be required for the haemodynamically unstable mother or if a coagulopathy prevents a regional technique.
- Antacid prophylaxis should be given and a standard rapid sequence induction performed.
- The halogenated volatile agents will assist placenta removal by providing greater uterine relaxation; however, they may precipitate increased postpartum bleeding.

Additional uterine relaxants

- Glyceryl trinitrate: During regional anaesthesia, aliquots of GTN are effective, i.e. sublingual spray or 50–100 micrograms IV as required.
- Beta-sympathomimetics: Salbutamol or terbutaline will assist uterine relaxation.

On placental delivery, administer 5IU oxytocin IV bolus (with caution if patient is hypotensive) and commence an infusion of 40IU oxytocin in 500mL normal saline over 4h.

Complications

- Primary PPH or secondary (delayed) PPH, due to retained placental fragments.
- Cervical shock—profound bradycardia and hypotension, precipitated by increased vagal tone, when the placenta sits in the open cervix.
- Uterine inversion.
- Postpartum sepsis. Prophylactic antibiotics are usually administered.

Suturing the perineum

Definition

Perineal trauma may occur spontaneously during vaginal birth or by surgical incision, i.e. episiotomy, where an incision is intentionally made to increase the diameter of the vulval outlet to facilitate delivery.

Episiotomy rates vary considerably according to individual practices and policies of staff and institutions. In the UK, an estimated 85% of women having a vaginal birth will sustain some degree of perineal trauma and, of these, 60–70% will require suturing.

Clinical classification of spontaneous tears

- 1st degree—injury to the skin only.
- 2nd degree—injury to the perineum involving perineal muscles but not the anal sphincter.
- 3rd degree—injury to perineum involving the anal sphincter.
- 4th degree—injury to the perineum involving the anal sphincter and anal epithelium.

Key issues

There are a number of recognized risk factors for perineal trauma:
- Primiparity.
- Fetal birth weight >4000g.
- Prolonged second stage of labour.
- Instrumental delivery.
- Direct occipito-posterior position.
- Maternal factors: age, nutritional status.
- Perineal trauma can be associated with significant post-delivery haemorrhage, which is often underestimated. Continuing vaginal bleeding should always be investigated. High vaginal or cervical lacerations may be missed and continuing bleeding falsely attributed to uterine atony.
- Perineal trauma causes significant pain and discomfort in the immediate postdelivery period and in the longer term.
- Examination and suturing should be performed as soon as possible to reduce bleeding, pain and the risk of infection.

Management

- Assess the mother for signs of hypovolaemia, establish IV access, and send samples for FBC, clotting studies, and group, and save or cross-match depending on measured blood loss.
- Perineal trauma is conventionally repaired in three layers; deep and superficial perineal muscle layers, vaginal tissue, and skin.

First- and second-degree tears

Superficial suturing of the perineum is usually performed with local infiltration instilled by the obstetrician or midwife, or an epidural top-up should be given if an indwelling epidural catheter is present, e.g. 10mL 0.1–0.25% bupivacaine to establish a perineal block.

Third- and fourth-degree tears

More extensive suturing of the perineum usually requires transfer to the operating theatre for further assessment, and both anaesthetic and surgical management.

To facilitate adequate anaesthesia of the sacral dermatomes, the anaesthetic options for management are:

Epidural top-up

- 10mL 0.5% bupivacaine with a short-acting opioid may be administered via an indwelling epidural catheter, preferably with the mother sitting up or with 45° head-up tilt.
- Always assess the sacral component of the sensory block prior to allowing suturing to commence.

Spinal anaesthesia

- 1.5–2mL heavy 0.5% bupivacaine with a short-acting opioid should be injected into the intrathecal space.
- Site the spinal with the mother in the lateral position if she is uncomfortable, and sit her up or with 45° head-up tilt as soon as possible thereafter.
- The postpartum uterus does not augment the extent of cephalad spread of LA to the same degree as the pregnant uterus.

General anaesthesia

- GA may be necessary to achieve adequate muscle relaxation and visualization for surgical repair of severe or complex lacerations, or for delayed or revision of suturing.
- GA may be required for the haemodynamically unstable mother or if a coagulopathy prevents a regional technique.
- Antacid prophylaxis should be given and a rapid sequence induction performed on all mothers requiring GA within 24h of delivery.

Complications

- Perineal trauma can cause significant PPH. Check FBC following the repair.
- Significant pain and discomfort can follow perineal tears or an episiotomy. Consider epidural diamorphine or morphine if an extensive repair has been performed. Prescribe balanced analgesia regularly for the postpartum period.
- Beware of opioid analgesia causing constipation and straining at defaecation. A regular laxative should be prescribed with all opioids.
- Urinary and faecal incontinence may be apparent in the early postpartum period.
- Urinary retention. A catheter is frequently left *in situ* for the first 24h. If this is not the case, then specific observations should be mandatory.

Chapter 15

Postpartum review and problems

Sarah Harries

Post-delivery ward round and documentation

- Documentation of all anaesthetic procedures performed in the delivery suite and obstetric theatre should be completed both in the patient's medical notes and as a separate anaesthetic register of work. This may be paper-based or more typically in electronic format.
- The surgical procedure, anaesthetic technique, obstetric indication and urgency, relevant medical history, and any complications should all be documented.

The anaesthetic register of procedures is an essential tool in maintaining continuity of care and effective communication between the doctors at handover times and during post-delivery ward rounds.

The post-delivery ward round should be informal, respecting the mother's privacy, and happen at least once a day.

The following can be reviewed:

- Maternal satisfaction.
- Any difficulties during the anaesthetic procedure explored.
- Consequences of problems encountered, e.g. inadequate analgesia, dural tap etc.
- Time interval between request and labour analgesia.
- Post-delivery analgesia.
- Fluid balance, blood transfusion, and post-delivery haemoglobin.
- Mobilization.
- Pruritis.
- Micturition.
- Neurological recovery and deficits.
- Thromboprophylaxis.
- Discussion regarding early discharge in line with enhanced recovery protocols.

The outcome of the post-delivery ward round and any action taken must be documented. The community midwife or GP should be informed of ongoing problems, e.g. headache, with written information in the mother's handheld notes or a letter. More serious problems can be communicated via the local community midwifery office.

- The ward round gives the anaesthetist an opportunity to continue care in the post-delivery phase and to address any concerns the mother may have.
- It is an excellent time for formal and informal feedback between a senior and trainee anaesthetist about techniques used.
- Information and feedback from the mother can be used as part of the anaesthetic trainee's workplace-based assessment.
- Documentation of appropriate levels of monitoring after operative delivery or administration of opioids can be checked.
- Adequacy of post-delivery analgesia, both caesarean and vaginal, can be verified.

Early identification of dissatisfaction

- It is an ideal time for a senior anaesthetist to identify and talk to the mother who has been less than satisfied with her anaesthetic care.
- Addressing issues at this early stage can avoid potential complaints or litigation later.
- The incidence of litigation is high in obstetric practice and is most frequently due to inadequate analgesia, but delay in providing analgesia is also a problem.
- Patients can expect an accurate and honest explanation of events, with an apology if there are shortcomings.
- All discussions with the mother should be formally documented.
- Some mothers may need more than one follow-up, and the anaesthetic register can be used to continue their follow-up care, e.g. persistent headache, neurological symptoms or signs.
- All documentation should be legible and complete, with a signature and surname in capitals.
- It is not uncommon for complaints to be received many months or years following the delivery, when reference to accurate documentation is essential.
- In addition, the anaesthetic register can also be used for purposes of clinical audit or as a reference guide for the anaesthetic management of rare medical disorders complicating pregnancy.
- The post-delivery ward round and accompanying documentation should form part of the anaesthetic care and be given the same importance as intrapartum care.

Maternal satisfaction

- Maternal satisfaction about the experience of childbirth is mentioned frequently, but poorly defined.
- Maternal satisfaction has many dimensions and is a complex, multifactorial psychological response to childbirth.
- Different methods have been used to quantify maternal satisfaction, e.g. post-delivery interviews, self-completed questionnaires with visual analogue scales, verbal numerical scales, and question and answers.
- Studies of maternal satisfaction have traditionally assumed good analgesia as the most important factor, but this view has been dispelled in many surveys.
- In some surveys, mothers with epidurals and the best analgesia were less satisfied, probably because of the complexity of their labour.

Factors that improve maternal satisfaction
- Support in labour.
- Listening to the woman's concern.
- Kindness and compassion of staff.
- Continuity of care.
- Antenatal class attendance.
- Vaginal delivery.
- Privacy.
- Requested and expected labour analgesia.

- Information and support are considered to be the most important factors for mothers.
- Labour analgesia is placed low on the indicators for maternal satisfaction.
- Women having a CS found the lack of control a less fulfilling experience.
- Maternal age, social class, income, marital status, support of the partner, planned vs unplanned pregnancy, previous terminations, depression, and ethnicity are other factors which influence maternal satisfaction greatly.
- Epidural analgesia for labour has been the focus for anaesthetists with regards to maternal satisfaction.
- Low dose epidurals have improved the quality and safety of anaesthesia, and retaining motor power improves satisfaction.
- PCEA confers no advantage over an intermittent bolus regimen in relation to maternal satisfaction.
- During elective CS, lower pre-operative anxiety is associated with greater maternal satisfaction and better recovery.
- Information provided by the anaesthetist and perceived emotional support is also of importance.
- It may be possible to identify women with high anxiety and facilitate satisfaction and recovery through additional support.

- The time of assessment of satisfaction is also very important as maternal satisfaction alters with time.
- The ideal time for satisfaction assessment is not known.
- Maternal satisfaction is multifactorial, therefore it is difficult to draw conclusions solely from anaesthetic studies as they usually concentrate on the dimension of pain relief.
- Effective pain relief may be the top priority for the anaesthetist, but not necessarily the priority of the mother.

Backache in pregnancy

Simple backache assessment and advice

Background
- Back pain affects 50% of women during pregnancy and 40% of women postpartum.
- One-third of pregnant women report that it is a severe problem, interfering with normal daily life and their ability to work.
- A multidisciplinary approach to management should be adopted.
- Advice and the treatment options provided by experienced obstetric physiotherapists are invaluable.

Postulated causes of back pain during pregnancy
- Rapid postural changes and altered biomechanics.
- Endocrine changes (relaxin) soften ligaments around the pelvis and increase joint laxity.
- Engorgement of epidural veins. There are case reports of distended epidural and paravertebral veins causing nerve root compression.

Risk factors
- Previous back pain (especially during previous pregnancies).
- Increasing parity.
- Physically strenuous and unrewarding employment.
- Repetitive lifting and bending.
- Young age.

Management of back pain

Prevention
- Maintaining a good level of fitness prior to pregnancy.
- Patient education early in pregnancy.
- Back care (correct posture, rolling and lifting techniques).
- Cessation of smoking is thought to reduce the severity of back pain and the risk of intervertebral disc prolapse.

Good back care
- *Lying*—Ensure comfortable sleeping and resting positions. May require extra pillows for support. Avoid positions of unsupported rotation.
- *Rolling techniques*—Roll with legs adducted and knees flexed. Turn head in direction of roll. Lead with top arm across chest and lay outside knee on inside leg to facilitate rolling of the mid and lower trunk, respectively.
- *Sitting*—Maintain good posture. Buttocks well back on seat, thighs fully supported for most of their length and hips and knees at 90°. Feet supported flat on floor. Spine fully supported allowing natural curvature.
- *Standing*—Weight evenly distributed over both feet. Feet apart and slightly angled, knees off stretch. Avoid trunk on hip flexion and twisting movements, particularly when load bearing.
- *Lifting*—Avoid heavy lifting. Hold load close to the centre of mass. Bend at the knees.

Analgesia options
See Chapter 5.

Physiotherapy management options
- Multi-disciplinary input is essential to manage mothers with significant backache or pelvic girdle pain in the postpartum period.
- Early involvement and assessment by an obstetric physiotherapist prior to discharge is very helpful.
- Physiotherapist led group post-natal classes to address postpartum recovery of abdominal muscle strength and conditioning also benefits mothers in the longer term.

Advice on long-term backache following epidurals
- It is very common to have localized tenderness and bruising at the site of epidural insertion, particularly if there were multiple attempts with the Tuohy needle.
- This will resolve spontaneously over a few days and is not a cause for concern.
- Simple analgesics such as paracetamol and NSAIDs should be prescribed in the postpartum period.
- Patients can be reassured that there is no association between epidural analgesia and long-term backache.
- Epidurals were implicated in the development of chronic backache in two retrospective studies in the early 1990s. These studies were criticized as the reported antenatal backache rates were much lower than expected.
- Multiple prospective studies have since failed to show an association between long-term backache and epidural analgesia.

Assessment of back pain
- If back pain presents during pregnancy or following delivery, a thorough history and neurological examination is essential before deciding whether further investigations or referral is appropriate.
- There are many causes of back pain that may be unrelated to pregnancy, delivery, or anaesthetic procedure and which must not be missed.

Red Flags—when to ask for help/further investigations
- Bladder or bowel dysfunction.
- Saddle anaesthesia.
- Progressive neurological deficit.
- Back pain associated with fever (especially in immunocompromised or diabetic patients).
- Suspected abscess/haematoma following epidural or spinal anaesthesia, usually indicated by severe deep-seated back pain or a sensation of 'electric shock' radiculopathy pain in the lower and mid-spine or legs.
- History of IV drug abuse.
- Suspected pyelonephritis.
- Recent significant trauma.
- Unexplained weight loss/systemic illness.
- Previous malignancy.

Investigations

- Plain radiographs are unlikely to be of diagnostic benefit in the investigation of lower back pain (with the exceptions of malignancy and trauma) and will expose antenatal mother and baby to ionizing radiation.
- If imaging is required the investigation of choice is MRI. If backache is associated with ANY neurological deficit, an urgent MRI should be requested.
- If there is a suggestion of an infective source, serial WCC, C-reactive protein, and blood cultures should be taken.

Further reading

Russell R, Reynolds F. Back pain, pregnancy and childbirth. *BMJ* 1997; 314: 1062–1063.
Reynolds F. Epidurals and backache: again? *BMJ* 2002; 325: 1037.
Howell CJ et al. Randomised study of long term outcome after epidural versus non-epidural analgesia during labour. *BMJ* 2002; 325: 357–359.

Headache

Headache is a common complaint in the postpartum period and there are many causes. It resolves spontaneously in the majority of cases; however, there is potential for considerable morbidity.

Differential diagnosis

- PDPH is one of the most common causes of headache in the postpartum period.
- In women receiving epidural analgesia, the incidence of dural puncture ranges from 0 to 2.6% and is largely dependent on operator experience.
- 30% of dural punctures are not recognized at the time of epidural insertion and first present in the postpartum period with a classical postural headache.
- After a dural puncture with 16G Tuohy needle, up to 70% of women will report symptoms of PDPH.
- It is always important to consider other causes of headache to avoid serious morbidity.

Surveys have reported that 39% of women suffer symptoms of headache unrelated to dural puncture following delivery.

> ### Other causes of postpartum headache
> - Non-specific (tension) headache frequently associated with fatigue.
> - Pre-eclampsia (30% of eclampsia occurs in the postpartum period).
> - Dehydration.
> - Migraine.
> - Sinus headache.
> - Viral, bacterial, or chemical meningitis.
> - Intracranial haemorrhage.
> - Cerebral venous thrombosis.
> - Intracranial tumour.
> - Cerebral infarction.
> - Drugs.
> - Benign intracranial hypertension.

Aetiology of PDPH

Following a dural tap, there is a leak of CSF and a lowering of CSF pressure. There are two possible explanations for the headache:
- The lowering of the CSF pressure causes traction on the pain-sensitive intracranial structures in the upright position and causes the classical postural headache.
- Monro–Kellie hypothesis states that the sum of volumes of the brain, CSF, and blood is constant. When the CSF volume decreases there is a compensatory increase in blood volume. The subsequent venodilatation stretches pain receptors in the vessel wall and causes the headache. There is radiological evidence for this and it forms the basis for some of the therapeutic drug treatments.

Diagnosis of PDPH

Clinical

- Headache is the predominant complaint; it is usually distributed over the frontal and occipital areas, radiating to the neck and shoulders, sometimes associated with neck stiffness.
- It can start almost immediately and is usually present within 72h of dural puncture.
- Headaches in the temporal, vertex, and nuchal areas are less commonly reported.
- The headache is exacerbated by an upright posture and relieved by lying down.
- Pressure over the upper abdomen can cause very temporary relief of PDPH and aid in diagnosis.
- Other associated symptoms are nausea, vomiting, hearing loss, tinnitus, vertigo, dizziness, paraesthesia of scalp, visual disturbances, light intolerance, and cranial nerve palsies.
- Subdural haematoma, cerebral venous sinus thrombosis, cerebral herniation, and death have been reported as a consequence of dural puncture.
- If the headache is not posture related, a diagnosis of PDPH should be questioned and other serious intracranial causes of headache excluded.

Risk factors associated with PDPH

- Female.
- Young.
- Lesser BMI.
- History of chronic or recurrent headache.
- Previous PDPH.
- Large needle.
- Quincke (cutting tip) spinal needles.

Investigations

- When a clinical diagnosis of PDPH cannot be made with certainty, additional tests may be used.
- MRI may demonstrate diffuse dural enhancement, evidence of a sagging brain, and enlargement of the pituitary gland.
- CT myelography or thin section MRI can be used to locate the CSF leak in severe persistent cases.

Management of PDPH

Prevention

The size of the dural perforation is the most important factor for the development of the headache.

Needle size

- A fine gauge spinal needle, 29G, produces a small dural perforation with a lower incidence of headache and a higher failure rate.
- A 25G probably represents the optimum balance between the risk of headache and technical failure.

Needle orientation
- A needle orientated with the cutting tip parallel to the dural fibres may reduce the incidence of PDPH (relevant to Tuohy and Quincke needles only).

Needle design
- Pencil point (atraumatic needles) needles produce fewer headaches than medium bevel cutting needles (Quincke). However, an increased incidence of paraesthesia has been observed with pencil point needles.

Operator skill and fatigue
- An inexperienced operator and fatigue may increase the incidence of inadvertent dural puncture.

Treatment
After diagnosis of a PDPH is made, a rational approach to management must be adopted. The severity of the headache should be assessed and a full explanation of the problem given to the mother.

The natural history of most PDPHs is that they will resolve with time, with anticipated improvement over 5–10 days. Some headaches if left untreated may become chronic. An epidural blood patch (EBP) is considered the optimal treatment for severe PDPH. However, other treatment options can be considered before an EBP is performed:

Simple
- Rehydration.
- Paracetamol, NSAIDs.
- Opioids and antiemetics.
- Comfortable posture—supine posture is not mandatory.
- Psychological support—reassure the mother that in most cases the headache is not harmful.

Caffeine
- Acts by vasoconstriction of the dilated cerebral vessels.
- Dose: 300–500mg oral or IV.
- One cup of coffee contains 50–100mg.
- Therapeutic doses may cause atrial fibrillation or seizures.

Sumatriptan, desmopressin
- Some small case series demonstrating benefit, but no strong evidence for use.

Synthetic ACTH
- Was popular but recent evidence showed it to be ineffective.

Epidural blood patch

The option of an EBP should be offered to women 24–48h after suspected dural puncture when other measures have failed. The benefits of delaying EPB are:

- Clarification of nature of headache.
- Observe for signs of maternal infection.
- Increased success rate after the first 24h. A hypothesis for this is that local anaesthetic has a very small antiplatelet action and may inhibit clot formation over the dural hole.

Contraindications
- Patient refusal.
- Fever associated with a raised WCC.
- Coagulopathy.
- Infection on skin of lower back.
- HIV-positive patients with other active bacterial or viral illness (blood patch has been safely reported in HIV patients without active signs of other infection).

Technique
- Review the anaesthetic record to determine the expected depth of the epidural space before starting.
- Two operators, strict asepsis with hat, gloves, mask, and gown for both.
- A clean, spacious environment is required.
- The lateral position is usually recommended, but the procedure can be carried out in the sitting position if technical difficulties are encountered in the lateral position or the mother finds it more comfortable.
- The Tuohy needle should ideally be inserted into the same intervertebral space as the dural puncture or the one below. Look for puncture marks on skin rather than estimate the intervertebral level.
- 2×20ml blood should be drawn from the antecubital vein under strict asepsis and handed directly to the epidural operator.
- Inject up to 30mL of blood into the epidural space slowly over several minutes. Stop when the mother feels that further injection is painful. Pain can be felt as a deep-seated fullness in the back or as a radiculopathy-type pain in her legs. Less than 10mL of blood can cause these symptoms, and the ability to inject less blood is not associated with a greater failure rate. However, 20ml is considered the optimal therapeutic volume to inject.
- Send remaining blood for culture and sensitivity.
- Bed rest for 1h, then try to mobilize as usual.
- There have been occasional reports of haemodynamic disturbance with EBP.

Mechanism of action of blood patch
- Initially, there is compression of the dural sac, followed by an increase in CSF pressure and cephalad movement of CSF. A dramatic rapid improvement in symptoms is characteristically seen.
- Clot formation follows in minutes to hours. The failure of clot formation over the dural puncture is thought to be the mechanism of secondary failure when the headache returns over hours to days.
- By 7 days, there is fibroblastic activity and collagen formation.
- There is no evidence of axonal oedema, necrosis, or demyelination.

Outcome
- There is a 70% complete and further 20–25% partial success rate if carried out >24h after the dural puncture.
- Further blood patches may be repeated with increasing success.

Complications
- Repeat accidental dural puncture.
- Immediate exacerbation of symptoms and radicular pain.
- Long-term complications are very rare.

Prophylactic blood patch
- Prophylactic blood patch has been performed when blood is given into a resited epidural catheter before removal.
- It cannot be performed if the epidural catheter has been placed intrathecally.
- It is an unnecessary intervention in the 20–30% of women who would not get a headache.
- It is generally thought to be less effective than a deferred blood patch, but the evidence is conflicting.

Additional treatment options
- Epidural saline, dextran 40, and fibrin glue have been utilized, but there is inadequate evidence to support their use.
- In unresponsive patients, surgical closure of the dural perforation may be required.

When to ask for further help
- Severe non-posture headache.
- Atypical presentation of symptoms and signs, especially if sudden and late.
- Other associated symptoms.
- Neurological symptoms or signs.
- Evidence of systemic infection with true meningism.
- Altered level of consciousness.
- Seizures.
- Headache persisting after two epidural blood patches.

Further reading

Russell R et al. Treatment of obstetric post-dural puncture headache. Part 1: conservative and pharmacological management. *International Journal of Obstetric Anesthia* 2018; 38: 93–103.
Russell R et al. Treatment of obstetric post-dural puncture headache. Part 2: epidural blood patch. *International Journal of Obstetric Anesthia* 2018; 38: 104–118.

Neurological complications

Neurological deficit after delivery

- Neurological deficit is well recognized after delivery. The overall incidence is between 11.0 and 27.9 patients per 10,000.
- Maternal obstetric palsy, often termed neuropraxia, is caused by compression or stretching of nerves and nerve roots by the fetal presenting part or abnormal posture adopted by the mother. It most commonly improves after ~72h, but can take months to resolve or occasionally be permanent.
- Maternal obstetric palsies are more common in primiparous women of short stature, a large baby, persistent posterior or transverse position of the fetal head, and in those requiring instrumental delivery, particularly following a prolonged labour.
- The incidence of neurological symptoms following regional anaesthesia has been quoted as 0–36 per 10,000 procedures after epidural and 35 per 10,000 procedures after spinal anaesthesia.
- However, the RCoA NAP3 survey in 2009 quoted a much lower incidence of permanent harm, i.e. following obstetric spinal anaesthesia 1 in 67,000, following obstetric epidural 1 in 161,550 and following CSE 1 in 25,350. Although reassuring for obstetric anaesthetists, there was concern that the obstetric central neural blockade complications in the survey year were under-represented.
- Neurological deficits caused by acute prolapsed intervertebral discs are associated with pregnancy and childbirth and are a reversible cause of injury. They are usually associated with pain, but not invariably. A high index of suspicion is needed to make a rapid diagnosis.

Maternal obstetric palsies

Lumbosacral plexus injury—L4/5, S1/5

- Caused by compression of the lumbosacral trunk against the sacrum by the head of the fetus.
- The classic injury is an L5 compression injury of the nerve root as it passes over the pelvic brim, as illustrated in Fig. 15.1.
- The more posterior L5 root fibres eventually form the common peroneal nerve and are more readily damaged.
- The distribution of the injury results in a foot drop and numbness on the lateral aspect of the lower leg and foot crossing to the great toe.
- It can be clinically difficult to differentiate from a more distal injury.
- The injury most commonly presents on the side of the fetal occiput with a persistent occipital-posterior presentation, as illustrated in Fig. 15.1.
- All forms of rotational delivery are associated with lumbosacral damage.
- Damage by forceps blades can result in injury on the opposite side to the occiput.

Common peroneal neuropathy—L4/5, S1/2

- Caused by compression of the common peroneal nerve as it turns around the head of the fibular.
- Is associated with lithotomy position but can be caused by persistent flexion of the knee and prolonged resting of the leg against a hard surface.

Femoral neuropathy—L2/4
- Forced flexion of the hips causes the femoral nerve to be compressed under the inguinal ligament.

Other neuropathies
- Obturator neuropathy—L2/4. Damaged by the fetal head or forceps.
- Perineal nerve injury—S3/5 caused by deep arrest of the fetal head. Presents with saddle anaesthesia and bladder disturbance.
- Sciatic nerve injury—L4–S1. Occasional reports of damage possibly at the sciatic notch. May be related to prolonged periods of sitting or the supine position with tilt.
- Meralgia paraesthetica—L2/3. Compression of the lateral cutaneous nerve of the thigh. Probably present in late pregnancy, but may be first noted after delivery.

Features of neuropathies
- Obstetric palsies can present with a very mixed picture, making accurate location of the site of injury difficult.
- Motor and sensory fibres may be differently affected within a single nerve.
- Reflexes may or may not be affected.
- Conventional nerve conduction studies can be difficult to perform and interpret because of the proximal site of some nerve injuries.
- In severe or persistent cases, an early neurology opinion is important.
- The neuropathy can be painful and will not respond to conventional analgesia. Neuropathic pain strategies may have to be used.

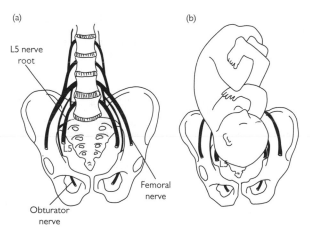

Fig. 15.1 Postpartum neuropathy. (a) The L5 nerve root is especially vulnerable as it emerges over the sacroiliac junction. (b) This is especially so when the fetus is in a persistent occipital-posterior position. The resulting neuropathy is nearly always on the side of the occiput.

Injuries related to regional anaesthesia

Nerve root damage
- Due to direct needle or catheter trauma or due to injection of local anaesthetic into the nerve.
- Pain or paraesthesia is felt at time of insertion.
- Frequently over the L3 dermatone across the front of the thigh.
- Persistent paraesthesia should never be dismissed and the needle or catheter should be removed.
- If severe or persistent pain is felt on inserting an epidural catheter, the catheter and needle should be removed.

Spinal cord damage
- Due to direct damage to the conus medullaris.
- High placement of spinal needle could be a causal factor or an abnormally low conus.
- Due to dural puncture during high epidural placement.

Other injuries
- Cranial nerve palsy—usually due to CSF leak following dural puncture; most common lesion is VIth nerve palsy.
- Epidural/spinal haematoma.
- Epidural/spinal abscess.
- Meningitis—bacterial or aseptic.
- Anterior spinal artery syndrome.
- Cauda equina syndrome.
- Arachnoiditis.

> The spinal cord usually terminates at the level of L1 and becomes the cauda equina below this. In up to 20% of the population, it may extend to the lower border of L2. It is therefore advisable to identify and use L3/4 interspace or lower for spinal anaesthesia.

Assessment and management
- Full history, with particular attention to pre-existing problems and the progress of labour and delivery.
- Careful documentation of paraesthesia at the time of spinal or epidural.
- Was there return of function after regional block before the development of symptoms?
- Have the symptoms and signs progressed?
- Full neurological examination and careful documentation of deficit, including both sensory and motor signs by a senior anaesthetist.
- No symptoms should be dismissed.
- Serial temperature recordings, blood for WCC and C-reactive protein if infection suspected.

Signs of serious pathology must be sought
- Pain, redness, or swelling at the site of injection.
- Pyrexia, raised WCC.
- Evidence of meningism.
- Persistent or progressive neurological deficit.
- Bladder or bowel dysfunction.
- Saddle anaesthesia.
- Back pain associated with fever (especially in immunocompromised or diabetic patients).
- Bilateral signs.

- Close observation and reassurance may be adequate as symptoms often resolve within 72h post delivery.
- Small areas of numbness across the buttocks after an apparently uncomplicated spinal anaesthetic is relatively common. If there are no associated bladder symptoms or other nerve injuries then the mother can usually be reassured that normal skin sensation will return.
- Urgent neurology opinion and MRI must be considered in all cases of suspected spinal injury, epidural, and spinal abscess or haematoma.
- If nerve injury is suspected, nerve conduction studies and out-patient neurological referral at 6 weeks post delivery is appropriate. Many cases of nerve injury (obstetric and anaesthetic related) will become the subject of a complaint. Early and close liaison with a neurologist may be helpful.

Further reading

Cook T et al. Major complications of central neuraxial block: Report on the Third National Audit Project of the Royal College of Anaesthetists *British Journal of Anaesthesia* 2009; *102* (2): 179–190
Loo CC et al. Neurological complications in obstetric regional anaesthesia. *International Journal of Obstetric Anesthesia* 2000; 9: 99–124.

Haematoma

- An epidural or spinal haematoma is rare, but potentially catastrophic if missed.
- It may occur spontaneously or after regional anaesthesia, particularly in patients with evidence of clotting dysfunction.
- Clotting dysfunction may be intrinsic, e.g. thrombocytopenia or haemophilia, or acquired, e.g. thromboprophylaxis.
- All obstetric units should have guidelines for the safe timing of regional anaesthesia and anticoagulation (see p. 189 for further guidance).

Signs

- Prolonged (>8h) effect of anaesthesia, with back pain and localized tenderness.
- Bilateral motor and sensory loss combined with disturbance of bowel or bladder function.
- Return of neurological function followed by a new progressive deficit.

Management

- Always follow-up regional blocks which appear to last longer than expected. There should be good if not complete return of function within 4-hours after spinal or epidural anesthesia.
- Perform urgent MRI if signs are suggestive of spinal haematoma.
- If epidural or spinal haematoma evident, emergency neurosurgical decompression is indicated to prevent permanent disability.
- The prognosis is poor if neurological deficit is >12h old.

Neurological infections

Meningitis

The incidence of meningitis following regional anaesthetic techniques ranges from 1 to 15 in 100,000 in spinal anaesthetics.

Septic meningitis

- Septic meningitis may be secondary to bacterial or viral infection.
- Bacterial infection, often due to *Streptococcus pneumoniae* or *Neisseria meningitides*, may be secondary to a bacteraemia and not related to regional anaesthesia.
- If secondary to spinal anaesthesia, *Streptococcus viridans* is frequently the causative organism.
- The causative organism is most probably a contaminant from the patient's own skin.
- For meningitis to occur following regional anaesthesia, there may have been a breach in the aseptic field.
- CSE technique has been associated with an increase in reported cases of meningitis and epidural abscess. The true incidence is not known, as there may be reporting bias.
- The breakdown in the protective barrier offered by the dura and introduction of the epidural catheter, which is continuous with the skin as part of the CSE technique, are the possible contributory factors.
- Viral meningitis may occur following regional anaesthesia in women with herpes simplex or herpes zoster infection.

Signs
- Fever.
- Headache.
- Neck stiffness.
- Photophobia.

Management

- Lumbar puncture to identify the causative organism.
- Aggressive antimicrobial treatment.
- Referral to neurology or general medicine.
- The prognosis for recovery is better following meningitis than an epidural abscess.

Aseptic meningitis

- Rare consequence of disinfectant from the skin preparation or contaminated syringes being introduced into the epidural or intrathecal space.
- Features mimic septic meningitis.

Arachnoiditis

- Rare inflammatory disorder where the membranes around the spinal cord and cauda equina become fibrotic.
- This causes constriction of the cauda equina with progressive painful neurology.

- Cause is not known.
- Spinal and epidural anaesthesia has been implicated, but there is no proved association, and most cases are not linked with regional anaesthesia.
- Preservatives within local anaesthetic solutions have been blamed.

Epidural abscess

- A rare but serious complication of regional anaesthesia.
- Incidence is 0.2–3.7 cases per 100,000 obstetric epidurals.
- May occur spontaneously or following a breach in sterile conditions during epidural or spinal anaesthesia.
- CSE technique has been associated with an increase in reported cases.
- The most common organism involved is *Staphylococcus aureus* (57%).

Signs

- Classically presents with severe deep-seated backache ± localized tenderness.
- Nerve root irritation with 'electric shock' or 'sparking' sensations into the buttock or legs are a Red Flag symptom and should not be dismissed.
- Pyrexia and signs of systemic sepsis occur late in the presentation.
- Localizing nerve root pain and sudden onset of weakness may follow after 2–3 days.
- This is a neurosurgical emergency.

Management

- Aggressive treatment with IV antibiotics and urgent neurosurgical decompression is paramount.
- If neurological symptoms present, prognosis for full recovery is poor.

Further reading

Rice I et al. Obstetric epidurals and chronic adhesive arachnoiditis (Review). *British Journal of Anaesthesia* 2004; 92: 109–120.

Grewel S et al. Epidural abscesses. *British Journal of Anaesthesia* 2006; 96: 292–302.

Reynolds F. Infection as a complication of neuraxial blockade. *International Journal of Obstetric Anesthesia* 2005; 14: 183–188.

Cauda equina syndrome

- Caused by damage to the sacral nerve roots (S2–S4) either due to direct needle trauma or after injection of large volumes of LA causing root compression.
- Continuous spinal infusions via a spinal microcatheter and high concentration lidocaine have also been implicated.

Signs

- Bowel and bladder dysfunction.
- Saddle anaesthesia.
- Residual sensory loss.
- Lower limb paralysis (varying degrees).

Management

- Urgent MRI to exclude a reversible cause, e.g. haematoma, abscess, prolapsed intervertbral disc.
- Neurological referral for assessment of signs.
- Ongoing management is largely supportive.

Further reading

Brooks H, May A. Neurological complications following regional anaesthesia in obstetrics. *British Journal of Anaesthesia CEPD Reviews* 2003; 3: 111–114.

Dealing with a complaint

Complaints against health service staff are increasing year on year, and the field of obstetric anaesthesia is no exception. Complaints are a source of great anxiety to all healthcare staff who may be implicated. If a complaint is being made against you, it is essential that you understand your hospital or Trust's process for dealing with it.

There are broadly three stages at which a complaint may be resolved:

- Local Trust response.
- Independent Review Panel.
- Health Service Commissioner or Ombudsman.

Many complaints relevant to childbirth are not forwarded for many months or sometimes up to 2yrs following delivery. It is essential that accurate, contemporaneous documentation is maintained at all times.

If a woman indicates in the immediate postnatal period that a complaint is likely, documentation in the contemporary notes should be reviewed. They must NOT be changed in any way, but supplementary comment is appropriate as long as it is absolutely clear when the additional notes were made.

Local response

- Written complaints are normally sent directly to the Trust Chief Executive and passed to a complaints team or department for further action.
- If a complaint is received directly, do not respond personally. It should be forwarded to the Chief Executive via the Clinical Director or the Directorate Manager.
- Complaints are handled by a team of experienced co-ordinators, who will request a response from all staff involved in the woman's care.

The complainant is entitled to the following:

- A full, detailed, and honest explanation of what happened, when, and why.
- An apology if there was an error or omission in their care.
- If an error or omission occurred, they should be advised about the Trust's action, or proposed action, to prevent a recurrence.
- Many complaints are resolved with a clear explanation and a timely apology, with the assurance that any failures will be rectified for the future.
- An open and sympathetic approach is recommended.
- A hostile and defensive reaction is more likely to lead to attempted litigation challenges later.
- A written response, signed by the Chief Executive, will be compiled based on the statements from all staff implicated, and forwarded to the complainant.
- The majority of written complaints are concluded with local resolution.
- A meeting with the complainant is sometimes arranged at an early stage. This involves a group discussion with senior doctors and managers involved in the case. The Trust's complaints manager usually chairs the meeting and is responsible for taking minutes. The complainant usually

comes with an advocate (often from a patients' advocate group). Any doctor who is asked to attend such a meeting is also entitled to an advocate (frequently a senior colleague).

The Independent Review Panel
- If the local response does not satisfy the complainant, referral for independent review is considered by a Convener.
- The independent review panel comprises the Convener, an independent lay chairman, a third lay person, and usually two independent clinical assessors to advise the panel.
- Its purpose is to establish the facts and make recommendations to improve the effectiveness of the service.
- Following review of all documentation, all parties are interviewed by the panel, and recommendations are sent to the parties concerned.

Health Service Commissioner
- If the complainant remains dissatisfied after receiving the report from the independent review, she has the right to take the matter to the Health Service Commissioner (Ombudsman).
- The Ombudsman is independent of the NHS and the government.

Legal action
- If a woman explicitly indicates an intention to take legal action, the complaints process should stop immediately.
- Legal action is taken out against the Trust not individual doctors.
- The Trust's legal department take over the case and request their own expert views.

Obesity in pregnancy

Huda Al-Foudri, Stuart Davies, and Abrie Theron

Definition, classification, and prevalence

Definition

- The World Health Organization define obesity as an abnormal or excessive accumulation of fat that may impair health.

Calculation/formula

- Obesity is quantified using the body mass index (BMI) which is defined as a person's weight in kilograms divided by the square of his/her height in metres:

$$BMI = Weight(kg) / (Height\ in\ metres)^2$$

- A BMI ≥ 30 is classified as obesity as per NICE / WHO definition set out in Table 16.1.
- Variations occur based on ethnicity, muscle bulk, age, and sex. The BMI may not correspond to a similar degree of fat in different individuals and should only be used as a guide.

Epidemiology and prevalence

- According to the WHO in 2008 more than 50% of men and women in the European region were overweight or obese, with 23% of women being obese.
- The CMACE (Centre for Maternal and Child Enquiries) report published in 2010, looked at obesity in pregnancy in the UK and showed an increase in maternal obesity: 5% (38,500 maternities per year) had a BMI of equal or more than 35, 2% of patient's BMI was equal or more 40 and 0.2% of women who gave birth had a BMI of equal or more than 50.
- The recent maternal mortality report (MBRRACE 2012–14) showed that more than half of the women who died were overweight (18%) and obese (33%).

Table 16.1 Classification of obesity

BMI	WHO/NICE	Other
<18.5	Underweight	
≥18.5–24.9	Normal weight	
≥25.0–29.9	Overweight / Pre-obesity	
≥30.0–34.9	Class I obesity	Obese
≥35.0–39.9	Class II obesity	Severe obesity
≥40.0	Class III obesity	Morbid obesity
≥50		Extreme obesity

Adapted with permission from World Health Organization, Body Mass Index -BMI http://www.euro.who.int/en/health-topics/disease-prevention/nutrition/a-healthy-lifestyle/body-mass-index-bmi

Physiology and associated morbidity

Pregnancy and obesity diminishes a patient's physiological reserve.

Respiratory system

- Tidal volume, respiratory rate, and minute ventilation increase and it is normal to see a drop in $PaCO_2$ in pregnancy.
- Lung compliance decreases and the work of breathing increases in obesity.
- A decrease in FRC and an increase in V/Q mismatch cause the PaO_2 to decrease easily in both pregnancy and obesity.
- Obesity is a risk factor for the development of obstructive sleep apnoea (OSA).

Cardiovascular system

- Blood volume increases and the haematocrit falls in pregnancy.
- HR, SV, and CO also increase in pregnancy and the LV dilates due to increased volume load.
- In obese women the LV mass increases.
- SVR and MAP decreases in normal pregnancy and aortacaval compression can cause hypotension.
- PIH is more common in obesity due to endothelial dysfunction caused by the increase in inflammatory mediators.
- There is an increased risk of IHD, cardiomyopathy, and heart failure in the obese.
- Pulmonary hypertension and RVF can occur in severe OSA.

Gastrointestinal system

- Gastric reflux increases in pregnancy and the presence of hiatus hernia is more common in the obese.
- This increases the risk of regurgitation and aspiration.

Renal system

- GFR increases in pregnancy, but renal blood flow can decrease due to high intra-abdominal pressure in the obese.

Endocrine system

- Insulin resistance in obesity increases the risk of gestational diabetes.

Haematological system

- There is an increased risk of venous thromboembolism.

Pharmacokinetic changes of obesity

- Volume of distribution increases.
- Retention of lipid-soluble drugs (opioids, propofol).
- Increased clearance of renally excreted drugs e.g. LMWH, increased doses may be required.

Maternal & fetal morbidity

Maternal
- Miscarriage rate is tripled.
- PIH and gestational diabetes increase 4-fold.
- PET increases (13.5% vs 3.9%).
- PPH risk is quadrupled.
- Thromboembolism increases.
- Induction and failed induction rates increase.
- Instrumental delivery/CS rate increases.
- Infection is more common: Urinary tract infection, endometritis and wound infection with wound breakdown.

Fetal
- Increased rate of fetal abnormalities (secondary to difficult ultrasound detection).
- Still birth rate increases 2-fold for mothers with a BMI>35.
- Macrosomia is seen more frequently.
- Intrapartum fetal distress and meconium aspiration are more common.
- Failure to progress, abnormal presentation, and shoulder dystocia increase.
- All the above increase neonatal unit admissions.
- Perinatal mortality rate is 4 times higher.

Antenatal management

Antenatal screening

- Weight should be recorded at booking, using bariatric scales and the BMI calculated.
- Risk assessment must be performed early in order to identify and address all risks (i.e. gestational diabetes, PIH, PET) and to identify the need for referral to consultant obstetrician led care, anaesthetic assessment, obstetric medicine, etc.

Criteria for Antenatal Anaesthetic referral

- The joint guideline from CMACE and Royal College of Obstetricians and Gynaecologists (RCOG) recommends that women with BMI more than 40 or BMI more than 35 with a co-morbidity should be assessed by an anaesthetist.
- Women with a booking BMI more than 40, but with previous normal deliveries, may not be routinely seen in some units. It is feasible to train specialist midwives to screen obese women, so that only those most likely to have problems are seen by an anaesthetist. See Fig 16.1 for a Midwife Obesity Assessment screening proforma to identify women at higher anaesthetic risk.
- Obese women with previous anaesthetic difficulties should all be reviewed in an anaesthetic clinic.

Antenatal review and assessment

The antenatal review of the obese parturient should focus on:

Anaesthetic assessment

History

- Presence of co-morbidities (e.g. gestational diabetes mellitus, PIH, PET, IHD etc.)
- Previous deliveries and anaesthetic interventions.
- Drug history: Dose frequency and duration, especially anticoagulants, as it has an implication on the regional block.
- Sleep apnoea.

Examination

- Veins for IV access.
- Palpable vertebra in lumbar spine.
- Full airway assessment.

Analgesic / anaesthetic advice

- Discuss the different analgesic options available and encourage open-mindedness; Entonox®, IM opioids, epidural analgesia, and remifentanil PCA.
- Early IV access should be advised if it is thought to be difficult.
- The consultation should cover all types of anaesthesia available should the patient require an operative delivery or CS.
- The preference for regional anaesthesia should be emphasized especially if potential airway difficulties exist, with encouragement to adopt epidural analgesia early in labour, if significant anticipated technical difficulties and to prevent the need for an emergency GA.

Midwife Led High BMI Clinic assessment at 28 weeks gestation

Name: _____
Hosp No: _____
DOB: _____
Address: _____

Weight: _____ kg Height: _____ m BMI: _____

EDD ___ / ___ / _____

Previous deliveries: SVD x ____ Instrumental x ____ LSCS x ____

Anaesthesia: Epi x ___ Spinal x ___ CSE x ___ Remi x ___ GA x ___

Airway		Risk
Excess adipose tissue around neck? No / Yes	No	Yes
Small jaw? No / Yes	No	Yes
Prominent upper incisors? No / Yes	No	Yes
Neck movement >90° Yes/No	Yes	No
Jaw protrusion: In front / At or Behind of upper incisors	Front	Behind
Mouth opening: 3 or more / less than 3 fingers	3	<3
Mallampati:	I - II	III - IV

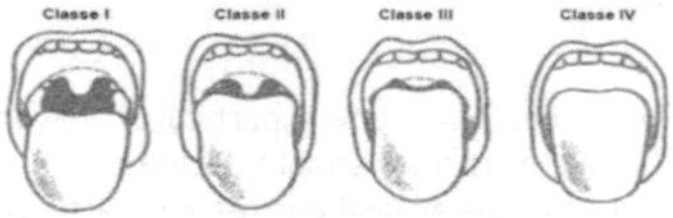

Classe I   Classe II   Classe III   Classe IV

Back		
Previous difficult spinal or epidural? No / Yes	No	Yes
Lumbar vertebra palpable? Yes / No	Yes	No
History of back surgery ? Yes / No	No	Yes

Discussion
☐ Explained increased risk of need for intervention
☐ Procedures (GA & Regional) may be more difficult
☐ OAA leaflets distributed

Outcome of Midwife Assessment

BMI > 45kg/m²	BMI > 35kg/m² with 1+ risk factor Potential difficult airway i.e. • Mallampati III-IV OR 3 airway risk factors Previous failed regional +/- conversion to GA Back surgery Any significant medical or pregnancy related problem	BMI < 45kg/m² No additional risk factors
Refer to Antenatal Anaesthetic Clinic 32/40 appointment		Early review by anaesthetist on admission to CLU

Midwife: Date:

Fig. 16.1 Midwife Obesity Assessment screening proforma.

Reproduced with permission from Dr Theron, Dr Harries and Dr Collis, University Hospital of Wales, Cardiff. Mallampati score: Reprinted by permission from Canadian Anesthesiologists: Springer Nature. *Canadian Journal of Anesthesia*. A clinical sign to predict difficult tracheal intubation; a prospective study. Mallampati S. Rao et al. © Canadian Anesthesiologists 1985.

Dietary advice

- Obese pregnant women should receive counselling about weight gain, nutrition, and healthy food choices during their antenatal reviews, ideally from a dietician.
- Dieting is not recommended during pregnancy as it may harm the fetus; however, healthy eating clubs are encouraged.
- Obese women should ideally gain less weight in pregnancy than the non-obese—it should be limited to less than 10kg.
- Encourage moderate activity.

Anaesthetic plan

Once the assessment is completed and the various options and their associated risks have been discussed, a plan for the anaesthetic management for labour and delivery should be made with the patient and clearly documented. It should include the following:

Preferred mode of delivery

In most cases there would not be a need to dictate a particular delivery purely due to maternal weight. The obstetric team should decide the most suitable mode of delivery, with input from the anaesthetic team if particular concerns. In some extremely obese women, when a caesarean section would be a particular challenge as an emergency, it may occasionally be necessary to opt for an elective caesarean section, to ensure the presence of experienced staff, both obstetric and anaesthetic, and specific equipment.

Analgesic/anaesthetic options for delivery

The planned analgesia/anaesthesia should be documented with the associated risks discussed.

Seniority of the anaesthetist

The seniority of the anaesthetist present to provide the analgesia / anaesthesia, depending on any anticipated difficulty, should be determined and documented. The CMACE and RCOG joint guideline recommends that obese patients should be managed by at least a senior trainee.

Thromboprophylaxis management

Obesity is a risk factor for venous thromboembolism in pregnancy, the risk being higher with increasing obesity. RCOG guidance strongly recommends thromboprophylaxis is initiated antenatally with low molecular weight heparin in the following dosage regime:

- 91–130kg: enoxaparin 60mg daily, dalteparin 7500 units daily, tinzaparin 7000 units daily.
- 131–170kg: enoxaparin 80mg daily, dalteparin 10,000 units daily, tinzaparin 9000 units daily.
- >170kg: enoxaparin 0.6mg/kg/day, dalteparin 75u/kg/day, tinzaparin 75u/kg/day—usually administered in divided doses.

The anaesthetic plan should include how to manage the anticoagulation the patient may be taking in relation to the administration of a regional block, with clear instructions on the safe dosing interval between the last dose of LMWH and safe timing of regional placement.

Current guidance for the safe interval is:

- Prophylactic LMWH >12 hours. (Once daily dose).
- Therapeutic LMWH >24 hours. (Usually twice daily dose).

OAA high BMI leaflet

The OAA has produced a useful information leaflet outlining the risks associated with increased BMI and delivery. It is a helpful adjunct to the anaesthetic consultation and a copy should be provided to the patient for reading following their antenatal visit. Copies are available form www.labourpains.com.

Peripartum management

Admission to labour ward

The duty anaesthetist should be informed of the admission of any obese parturient to the labour ward, regardless of whether anaesthetic intervention is needed or not. This allows early assessment of the patient and for plans made in the antenatal assessment to be identified. Some patients may not have been identified antenatally and may see the anaesthetist for the first time when admitted to labour ward. A full assessment of the patient should be made at this stage.

There should be a system for alerting staff of the admission of obese patients. Systems in use include:

- Alert sticker on the patient notes.
- Obesity/high risk card inside the notes.
- Writing the BMI on the handover board in labour ward.

Labour analgesia

Epidural

Advantages of an epidural
- Analgesia to facilitate a difficult vaginal delivery as there is a greater risk of fetal macrosomia and shoulder dystocia.
- Can be extended to provide anaesthesia for instrumental delivery and CS and hence avoid the risks associated with a GA.
- Use for post-op analgesia which avoids systemic opioids.

Risks with the epidural analgesia
- Higher initial failure rate.
- Multiple attempts increase risk of complications.

Remifentanil PCA
- Indicated if epidural analgesia was not possible or is contraindicated, e.g. recent dosage of thromboprophylaxis.
- The patient must have continuous SpO_2 monitoring, and if necessary be given supplementary oxygen.

Anaesthesia for caesarean section/operative delivery

Regional anaesthesia

Spinal anaesthesia
Spinal anaesthesia is considered safer than a GA, with less associated mortality and morbidity; however, the following problems may occur:
- Technical difficulty: it may be challenging to accurately identify the midline and intervertebral spaces.
- Increased cephalad spread with possible high spinal block due to:
  - Reduced CSF volume in obesity due to epidural venous engorgement. Consider using a smaller volume of LA.
  - Excess adipose tissues in the buttock resulting in a Trendelenberg position when lying flat.
  - Inadequate duration of block if surgery is prolonged. A CSE technique should be considered if there is potential for prolonged surgery.

General anaesthesia

Airway assessment

Predictors of difficult intubation include:

- Large breasts.
- Greater anterior-posterior diameter of the chest.
- Short sternomental and thyromental distance.
- Short neck with increased fat in the neck.
- Neck circumference/thyromental distance ratio ≥ 5.
- Fat pads on the back and shoulders (positioning).
- History of a previous difficult intubation.
- Weight gain of more than 15kg in pregnancy.

Difficult intubation is more frequent in obese patients than in non-obese patients (13.8% vs 4.8%). Failed tracheal intubation rate in the general population is 1:2230 compared to 1:224 in the obstetric population. Obese obstetric patients have an even higher incidence of difficult and failed intubation.

Positioning

- Consider using the **ramped** position (see Chapter 12, p. 339) with left uterine displacement, even if a regional block is in place, as the patient will be in an optimal position if a GA is required urgently.
- Position the operating table in the reverse Trendelenberg position, preferably on an Oxford HELP® pillow.
- The patient has to be secured to the operating table before it is moved to ensure patient safety. Use lateral table extenders if necessary.
- Ensure that the patient weight does not exceed the maximum weight limit of the table in all positions.
- Cephalad retraction of the large panniculus may result in hypotension, respiratory compromise, and fetal distress.

Ramped position (see page 339)

- There is evidence it improves the view during laryngoscopy in morbidly obese patients undergoing bariatric surgery.
- It involves achieving a horizontal alignment between the external auditory meatus and the sternal notch, which aligns the oral, pharyngeal, and tracheal axis better.
- Achieved by placing folded blankets under the chest and head, but can also be done with the aid of the Oxford HELP® Pillow and positioning of the table.
- Can also improve the cardio-respiratory parameters.

Anaesthetic management

- Equipment for difficult intubation should be available.
- Maximize the patient's oxygen reserves prior to intubation and extubation by means of thorough pre-oxygenation, apneic oxygenation, CPAP, Transnasal Humidified Rapid-Insufflation Ventilatory Exchange (THRIVE) and by keeping the patient as upright as possible.
- Use a rapid sequence induction. A video-laryngoscope is considered the most appropriate first-line laryngoscope for intubation if available, provided the operator has been trained in its use.

- Drugs:
  - Sodium citrate 0.3 M 30ml.
  - Omeprazole 40mg PO or IV.
  - Thiopental up to a maximum dose of 500mg.
  - Suxamethonium, use total body weight to a maximum dose of 200mg.
  - Atracurium metabolism is independent of hepatic metabolism and the time required for its reversal does not depend on the patient's total body weight or BMI.
- MAC is not altered by obesity; however, the increased body fat will act as a reservoir for the inhalational agents and may lead to delayed recovery.
- Nitrous oxide allows for a lower MAC of inhalational agents, but may not be possible as the obese patient is more prone to intra-operative hypoxaemia.
- Two anaesthetists should ideally be present at induction.
- A second-generation supraglottic airway device may be more appropriate for oxygenation during failed intubation.
- Difficult mask ventilation may result in gastric distension and increase the risk of aspiration and regurgitation.
- Use positive end expiratory pressure (PEEP) to improve intra-operative oxygenation and compliance and recruitment manoeuvres especially before extubation.
- Extubate the patient awake, sitting upright as much as possible.
- Avoid the nasal route if an awake fibre-optic intubation is performed as mucosal engorgement may result in bleeding.

Postpartum management

Postpartum analgesia

Regular paracetamol combined with high dose NSAID reduce opioid requirements.

Postpartum complications

- Hypoxaemia due to respiratory depression, atelectasis, and pneumonia.
- Thrombo-embolism.
- Wound or respiratory infection.
- PPH.
- Exacerbation of OSA.

Practical considerations and technical challenges

Manual handling
- Ensure mandatory manual handling courses for all staff and pay attention to the patient's pressure points.

IV access
- Establish IV access early in labour as it may be difficult.
- Consider ultrasound to aid cannulation.
- If peripheral cannulation is not possible, achieve central venous access.

Monitoring
- It may be impossible to obtain an interpretable external fetal heart rate and uterine contraction patterns in obese women.
- ECG complexes may be small.
- Non-invasive blood pressure measurement can overestimate the patient's BP. The width of the BP cuff has to be 40% and the bladder length 80% of the circumference of the patients' arm. Give consideration to using a thigh cuff.
- Invasive BP is recommended if it is difficult to measure BP with a non-invasive technique and if frequent ABG and blood sampling is required (i.e. pre-eclampsia, Hb for blood loss).

Regional techniques
Difficulty identifying the midline may result in lateral projection of the needle and misplacement. This can be avoided by:

- Using ultrasound (see Chapter 8).
- Identify the C7 spinous process as a body landmark of the midline.
- Ask the mother on manual palpation if it feels like you are palpating the middle of her back.
- Position the patient in the sitting position.

The depth of the epidural space may be greater, ultrasound guidance maybe helpful but it is dependent on the skill of operator.

- Long epidural needles are rarely required as very few patients have an epidural space deeper than 8cm.
- Long spinal needles are more likely to be needed. It may be better to use a CSE kit where the large and stiff epidural needle can be used as an introducer to identify the space better if the spinal needle introducer does not reach the spine.
- Leave extra catheter length in the space for possible catheter migration with patient movement.
- Fix the epidural catheter after the patient has straightened her back to avoid dislodging the catheter from the epidural space.

Previous bariatric surgery

- In patients who have had gastric banding surgery, the band may need to be deflated during pregnancy, because of the risk of poor nutrition.
- Excessive weight loss after bariatric surgery may increase the risk of IUGR and pulmonary aspiration due to decreased oesophageal-gastric peristalsis and reduced lower oesophageal sphincter tone.

Equipment and facilities

- The AAGBI recommends that each maternity unit should have a central list of all equipment and facilities required for the obese patient with their location and access, and that there should be a named consultant anaesthetist/team member who is responsible for the peri-operative management of the morbidly obese patient.

The equipment recommended to be available

- Adjustable intermittent pneumatic compression boots.
- Extra-large BP cuffs or thigh BP cuffs.
- Extra-long spinal and epidural needles.
- Wide theatre trolleys.
- Wide chairs.
- Lifting and lateral transfer equipment (e.g. HoverMatt® mattress).
- Arm extensions.
- Theatre table suitable for patients up to 250kg.
- Weighing scale or weighing bed taking up to 250kg.
- Ultrasound scan for central venous access and neuro-axial block guidance.

Further reading

CMACE. Maternal obesity in the UK: findings from a national project. Centre for Maternal and Child Enquiries (CMACE). London; 2010.

Knight M et al (eds) on behalf of MBRRACE-UK. Saving Lives, Improving Mothers' Care—Surveillance of maternal deaths in the UK 2012–14 and lessons learned to inform maternity care from the UK and Ireland Confidential Enquiries into Maternal Deaths and Morbidity 2009–14. Oxford: National Perinatal Epidemiology Unit, University of Oxford 2016.

Cook TM et al. 4th National Audit Project of the Royal College of Anaesthetists and The Difficult Airway Society, Major complications of airway management in the UK, Report and findings, March 2011.

Theron A et al. Introduction of a midwife led anaesthetic obesity clinic. *International Journal of Obstetric Anesthia* 2011; 20: S33.

Kim WH et al. Neck circumference to thyromental distance ratio: a new predictor of difficult intubation in obese patients. *British Journal of Anaesthesia* 2011; 106:743–748.

Hamilton CL et al. Changes in the position of epidural catheters associated with the patient movement. *Anaesthesiology* 1997; 86: 778–784

Chapter 17

The sick and septic mother

Lucy de Lloyd and Sarah Bell

Assessment of the critically ill mother

General principles

The critically ill obstetric patient poses many problems during clinical assessment and management:

- The physiological changes of pregnancy and the large physiological reserve in younger mothers can complicate clinical assessment. A high index of suspicion is required.
- Medical conditions might present differently during pregnancy and pregnancy itself may alter the disease state.
- Simultaneous assessment and management of both mother and fetus, who have differing physiological profiles, are paramount.
- The treatment of the mother will have an impact on the fetus, but the treatment of the mother takes priority.
- Good communication and multidisciplinary management involving senior obstetricians, anaesthetists and intensive care specialists is essential. There should be a formal escalation plan in place.

The assessment of the critically ill mother should consider the following differential diagnosis:

Specific pregnancy-related problems, e.g. haemorrhage, eclampsia, pulmonary embolus, amniotic fluid embolus.

Non-pregnancy-related problems, e.g. trauma, sepsis, diabetic ketoacidosis, respiratory failure due to asthma or infection.

- The use of an obstetric specific early warning chart, with modifications for the altered physiology of pregnancy, is helpful. Persistent red or amber triggers should mandate a careful clinical evaluation.
- The **ABCDE** approach will help systematic assessment:
  - *A: Airway assessment*—the airway may pose difficulties due to anatomical, physiological, or pathological changes, e.g. airway oedema due to pre-eclampsia.
  - *B: Breathing*—100% oxygen should be administered as there is decreased vital capacity and an increased oxygen requirement in pregnancy. A high oxygen requirement in a previously healthy woman is an ominous sign. Tachypnoea is an early sign of an underlying medical problem. Auscultate the chest for any added sounds, e.g. crepitations in pulmonary oedema secondary to pre-eclampsia.
  - *C: Circulation*—assess capillary refill (normally <2s and usually shorter in pregnancy), colour, conscious level, jugular venous pressure, urine output, and any evidence of concealed or overt haemorrhage. Check a venous or arterial lactate. If >2mmol / L establish the cause. Check pulse and BP. Avoid aorto-caval compression. Establish large-bore IV access.
  - *D: Disabilty*—rapid assessment of neurological status includes AVPU system (A alert, V response to vocal stimuli, P response to pain, U unresponsiveness), GCS, and pupillary assessment. A low AVPU score in pregnancy is a late sign and is always very serious.

Recommendations from Confidential Enquires into Maternal Deaths

- Intensive care should start as soon as it is needed and does not need to wait for admission to an ICU. It is possible to provide the majority of immediate intensive care treatment in an obstetric theatre.
- A HDU chart with obstetric early warning parameters, fluid balance and infusions should be used.
- FBC, electrolytes, coagulation and venous lactate should be tested on a regular basis.
- Hourly urine output should be monitored.
- An arterial line should be inserted early. Blood gas analysis should be performed and a metabolic acidosis should always be investigated further. There is a normal increase in metabolic acidosis in pregnancy and labour, but this is not associated with a lactic acidosis.
- Consideration should be given to improved stabilization and elective intubation prior to transfer.

Identifying the septic mother

Introduction

The worldwide incidence of sepsis in both the general and obstetric population is increasing. Sepsis remains a leading overall cause of direct and indirect maternal death.

- The maternal immune system undergoes complex changes during
  pregnancy in order to support the feto-placental unit.
- A state of maternal immunomodulation is observed, altering the
  susceptibility to infective organisms depending on the stage of
  pregnancy and the type of organism.
- Sepsis causes the release of pro-inflammatory cytokines which have
  multiple widespread actions, some of which may mimic the normal
  physiological changes of pregnancy.
- Deaths related to sepsis increased in the MBRRACE 2009–12 report,
  predominantly due to genital tract sepsis and influenza. Sepsis deaths
  since then have fallen.
- With reference to group A streptococcal genital tract sepsis—it is
  unclear whether the observed reduction is due to initiatives to improve
  care, or cyclical rates of disease, relating to the population burden of
  streptococcal infections.
- The H1N1 influenza pandemic was responsible for the peak in maternal
  mortalities observed. The importance of immunization in pregnant
  women is emphasized and immunization strategies are ongoing.

> ### The 2012–2014 **MBRRACE-UK report** describes deaths due to sepsis
> - Direct.
>   - Genitourinary: 0.29 per 100,000 maternities.
> - Indirect.
>   - Influenza: 0.04 per 100,000 maternities.
>   - Pneumonia (and other sources): 0.6 per 100,000 maternities.
>
> Data from Saving Lives, Improving Mothers' Care—Surveillance of maternal deaths in the UK
> 2012–14 and lessons learned to inform maternity care from the UK and Ireland Confidential
> Enquiries into Maternal Deaths and Morbidity 2009–14.

Recognition

- Pregnant women are often young and fit, with considerable physiological
  reserve and capacity for compensation. Consequently, illness may only
  cause clear deterioration in vital signs late in the course of the illness,
  when the body has reached the limits of its reserve and begins to
  decompensate.
- The importance of identifying vulnerable pregnant women early is
  highlighted in the findings of successive confidential enquires into
  maternal mortality.
- In the 2014 MBRRACE-UK report, lack of early recognition of the sick
  mother resulting in suboptimal care was identified as a contributory
  factor in 70% of deaths.

- A key element of strategies to improve recognition of the sick parturient is the use of Modified Early Obstetric Warning Score (MEOWS) charts. These are tailored to chart the physiological parameters of pregnant women, using coloured bands (white, amber, or red) to visually flag abnormal observations.
- These charts should be used in all clinical environments where pregnant women may be cared for, including obstetric triage/assessment units, emergency departments, medical and surgical assessment units, as well as delivery suite and the maternity wards.
- Deterioration noted should prompt urgent review and action, including senior advice and support and early critical care referral where appropriate.
- The use of a Sepsis Six pathway, which identifies Red Flag symptoms and signs, plus a 'first hour' sepsis checklist, i.e. blood tests including lactate, microbiology samples, early IV antibiotics, IV fluids, and ensuring oxygen delivery, can enhance and expedite care delivered to septic mothers.

Red Flag symptoms and signs of maternal sepsis
- Responds only to voice or pain or unresponsive.
- Systolic BP ≤ 90mmHg or drop of > 40 mmHg.
- HR > 130 beats per minute.
- Respiratory rate ≥ 25 breaths per minute.
- Oxygen saturations ≤ 92% on room air.
- Rash, mottled, ashen, cyanotic.
- Not passed urine in last 18 hours.
- Urinary output < 0.5ml/kg/hr.
- Lactate ≥ 2.0mmol/L.
  Red Flags may be a late presentation.

Amber Flags, especially with obstetric risk factors and fetal signs of sepsis, require urgent medical assessment, early blood-tests including lactate, and early consideration of antibiotics

Factors which may increase difficulty in recognition of the sick pregnant woman
- **Social and language difficulty** may hinder subjective expression of the woman's illness.
- **Dark skin pigmentation and obesity** may mask subtle changes in skin hue reflecting underlying poor perfusion.
- **Beta blockade and pre-eclampsia** may alter the early signs of hypovolaemia.
- **Repeated presentations to medical staff is a 'Red Flag'** and warrants a thorough assessment for signs of sepsis.

Causes of sepsis in obstetrics
For the purposes of the confidential enquiries into maternal death, the causes of sepsis in obstetrics are divided into infections which are caused by the pregnancy (direct), and other infections that are felt to be unrelated (indirect).

Direct
- Genital tract sepsis.
- Urosepsis.
- Mastitis.

Indirect
- Influenza.
- Pneumonia.
- Neurological infections.
- Other (including malaria, TB, and HIV).

Physiological changes in sepsis

Respiratory
- Increased respiratory rate is often the first sign of a systemic inflammatory response. This occurs on the background of the rise in respiratory rate seen in normal pregnancy.
- In sepsis, neutrophil adhesion to the pulmonary capillary endothelium increases permeability leading to interstitial oedema.
- The reduction in colloid oncotic pressure observed during normal pregnancy further increases this risk.

Cardiovascular
- The initial tachycardia, increased cardiac output, and modest reduction in systemic vascular resistance observed in septic patients mimics the normal physiological changes of pregnancy.
- As sepsis worsens cardiac contractility, vasomotor tone, and cardiac output all decrease.
- Microcirculatory damage leads to anaerobic metabolism and lactic acidosis.

Immune system
- Pyrexia is common in sepsis, although the absence of pyrexia does not exclude infection as a diagnosis.
- Fever is also associated with prostaglandin administration and epidural analgesia.
- Hypothermia may occur in severe sepsis.
- An elevated white blood cell count (WCC) occurs in sepsis but is also seen in late pregnancy and labour.
- Leucopenia (WCC less than 4×10^9) is a significant finding that may reflect an overwhelmed immune system.
- Disseminated intravascular coagulation with thrombocytopenia, consumptive coagulopathy, and microvascular emboli may occur in severe sepsis.

Renal
- Pregnant women are susceptible to urinary tract infections, including pyelonephritis, due to hormonally induced reduced ureteric tone, compression of ureters by the gravid uterus, reduced bladder tone, and increased risk of glycosuria.
- Sepsis can also cause renal dysfunction due to pre-renal and or renal causes.

Clinical presentation

The time taken to complete an assessment of the mother and fetus should be tailored to the gravity of the situation. Sepsis can be insidious in onset, variable in manifestation, and difficult to identify.

Clinical history

General

- Identify patient factors increasing vulnerability to sepsis including: impaired immunity (steroids, sickle cell disease), anaemia, diabetes, and obesity.
- Symptoms: feeling generally unwell, abnormal temperature.

Respiratory

- History of sore throat, respiratory infection, or contact with symptomatic individuals, particularly children.
- Symptoms: dyspnoea, cough, sputum, pleuritic pain, sore throat.

Cardiac

- History of previous cardiovascular disease.
- Symptoms: dyspnoea, palpitations, chest pain, ankle swelling.

Gastrointestinal

- Diarrhoea, vomiting and abdominal pain occur in genital tract sepsis.
- Symptoms: diarrhoea, vomiting, and abdominal pain.

Renal

- Known previous urological infection or congenital abnormality.
- Symptoms: dysuria, haematuria, renal angle, or back pain.

Neurological

- History of recent neuroaxial blockade should be sought.
- Symptoms: confusion, anxiety, deficit, headache, rash, neck stiffness, back pain, and any radicular features.

Breasts

- Symptoms: pain, swelling, redness, or discharge.

Obstetric

Identify obstetric risk factors increasing vulnerability to sepsis:

- Antenatal: group B streptococcal disease, vaginal discharge, trauma, pelvic infection, invasive intrauterine procedures, or cervical suture.
- Labour: prolonged rupture of membranes, long labour with > 5 vaginal examinations.
- Delivery: caesarean section, retained products of conception.
- Symptoms: altered fetal movements, perineal or pelvic pain/discharge/bleeding, preterm contractions.

Examination

General condition

- Looks unwell.
- Disproportionate pain.
- Temperature.
- Rash.

Respiratory
- Respiratory rate, SaO_2.
- Sputum—production and features.
- Chest expansion, palpation, percussion, auscultation.

Cardiovascular
- Heart rate and rhythm, blood pressure.
- Skin colour, temperature, and perfusion.
- New murmurs or peripheral stigmata of endocarditis.

Gastrointestinal
- Abdominal distension.
- Abdominal tenderness and rigidity.
- Jaundice.

Renal
- Renal angle pain, dysuria, foul smelling urine.

Neurological
- Neurological deficit, neck stiffness, photophobia.
- Assess back if recent neuroaxial blockade: tenderness, swelling, erythema.

Obstetric
- Lochia, discharge, or perineal swelling.
- Uterine pain and tenderness.
- Breast erythema, pain, swelling, or discharge.

Fetal wellbeing
- Fetal distress may be the first manifestation of maternal shock.
- Reduced fetal movements or fetal tachycardia (>160 beats/min).

Investigations
Investigations should be performed in parallel with initial treatment.

Blood tests
- Blood cultures (BUT do not delay administration of antibiotics).
- Full blood count.
- Urea and electrolytes.
- Liver function tests.
- Clotting profile (including fibrinogen level).
- CRP.
- Lactate—values can increase during end of the 1st stage of labour and throughout the 2nd stage. Trends may therefore be more meaningful than isolated values.
- Glucose.

Microbiological samples
- Consider: throat, sputum, vaginal, wound, urine, stool, placental, breast, and breast milk. If pus is present, collect and send it in a sterile container rather than a swab wherever possible.
- Fetal samples may also assist diagnosis, including ear, throat, and skin swabs.
- Review all previous samples taken during the pregnancy.

Arterial blood gases
- Consider ABGs if any respiratory compromise.

Imaging
- Chest X-ray if chest signs are identified.
- Consider USS, CT, or other appropriate imaging as required to ascertain the source of sepsis and inform management.

Management of the septic mother

As with any sick patient, management should follow a structured approach:

- **Airway** (with lateral tilt until delivery of the fetus).
- **Breathing.**
  - Titrate oxygen therapy to achieve target O_2 sats of >94%
- **Circulation.**
  - Obtain intravenous access and blood samples together.
  - Administer intravenous antimicrobial therapy.

> **Appropriate intravenous antimicrobial therapy administered within one hour** of identification of sepsis is crucial in improving outcome.
>   Delay beyond this time is associated with demonstrable increase in mortality.

- Give judicious fluid boluses (10ml/kg) under close observation.
- Consider invasive monitoring as appropriate.
- Catheterize and aim for urine output of >0.5ml/kg/hr.
- Optimize haemoglobin—aim for Hb >70g/L.
- If intra-abdominal, pelvic or uterine infection is suspected, operative source control may be required. This may include CS if intrauterine infection is suspected.
- Fetal condition will be optimized by maternal resuscitation. If sepsis has been diagnosed in the mother the neonatal team should be made aware as the neonate may also be at risk of developing sepsis.
- Prompt senior clinical review is necessary to recognize patients requiring referral to critical care.
- Effective teamwork between all professionals involved in a mother's care is vital in achieving a successful outcome.
- A patient who is clearly critically ill, continues to deteriorate, or fails to improve (despite initial resuscitation measures) should receive prompt critical care review.
- The following parameters should alert staff and trigger referral to critical care:
  - Persistent tachypnoea (RR > 25 breaths per minute).
  - Hypotension (systolic blood pressure < 90 mmHg).
  - Reduced level of consciousness.
  - Failure to return lactate to normal range.

Specific infections

Genital tract infection
In the recent MBRRACE-UK report, the organism Group A Streptococcus (GAS) was associated with genital tract infections in early pregnancy and peripartum, whereas coliforms were predominantly associated with second trimester ascending infections.

Group A β-haemolytic streptococcus
- 5–30% of population are asymptomatic carriers.
- Streptococcal sore throat is a common childhood infection.
- Mothers may have a history of respiratory infection or sore throat and may be in contact with small children.
- Spread is via person-to-person contact/droplets.
- The organism is transferred via the hands to the perineum.
- **Deterioration can be rapid and catastrophic.**

Respiratory tract infection
- A throat swab should be taken whenever a pregnant or recently delivered woman presents with sore throat or flu symptoms.
- There should be a lower threshold for antibiotic prescription in pregnant women with sore throat, due to the risk of Group A Streptococcal infection.
- This is described by the Centor Criteria, if any 3 criteria are present with a sore throat, appropriate antibiotics should be prescribed:
  - History of fever.
  - Tonsillar exudate.
  - No cough.
  - Tender anterior cervical lymphadenopathy.
- Consider influenza if a woman presents with sore throat and fever in the flu season. Advice should be sought from on-call virology regarding immediate treatment with anti-viral therapy where influenza is suspected. Immunization should be encouraged to reduce risk.

Anti-antimicrobial therapy
- **Liaison with microbiology for specialist antimicrobial advice should occur early.**

Suggested empirical therapy (organism unknown)
- Co-amoxiclav 1.2g tds/cefuroxime 1.5g tds/cefotaxime 1–2g qds-bd PLUS metronidazole 500mg tds.
- Penicillin allergy: clarithromycin 500mg bd or clindamycin 600mg–1.2g tds qds PLUS gentamicin.

In severe sepsis
- Piperacillin-tazobactam 4.5g tds/ciprofloxacin 600mg bd PLUS gentamicin 3–5mg/kg daily in divided doses tds.
- Meropenem 500mg–1g tds PLUS gentamicin.
- Metronidazole 500mg tds may also be added.
- If Group A streptococcal infection is suspected, clindamycin is more effective than penicillin because it inhibits exotoxin production.

If there are risk factors for MRSA, add teicoplanin or linezolid.

Transfer of the critically ill mother

The principles of transfer either intra-hospital or inter-hospital of the critically ill mother are the same as that of any adult critically ill patient, but with additional specific issues related to pregnancy.

- Good multidisciplinary preparation, planning, and communication are essential for a safe transfer.
- Essential obstetric information about the pregnancy, fetal viability, and delivery plan should be documented.
- Pregnancy specific problems such as PET should be clearly documented with an appropriate management plan. Not all intensivists are experts in pregnancy specific disorders.
- Once the mother is stable, ensure ongoing treatment, e.g. fluids, antihypertensive drugs, oxytocics are all continued during transfer.
- Avoid any aorto-caval compression in the antenatal patient and ensure monitoring of both the mother and the fetus during transit.
- Essential maternal monitoring should include ECG, pulse oximetry, BP, and urine output.
- Consider invasive BP and CVP monitoring in any haemodynamically unstable patient.
- All monitors and the ventilator should be checked for function, battery status, and whether the oxygen required for a safe transfer is available.
- End-tidal capnography is recommended in all ventilated patients.
- Resuscitation equipment and drugs should be checked and ready.
- Consideration should be made for the unexpected delivery of the baby during transfer if viable.
- Appropriate personnel who are experienced and trained in transfer procedures should accompany the patient.
- Ensure notes and investigations go with the patient.

Transfer checklist

It may help to consider the issues in a systematic way:

Mother

- Airway—endotracheal tube, laryngoscope, mask, oropharyngeal airway, laryngeal mask airway.
- Breathing—sufficient oxygen, Ambu-bag, transport ventilator.
- Circulation—cannulae, fluids, vasopressors, and never forget to tilt the antenatal mother.
- Disability—consider possible deterioration during transfer.
- Full monitoring, including end-tidal CO_2 if ventilated.
- Drugs—emergency drugs, IV sedation, muscle relaxants.
- Other equipment—spare batteries, infusions, pumps, oxygen, electrical leads, resuscitation equipment.
- Firmly secure all patient lines that are at risk of getting dislodged on movement.

Fetus

- Monitoring.
- Drugs.
- Equipment.

Communication
- Contact all relevant staff. This includes obstetricians, midwives, the neonatal team, anaesthetists, and any other specialists who may be involved in the mother's care.
- Decide who is required to transfer the patient (midwife, ODP, anaesthetist).
- Prepare a patient summary sheet and copy the notes.

Transport
- Vehicle required and whether an escort is appropriate.

Destination
- Identify where to go on arrival (hospital entrance, A&E, labour ward).
- Provide departure and expected arrival times and keep contact details of receiving staff.

Documentation
- Record patient observations, drugs administered, and other details of the transfer.

Personal
- You may require money, a phone, a coat, food, and drink and an anti-emetic if you experience travel sickness whilst travelling.

Further reading

AAGBI Safety Guidelines: Inter-hospital Transfer 2009 www.aagbi.org/sites/default/files/interhospital09.pdf

Appelboam R et al. Time to antibiotics in sepsis. *Critical Care* 2010;14:50.

Inpatient maternal sepsis tool, published by the Sepsis Trust–https://sepsistrust.org/wp-content/uploads/2018/06/Inpatient maternal NICE-Final-1107-2.pdf

Lucas DN et al. Sepsis in obstetrics and the role of the anaesthetist. *International Journal of Obstetric Anesthia* 2012;21:56–67.

Mor G et al. Inflammation and pregnancy: the role of the immune system at the implantation site. *American Journal of Reproductive Immunology* 2010;63:425–33.

NICE guideline [NG51]. Sepsis: recognition, diagnosis and early management. Updated September 2017.

Providing equity of critical and maternity care for the critically ill pregnant or recently pregnant woman July 2011 www.rcog.org.uk/globalassets/documents/guidelines/prov_eq_matandcritcare.pdf

Major obstetric haemorrhage

Rachel Collis

Definition, incidence, and impact

- Haemorrhage that occurs after delivery is called postpartum haemorrhage (PPH).
- Bleeding that started before delivery is called antepartum haemorrhage (APH).
- Obstetric haemorrhage is defined as a single blood loss of more than 500mL after vaginal delivery, or more than 1000mL after CS.
- Major obstetric haemorrhage (MOH) is defined as moderate if between 1000 and 2000mL, and severe if over 2000mL.
- Other definitions used to define major morbidity:
  - Haemoglobin drop of ≥40g/L.
  - Transfusion requirement of ≥4 units of red cells.
  - Need for invasive procedure such as brace sutures, uterine tamponade balloon, or interventional radiology to control bleeding.
- In women with lower body mass (e.g. less than 60kg), a lower level of blood loss may be clinically significant.

- Around 10% of deliveries are complicated by a 1000mL PPH.
- Massive obstetric haemorrhage >2500mL blood-loss occurs in around 6 per 1000 deliveries.
- Most of the severe maternal morbidity associated with haemorrhage occurs in this group.
- A medium sized delivery unit delivering ~3500 women per year would therefore expect to manage 21 cases every year, or 1–2 per month.
- Therefore, this is not a rare condition.

- 80% of parturients admitted to ICU are secondary to PPH.
- There has been no reduction in maternal deaths secondary to haemorrhage from 2009 to 2018.
- From a global perspective, although maternal mortality is improving, PPH remains a major contributing factor. The risk of death from PPH in sub-Saharan Africa is 1per 1000 maternities.

Organizational aspects

Planning

- A clear antenatal plan should be documented for high risk women including place of delivery, so appropriate facilities are available. In very high risk patients, delivery is best performed at a unit that can provide all the necessary interventions, i.e. interventional radiology, cell salvage, obstetricians familiar with brace sutures and tamponade balloons, specialist obstetric anaesthetists, on-site critical care facilities, and blood bank provision.
- Multidisciplinary antenatal care should include a referral pathway to a consultant-led anaesthetic assessment clinic at an early stage for any parturient considered 'high risk' for PPH at delivery.
- Identify known risk factors for haemorrhage:
  - Increasing maternal age (becoming more common).
  - Obesity.
  - Multiple pregnancies (increasing from assisted conception).
  - Previous PPH (especially from atony).
  - Previous abruption.
  - Pre-eclampsia or gestational hypertension.
  - Previous CS (all women who have had a previous CS must have their placental location identified). Beware the previous CS with placenta praevia. There is an increased risk of placenta accreta which is a cause of massive haemorrhage.
  - Women with pre-existing bleeding disorders and those on therapeutic anticoagulants.
- The unpredictable nature of obstetrics can make this simple rule complex in practice; high risk patients booked for delivery at a specialist centre can go into labour or bleed near the local unit. Every maternity unit with obstetric and anaesthetic staff should be equipped to manage most causes of PPH.
- Good antenatal care with early identification and treatment of antenatal anaemia is essential.
- Women with known placenta previa should have a group and save stored in blood bank, and suitability for electronic issuing of blood recorded.

Preparation

- A team approach is essential. CEMD repeatedly emphasizes the need for robust, multidisciplinary systems for communication and effective action. These must be clearly understood and regularly rehearsed by every member of the labour ward team.
- The importance of the team approach has led to the development of a number of multidisciplinary 'scenario-based' joint training courses for anaesthetists, obstetricians, and midwives. Regular attendance on one of these courses is beneficial.
- Teams require leadership, and the lead consultants in obstetrics and anaesthetics should work together with midwives to develop the necessary team skills in every unit. Locally based MOH protocols are beneficial as they take in to account local issues. Problems and systems failures are often only identified during an emergency, so 'fire drills' and simulations are essential.

- Analysis of the SaFE (Simulation and Fire drill Evaluation) study from the South West England region has provided evidence that after appropriate training and drills, improvement is seen in both knowledge and communication skills. This study has demonstrated that this can be achieved with in-house training.

Planning, protocols, practice, and audit

- Senior midwives, obstetricians, and anaesthetists should meet regularly to develop local protocols dealing with the clinical management and the organization/processes needed to cope with a major haemorrhage on their own unit.
- The issues will differ in each hospital, and the following questions should be addressed:
  - How are blood samples sent to the laboratories and blood bank?
  - How is portering organized to transport blood?
  - Where is the blood fridge and who has the key?
  - Do switchboard and blood bank understand the level of urgency of the requests made to them?
- There should be a clearly agreed 'code' via the hospital bleep system to alert the whole team to a MOH on the delivery suite.
- Planning should involve haematologists, laboratory staff, porters, ward clerks, healthcare support workers, etc. as necessary.
- Necessary equipment, e.g. blood warmers, pressure infusers, and monitoring devices, should be available.
- Copies of the local protocols should be issued to all relevant staff and be prominently displayed on the labour ward.
- Protocols which are written as a verbal check list are useful to improve compliance in a fast moving clinical situation.
- Measuring on-going blood loss after all deliveries, using a gravimetric technique in addition to blood collected in suction containers, can aid appropriate escalation policies. A number of quality improvement initiatives have advocated a step-wise 4-stage approach: 0=risk assessment, 1=PPH>500mL, 2=1000–1500mL, and 3=>1500mL. Appropriate actions are then designated to each step.
- Appropriate escalation policies should include the personnel and seniority of those attending the mother's bedside.
- All aspects of the agreed major PPH protocol must run well inside and outside normal working hours. There should be clear lines of communication between junior and senior staff outside normal working hours so appropriate help is rapidly available during a major PPH.
- Compliance with the local protocols should be the subject of regular multidisciplinary audit, with identified failings being promptly addressed.

Clinical management overview

Overview
The aim is to prevent haemorrhage escalating to the point where it is life-threatening by early recognition. Denying there is a problem and delaying definitive treatment can lead to escalation to the point where haemorrhage is life-threatening.

- The midwife in charge and the front-line obstetric and anaesthetic staff should be alerted when women present with minor PPH (blood loss 500–1000ml) without clinical shock.
- A multidisciplinary team should be summoned to attend at the bedside for major PPH (blood loss of more than 1000ml) with ongoing bleeding or clinical shock. This should include an obstetrician, midwife in charge of the delivery suite, and an anaesthetist.
- The cause of the bleeding should be identified and appropriate treatment instigated. Almost all bleeding early in an obstetric haemorrhage has an obstetric cause requiring obstetric intervention.
- There should be a clear escalation policy if bleeding continues with an accumulative measured blood loss of more than 1500mL. If the mother is not already in theatre, she should be moved there so definitive treatment can be instigated, which usually requires examination under anaesthesia at this stage.
- CEMD emphasizes that major haemorrhage requires consultant anaesthetist(s), consultant obstetrician(s), and senior midwifery staff to be involved.
- Blood bank should have a specific policy to deal with major obstetric haemorrhage. The advice of a consultant haematologist may be required if bleeding is on-going.
- Other specialists are occasionally required such as general, urology and vascular surgeons, and interventional radiologist.
- The operating obstetrician should be confident that she/he can perform a caesarean hysterectomy—not all obstetricians have this experience, and the involvement of more than one operating surgeon is often appropriate.

Directed therapy

The 4Ts pneumonic usefully divides the majority of causes of obstetric haemorrhage into groups allowing a swift differential diagnosis and directed treatment. 80% of PPH is caused by lack of tone and/or trauma.

- **T**one, e.g. uterine atony.
- **T**rauma, e.g. tears, lacerations, uterine rupture or inversion.
- **T**issue, e.g. retained placental fragments, clots, or membranes.
- **T**hrombin, e.g. DIC, dilutional coagulopathy, or severe thrombocytopenia.

Atony

Immediate management
- Empty the bladder as a full bladder will exacerbate atony.
- Rubbing-up' of a contraction is an effective skill which should be used early.
- Bi-manual compression: Can be a first-line life-saving measure for severe atony. One hand makes a fist in the vagina, whilst the other compresses the uterus downwards on the mother's abdomen. It can be used until uterotonics are effective, or if blood loss is on-going and the mother is being transferred to theatre.

Pharmacological management
- *Oxytocin:* A hormone which causes uterine contraction and peripheral vasodilation. Administered as a slow IV diluted bolus of 5 units and repeat once, followed by a continuous infusion of 10 units/hour if required. Give slowly as it can cause significant hypotension and give cautiously in women with cardiac disease. Carbetocin is a long-acting oxytocin analogue and is given as a one off IV or IM injection.
- Syntometrine®: Ergometrine 500 micrograms/oxytocin 5 IU is a combined preparation for deep IM injection. It is commonly given as a prophylactic measure to reduce the risk of uterine atony. It can be repeated and is useful as a first line treatment of uterine atony as IV access is not necessary.
- Ergometrine: An ergot alkaloid, which causes uterine and vascular smooth muscle contraction. Administered as 250–500 micrograms IV or IM. The IV dose should be diluted to at least 10mL and given slowly to a maximum dose of 1mg. It causes hypertension and vomiting and should be avoided in pre-eclampsia and essential hypertension.
- Carboprost: A 15-methyl prostaglandin F2-α is a third line uterotonic which is given as a 250 microgram intramuscular or intramyometrial injection (**never IV**). It can be repeated every 15min, to a maximum dose of 2mg. It can cause nausea, vomiting, diarrhoea, and severe bronchospasm, and should be avoided in patients with asthma.
- *Misoprostol:* A synthetic prostaglandin E1 analogue and effective uterine constrictor. Give 800–1000 micrograms sublingually or rectally as a tablet. May cause nausea, vomiting, or diarrhoea. Can also cause bronchospasm (less severe than carboprost). Its advantage is that it does not need to be refrigerated or given as an injection.

Surgical management

- Although pharmacological management is the mainstay of early atonic PPH management, repeated doses of the same drug is futile and causes delay. If the bleeding is on-going >1500mL after the step-wise escalation of uterotonics, surgical intervention must be rapidly considered.
- Examination under anaesthesia: Retained blood clots and placental tissue are potent causes of persistent atony.
- Uterine tamponade: Either with ribbon gauze or a tamponade balloon inserted vaginally into the uterine cavity is effective.
- Compression sutures: Give external mechanical compression of the uterus (Fig 18.1). This involves a laparotomy where two sutures compress the upper segment of the uterus. Absorbable sutures mean subsequent pregnancies are unlikely to be affected.
- Vascular control: Aortic compression in an extreme emergency can be a life-saving manoeuvre. Direct compression of the aorta against the spinal column is applied at laparotomy and can reduce haemorrhage by around 40%. Clamping of the aorta by an experienced vascular surgeon may also be required.
- Bilateral uterine artery ligation can be performed at laparotomy and does not affect future pregnancies due to collateral circulation. This is reported as successful in 95% of cases.
- Bilateral internal iliac artery ligation is reported as successful in 50% of cases of atony and placenta accreta. The complications include ligation of external iliac artery, trauma to iliac veins, ureteric injury, and retroperitoneal haematoma.
- Hysterectomy can be live-saving but the decision and surgery should be carried out by a consultant, and in many circumstances by two. It should, however, be carried out promptly, if the patient has severe cardiovascular compromise and if other methods have failed.

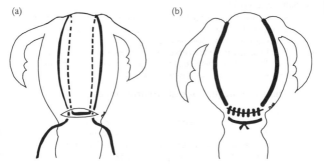

Fig. 18.1 B-Lynch suture. (a) A single suture is inserted as shown. (b) As it is drawn tight, the fundus of the uterus is compressed against the lower segment. The uterus is now physically unable to relax.

Trauma

- Lacerations and tears to the uterus or lower genital tract are a common, are frequently an underestimated cause of haemorrhage, and must be carefully explored and repaired.
- Surgical procedures will require adequate anaesthesia, which may require GA.
- Regional anaesthesia should only be considered if the patient is fully resuscitated, haemodynamically stable, and has normal clotting.

Tissue

- The uterus must be empty for effective contraction to occur. Remaining fragments of placenta, blood clot, or membranes must be removed.
- This can sometimes be done gently after a vaginal delivery without anaesthesia, but frequently requires more detailed examination and adequate anaesthesia.
- Abnormally adherent or invasive placenta (accreta, percreta) can pose particular problems necessitating hysterectomy, but in extreme cases the placenta may invade outside the uterus and have to be left in situ.

Thrombin

- This part of the pneumonic is the least common of the causes of PPH, i.e. <5% of PPH, but can exacerbate haemorrhage associated with other causes making haemorrhage very difficult to control.

Dilutional coagulopathy

- Occurs when there has been a delay in recognition or treatment of haemorrhage or if bleeding has been rapid and uncontrolled, such as with placenta previa/accreta.
- It occurs if haemorrhage has exceeded ~2500mL, is on-going, and blood volume has been replaced with clear IV fluids.

Consumptive coagulopathy

- Is associated with placental abruption, amniotic fluid embolus, and severe sepsis. It occurs early in the bleed with an apparent consumption of coagulation factors, especially fibrinogen.
- Initially bleeding can be concealed or not severe especially prior to delivery. It can then rapidly lead to severe and uncontrolled bleeding from other causes, such as atony or trauma.

Major haemorrhage: Special circumstances

Placenta praevia/accreta

- Placenta praevia occurs when the placenta covers the cervix necessitating delivery of the fetus by caesarean section.
- Anterior placenta praevia is associated with more blood loss as the placenta is cut before the delivery of the baby.
- Posterior and anterior placenta praevia are both associated with major PPH, because of a poorly contracted lower segment which does not respond to uterotonics.
- Balloon tamponade or brace sutures can be helpful.
- Placenta accreta occurs when there is abnormal placentation in a previous uterine scar, where there is no natural plane for uterine separation.

- The placenta can sometimes be cut away but if bleeding is severe, if the abnormal placental tissue extensive or invading other pelvic organs (percreta), then a hysterectomy is required.
- In patients who have had previous CS, ask the obstetrician about placental site (on ultrasound). If anterior, prepare for potential sudden major blood loss and make a plan if large transfusion required.

Uterine rupture

- Is more common in the developing than the developed world. It is associated with previous CS, uterine surgery, or uterine perforation associated with termination of pregnancy, which may have been illegal and therefore concealed. It can rarely be associated with very prolonged and obstructed labour, without previous uterine surgery.
- The condition is rapidly fatal for the baby and associated with major concealed haemorrhage which is difficult to quantify. Fetal demise, maternal cardiovascular compromise, and a distended tense abdomen are the only findings.
- Uterine rupture through a previous CS scar can be associated with less bleeding than rupture through the body of the uterus as the old scar is relatively avascular.
- In all cases the mother will require an urgent laparotomy, which must not be delayed as the cause of the haemorrhage is traumatic and will not improve until surgically treated.

Abruption

- Is caused by premature separation of the placenta leading to fetal demise.
- It is associated with PET and can be very difficult to treat, as the mother may have severe hypertension as well as major haemorrhage.
- Bleeding occurs between the placenta and the uterus. Clot forms causing a localized consumption of fibrinogen and platelets.
- The mother can seem stable as blood-loss is usually not severe at this stage. Major PPH then occurs after delivery (vaginal or caesarean) due to coagulation deficiency.
- If the baby is still alive then caesarean delivery should be performed. This usually indicates that the abruption is small or early in its development and severe coagulation problems are unusual.
- If the baby is dead, delivery should be expedited to reduce the time over which consumption occurs. Vaginal delivery is probably safer.
- If there is a coagulopathy present, coagulation products should be given to correct clotting factors before delivery.

MOH: Role of the anaesthetist

- The anaesthetist is as an essential part of the multidisciplinary team (MDT) who should attend the mother's bedside during a PPH.
- The whole team should attend the mother when the measured blood loss is 1000mL with on-going bleeding.
- Almost all MOH can be prevented if the MDT attends the bedside and instigates appropriate directed treatment.
- The anaesthetist should lead on establishing IV access, taking blood for laboratory and VHA testing, point of care Hb and lactate, and in addition administering IV fluids.
- With on-going MOH of more than 1500mL, the mother should be moved to theatre, if not already there, and the anaesthetist should liaise with all theatre staff.
- A second anaesthetist should attend if possible to optimize resuscitation and ensure theatre drugs and equipment are ready.
- Having assessed the mother, the anaesthetist should liaise with blood bank to order blood and blood products as required preferably aided by VHA testing.

Initial resuscitation and stabilization

Resuscitation should follow the obstetric ABC principle as follows:
- Tilt.
- 100% oxygen.
- ABC with rapid initial assessment and correction as found.
- Diagnosis and definitive treatment.

Tilt (if undelivered)
- Avoid supine aorto-caval compression by either placing the patient in the left lateral position, or providing 15° degrees left lateral tilt with a wedge under the right hip.

Oxygen
- Administer 15L/min oxygen via a tight-fitting face mask with a reservoir bag.
- Turn the wall oxygen flowmeter to maximum—this will achieve optimal oxygen saturation of the blood remaining in the circulation and help to prevent tissue hypoxia.

Airway
- A severely shocked patient may lose consciousness due to hypotension and require tracheal intubation to protect the airway from gastric acid aspiration, and to maintain adequate oxygenation/ventilation.

Breathing
- This may become inadequate and the patient may require ventilation as consciousness is lost, and severe tissue hypoxia and metabolic acidosis supervene.

Circulation
- Rapid assessment of the estimated blood volume lost should be performed while simultaneously:
  - Infusing 500–1000mL of crystalloid (Hartmanns/normal saline) rapidly and set up blood warmers and pressure infusors as soon as available.
  - Keeping the patient warm—use active heating as soon as practicable, e.g. warm air blower (Bair Hugger), warming mattress, fluid warmers. Coagulopathy is exacerbated by hypothermia.

Common pitfall
- A normal BP does not exclude major blood loss in the pregnant patient.
- The physiologically increased plasma volume and red cell mass of pregnancy means total blood volume can be increased by up to 40%. Up to 40% blood volume can be lost (1500–2000mL) before hypotension appears, due to blood being shunted away from the feto-placental unit (750mL/min) to maintain flow to vital organs.

Early signs of impending decompensation occur with a normal blood pressure
- Tachycardia >100bpm.
- Fetal distress.
- Skin pallor with increased capillary refill time (>2s, which is the time it takes to say 'capillary refill').
- Decreased/absent urine output (this is not usually known in the acute situation).

Signs of life-threatening hypovolaemia, i.e. >50% blood volume loss include
- Hypotension.
- Tachypnea.
- Mental clouding, progressing to unconsciousness.

Assess the response to initial volume replacement
- 15–30% blood loss (750–1500mL) will respond to crystalloids alone; tachycardia will improve and remain improved.
- 30–40% blood loss (1500–2000mL) will have a transitory response to crystalloids and will require colloid infusion while waiting for cross-matched or group-specific blood.
- >40% blood loss (>2000mL) is life-threatening and requires immediate transfusion; use O-negative blood if group-specific is not available. Avoid excessive amounts, i.e. >2000mL, of clear IV fluids.

Assess the need for additional/invasive monitoring
- Invasive monitoring can be a very helpful adjunct to the management of the mother with a major haemorrhage, but fluid resuscitation **MUST NOT** be delayed during attempts to place CVP and arterial lines. **Wait until a second anaesthetist can aid insertion.**
- An arterial line is required for most cases where blood loss is >2000mL or rapid enough for the mother to be haemodynamically unstable, both for accurate real-time invasive BP monitoring and sequential blood gas

analysis (including point of care Hb and lactate monitoring), VHA, and repeated laboratory testing.

- A CVP line gives some useful extra information on volume status. If one is considered necessary, an internal jugular line should be placed under ultrasound guidance whenever possible. Pregnant women are prone to fluid overload and pulmonary oedema especially if pre-eclamptic and a CVP line may aid resuscitation.
- A urinary catheter is mandatory with any blood loss >1500mL as urine output is an important indicator of the adequacy of volume replacement.

Anaesthesia

- If the mother does not already have a regional anaesthetic, consider a GA if:
  - Haemorrhage is severe.
  - There is ongoing haemodynamic instability.
  - Diagnosis is uncertain.
- If there is a spinal or epidural *in situ,* then it may safely be continued, as a GA induction may make haemodynamic instability significantly worse.
- There are many case reports of caesarean hysterectomies performed solely under regional techniques.
- A regional technique de-novo is generally safe if blood loss is <2000mL, and the mother is well fluid resuscitated.
- The standard rapid sequence obstetric GA technique may have to be modified in the patient who has suffered a MOH, where a bolus of thiopental or propofol/suxamethonium could cause significant hypotension.
- Alternatives include induction with ketamine 1–5mg/kg, opiate–benzodiazepine mixtures, etomidate, or volatile agents; this will be a decision for a senior anaesthetist, with the risk of acid aspiration balanced against the risk of haemodynamic decompensation.
- Indications for converting a regional to a general anaesthetic are:
  - Maternal unconsciousness due to hypotension.
  - Severe maternal anxiety.
  - Inadequate anaesthesia, especially during prolonged surgery.

Blood transfusion, coagulation factors, and tranexamic acid

Red cell transfusion

- Transfusion should aim for a Hb of 80g/L; over transfusion is unnecessary although with acute severe bleeding the initial Hb can be artificially high.
- All clinicians involved in blood transfusion should be aware of the potential adverse effects of transfusion and signs and symptoms of transfusion-related complications.
- The blood bank provides red cells in additive solution, and there is a hierarchy of transfusion choices depending on urgency. Local blood banks have varying protocols and procedures which should be clearly publicized on the major haemorrhage protocol.
  - O-negative blood for emergency use should be available on labour ward or within 5min distance.
  - Fully cross-matched blood will take 30–50min.
  - 'Electronic issue'—if the patient has had two recent 'group and screen' samples processed through the same laboratory, the electronic issue system allows the release of an unlimited number of units of blood immediately. Blood can be available in 10min. Electronic issue blood is not available for antibody positive samples which will include most Rh negative mothers who have had anti-D prophylaxis.
  - For very high risk women, cross-matched blood should be held in the blood bank.

Cell salvage

- Cell salvage can provide a useful source of red cells to reduce the patient's exposure to allogeneic blood and conserve the supply in massive bleeding.
- It is not cost effective to set up cell salvage for all CSs.
- It is now being used widely in the UK, and initial fears about possible contamination with amniotic fluid have not been borne out in practice.
- It was initially thought that the use of cell salvage in obstetrics mandatorily required the use of a leucocyte depletion filter (LDF) to ensure effective removal of all elements of amniotic fluid. More recently, the use of the LDF has been questioned, as there have been a small number of reports of unexplained hypotension apparently associated with its use. While the cause of the hypotension remains under investigation, many units have chosen to use cell salvage without the LDF, and there have been no reports of adverse effects. LDF slows down the rate of salvage blood replacement, and it is acceptable to remove it if necessary.
- The practice of using 2 separate suckers and wasting the initial blood loss prior to placental removal has also been shown to be unnecessary in terms of the quality of salvaged blood.
- If the mother is Rhesus negative there is a potential for fetal red cell exposure, and a Kleihauer test should be performed within 72h and an appropriate calculated dose of anti-D given.
- Because of the risk of allo-immunization of the mother from fetal cells (not only Rh antibodies), collected blood should not be returned unless it will substantially make a difference to the mother's haemoglobin.

Replacement of coagulation factors

- There is increasing recognition that coagulation deficiency occurs late during most MOH.
- Pregnant women have a high level of fibrinogen and other coagulation factors which are a physiological buffer to prevent coagulopathy in the majority of MOH.
- APTT and PT will remain normal in most cases of MOH until blood loss exceeds 3000mL.
- Plasma fibrinogen of 3g/L early during a PPH is a biomarker for severity.
- Fibrinogen falls earlier than other coagulation factors and should be replaced if below 2g/L (Clauss fibrinogen)
- There is no advantage of replacing fibrinogen above this level.

Fresh frozen plasma (FFP)

- Is derived from non-pregnant donors and contains 2–3g/L of fibrinogen.
- In the majority of MOH, FFP will contain less fibrinogen and other important coagulation factors, such as factor VIII and Von-Willebrand factors, than the plasma of the mother.
- The current recommendation is to give RBC and FFP as a 1:1 fixed ratio if clotting results are not available in an on-going haemorrhage, when 4 units of RBC have ALREADY been given.
- FFP should be given to keep the APTT and PT within the normal range.

Cryoprecipitate

- This is a pooled blood product. The usual dose is 1 pool (5 bags), which contains 1625mg fibrinogen and high levels of Factor VIII and von Willebrand factor.
- In a 70kg patient, 1 pool of cryoprecipitate will raise fibrinogen 35mg/dL if there is no further dilution or consumption.
- It is an effective treatment for hypo-fibrinogenaemia associated with MOH.

Fibrinogen concentrate

- Each vile contains 1 g of fibrinogen and its effect can be reliably titrated against the patients fibrinogen levels.
- A dose of 4 g is usually effective, although this will depend on the starting plasma fibrinogen levels, the size of the patient, and the rate of haemorrhage.
- It is a concentrated lyophilized protein that is easily reconstituted in water, and can be administered in minutes during an emergency.
- It goes through a process of virus inactivation, therefore reducing the risk of transmission of infective agents.
- There is a low risk of allergic reactions.
- Case reports, case series, and RCTs have shown it can reduce bleeding during PPH in the presence of Clauss fibrinogen <2g/L)

Recombinant factor VIIa

- New models of coagulation emphasize the interaction of tissue factor and factor VIIa in initiation, amplification, propagation, and localization of fibrin clot. This reaction bypasses all the other 'classical' coagulation cascade elements and generates thrombin on the platelets at the site of bleeding.

- Case reports have described its effectiveness in preventing hysterectomy when other coagulation products have failed, although there are no randomized trials to verify its effectiveness.
- It is ineffective if the patient is acidotic or hypothermic or if insufficient coagulation products have been given. Fibrinogen levels should be corrected to >1g/L prior to administration.
- Given by bolus IV injection over 5–10min, 2h half-life, dose 90 micrograms/kg repeated every 2–3h.
- It is very expensive and is not licensed for use in PPH. The manufacturers have said it should not be used for this indication and it can cause severe thrombosis.

Platelets
- Maintain platelet count above 50×10^9 by transfusing if numbers fall below 75×10^9.
- Platelet transfusions are rarely required, unless there is a 5000mL PPH, thrombocytopenia prior to delivery or DIC associated with abruption, severe sepsis or AFE.
- Platelets are stored in the transfusion centre, not necessarily at the local hospital blood bank—anticipate the need for platelets early and liaise with the haematologist.
- Most formulaic transfusion practices where platelets are given with a fixed ratio of RBC and FFP will lead to over-transfusion. Most laboratories will process a FBC within minutes in an emergency, therefore titrating platelet transfusion on actual platelets numbers should be practiced if possible.

Tranexamic acid

- Is an anti-fibrinolytic agent, and can be given by slow IV injection at a dose of 0.5–1.0g every 4 hours for 12 hours.
- It competitively inhibits the conversion of plasminogen to plasmin, thereby preventing fibrin degradation and stabilizing clot formation.
- In a double blind randomized trial predominantly conducted in developing world countries, it was shown to reduce the rate of maternal death and hysterectomy if given early in the bleed and within 3 hours of the start of the bleed.
- It is now recommended that 1g should be given if PPH exceeds 1000mL and has not stopped, and repeated after 30min if bleeding is on-going.

MOH: Role of point of care testing

Point of care testing in MOH includes
- Near-side Hb measure (blood gas or Haemcue).
- Venous lactate.
- Ionized calcium.
- Blood glucose.
- VHA assays for coagulation.

Haemoglobin
- Hb should be kept above 80g/L with active bleeding.
- A single Hb can be falsely reassuring early in the MOH, before adequate resuscitation has occurred. It should be repeated if bleeding continues or there is any clinical concern.

Venous lactate
- Can help assess resuscitation status of the mother. A venous lactate >2mmol/L is a cause of concern, and careful evaluation of the cardiovascular status of the mother should be carried out.
- The combination of a falling Hb and a raised lactate may indicate concealed bleeding, such as an abruption or intra-abdominal bleeding after caesarean delivery.

Ionized calcium
- Should be monitored during massive RBC transfusion.
- Hypocalcaemia exacerbates coagulopathy and myocardial dysfunction, and is a consequence of massive rapid RBC transfusion. It can be accurately measured on many blood gas analysers. Keep ionized Ca >1.0 mmol/L by giving 10ml of 10% calcium gluconate IV.

Viscoelastometric haemostatic assays
- VHAs are an effective bed-side tests of coagulation and have increasingly been used safely in the management of MOH.
- The new automated cartridge machines from ROTEM® and TEG (Haemonetics) have made this technology more readily accessible with basic level training.
- Both devices readily identify hypofibrinogenaemia and clotting deficiencies associated with MOH and have been successfully used in large patient cohorts to guide treatment.
- Replace fibrinogen when below 2g/L, which correlates with:
  - ROTEM equivalent FIBTEM A5 = 10–12mm.
  - TEG equivalent CFF of MA = 17–19mm.
- FFP should be given if there is prolongation of the clot initiation time, as this indicates an overall clotting factor deficiency i.e.:
  - ROTEM CT EXTEM >80seconds.
  - TEG Kaolin R of >8min.

- Fibrinogen (fibrinogen concentrate or cryoprecipitate) should be replaced initially and will usually correct slight prolongation in the CT or Kaolin r time.
- In severe DIC with very low initial fibrinogen and prolonged clot initiation time at 1.5× normal, then FFP should be given with fibrinogen replacement therapy.
- VHA should be repeated with every additional 500mL of blood loss, if ongoing clinical concern and after coagulation products have been administered.

Continuing care

- All mothers who has suffered a major haemorrhage (PPH>1500mL) must have continuing care in an appropriate environment. Once haemostasis is achieved, the patient should be transferred to an appropriate critical care, i.e. HDU/level 2 or ICU/level 3 setting for further management. Maternal deaths have been attributed to substandard care in the postpartum period.
- The length of time on HDU will depend on haemodynamic stability over the first 6 hours after delivery.
- Observations should be made on a HDU chart with frequent measurements of BP and pulse, urine output, respiratory rate, and fluid balance.
- In all settings, there must be close ongoing liaison between obstetricians, obstetric anaesthetist, and ICU/HDU staff.
- Regular Hb and coagulation studies will need to be performed every 4–6 hours.
- Once bleeding has stopped, thromboprophylaxis must be commenced.
- Stand down the MOH protocol, and return unused blood and blood products to blood bank.

Indications for transfer for ventilation in an ICU

- Ongoing bleeding—especially if associated with coagulopathy.
- Hypothermia.
- Severe oliguria/anuria.
- Evidence of pulmonary oedema or increased oxygen requirements.
- Poorly corrected metabolic acidosis with an increased lactate.

Review

- Cases of major haemorrhage >1500mL should be reported to the local hospital critical incident reporting system.
- All staff involved should ideally conduct a 'rapid review' of the case within 48h to examine the effectiveness of the systems involved, to define lessons learned and to organize/provide counselling as necessary in the event of a bad outcome.
- A review of the causes and management of the haemorrhage should be made at the local critical incident meeting.
- Maternal deaths should be reported to the coroner and CEMD in due course.

Further reading

https://www.transfusionguidelines.org/transfusion-handbook

Mavrides E et al on behalf of the Royal College of Obstetricians and Gynaecologists. Prevention and management of postpartum haemorrhage. *British Journal of Obstetrics and Gynaecology* 2016; 124: e106–e149.

Catling, S. Blood conservation techniques in obstetrics: a UK perspective. *International Journal of Obstetric Anesthesia* 2007;16: 241–249.

Shakur H et al. Effect of early tranexamic acid administration on mortality, hysterectomy, and other morbidities in women with post-partum haemorrhage (WOMAN): an international, randomised, double-blind, placebo-controlled trial. *Lancet*, 2017; 389: 2105–2116.

Hunt BJ et al. British Committee for Standards in Haematology. A practical guideline for the haematological management of major haemorrhage. *British Journal of Haematology* 2015; 170: 788–803.

Collins PW et al on behalf of OBS2 study collaborators Viscoelastometry guided fresh frozen plasma infusion for postpartum haemorrhage: OBS2, an observational study. *British Journal of Anaesthia* 2017; 119: 422–434.

Mallaiah S et al. Introduction of an algorithm for ROTEM- guided fibrinogen concentrate administration in major obstetric haemorrhage. *Anaesthesia* 2015; 70: 166–75.

Shields LE et al. Comprehensive maternal hemorrhage protocols reduce the use of blood products and improve patient safety. *American Journal of Obstetrics and Gynaecology* 2015; 212: 272–280.

Hypertensive disease

Eleanor Lewis and Stuart Davies

Introduction

- Hypertension will affect approximately 1 in 10 pregnant women in the UK, whilst pre-eclampsia (PET), which is a pregnancy specific disease, complicates between 2–8% of pregnancies.
- Hypertensive disease is currently the 4th leading cause of direct maternal deaths in the UK, with a mortality rate of <1 per million maternities. This rate has markedly reduced between 2006–8 and 2012–14. The majority of deaths in the recent triennium are due to cerebral causes, most commonly intracerebral haemorrhage, related to high systolic blood pressure. Anoxia associated with seizures is an increasingly significant cause of mortality.
- Substandard care has been identified as a contributing factor in many deaths. It is hoped that increased emphasis on screening, early diagnosis, early involvement of senior clinical staff, and increasing use of management protocols will reduce the number of deaths.
- Pre-eclampsia in resource poor countries is rarely diagnosed early, and as many as 50,000 deaths a year are attributable to eclampsia alone.
- Placental abruption/haemorrhage, fetal IUGR, and risk of early delivery cause increased perinatal morbidity and mortality. It accounts for 5% of still births not linked to congenital abnormalities in the UK.

CEMACE Key Recommendations: 2006–2014

- All women with a headache or epigastric pain should have their blood pressure measured and proteinuria assessed. New epigastric pain after 20 weeks of pregnancy is PET until proven otherwise.
- Systolic blood pressure must be effectively controlled as it is directly linked to an increased risk of cerebral haemorrhage.
- Systolic BP >180mmHg is a medical emergency. Systolic BP>160 mmHg is associated with an increased risk of cerebral haemorrhage and requires immediate antihypertensive treatment. Target systolic BP <150 mmHg.
- Ergometrine should be avoided in the 3rd stage of delivery in hypertensive women.

MBRRACE Key Recommendations: 2014–2016

- BP and urinalysis should be checked at every antenatal visit.
- All women who develop PET should be referred promptly to consultant led care and have a clear plan for the remainder of their pregnancy.
- BP <150/100mmHg should be the target for adequate control.
- Beware of agitation and restlessness. They are important clinical signs of severe PET.
- Blood pressure must be controlled before intubation is attempted when administering a GA. Intubation is associated with a surge in blood pressure which has led to fatal cerebral haemorrhage in women with PET.
- Neuro-imaging should be undertaken urgently in any woman with PET who also has focal neurological signs or who fails to rapidly recover fully from an eclamptic seizure.

Classification and diagnosis

Hypertension is a common complication of pregnancy affecting between 10 and 15% of pregnancies. It is important to differentiate between pre-existing (chronic) hypertension, pregnancy induced (gestational) hypertension, and pre-eclampsia, as the treatment, outcomes, and timing of delivery differ significantly. In addition women with hypertension, particularly pre-existing hypertension, are at greater risk of developing pre-eclampsia.

Hypertension in pregnancy is defined as a manual BP reading >140mmHg systolic and/or 90mmHg diastolic on two consecutive occasions. It can be subdivided into mild, moderate or severe:
- **Mild**: systolic BP 140–149mmHg and/or diastolic 90–99mmHg.
- **Moderate**: systolic BP 150–159mmHg and/or diastolic 100–109mmHg.
- **Severe:** systolic BP >160mmHg and /or Diastolic >110mmHg.

Classification of hypertensive disorders of pregnancy

Pre-existing/chronic hypertension
- Occurs in 5% of pregnancies.
- Hypertension diagnosed before pregnancy or before 20 weeks gestation, which may be essential or secondary hypertension.
- Essential hypertension has no known underlying cause.
- Secondary hypertension is associated with chronic disease, e.g. renal disease.
- Chronic hypertension is associated with a 25% increased risk of PET.

Pregnancy induced (gestational) hypertension
- Occurs in 6–7% of pregnancies.
- Hypertension diagnosed after 20 weeks gestation with a normal booking BP.

Pre-eclampsia de novo
- 2–8% of pregnancies.
- Hypertension occurring with significant proteinuria after 20 weeks gestation.

Pre-eclampsia superimposed on pre-existing hypertension
- Occurs in 25% of women with pre-existing hypertension.

Eclampsia
- A convulsion in a pregnant woman with hypertension or who develops hypertension after the convulsion.
- Incidence: 1 in 2000 deliveries in developed countries.

Risk factors for PET
- First pregnancy or >10yrs since last pregnancy: 10-fold increase.
- New paternity multigravida pregnancy: 10-fold increase.
- Previous PET requiring early delivery: 20% risk of recurrence.
- Family history of PET in 1st-degree female relatives: 4–8× increase.
- Partner previously fathered an affected pregnancy: 2-fold increase.
- Age >40 years.
- BMI >35 at 'booking': 4-fold increase.
- An increase in BMI between pregnancies.
- Chronic hypertension (BP >140 systolic at 'booking'): 20% risk.
- Multiple pregnancy: 2-fold increase.
- Hydropic fetus.
- Associated medical conditions:
  - Diabetes mellitus.
  - Renal disease.
  - Antiphospholipid syndrome/other connective tissue disorders.

Doppler/ultrasound assessment
- Early identification of the high risk pregnancy can be performed using Doppler assessment of the utero-placental circulation.
- By 20 weeks gestation, a normal pregnancy should develop a low resistance Doppler waveform.
- In a low risk population at 20 weeks gestation, 20% of pregnancies will go on to develop pre-eclampsia if a low resistance circulation has not developed.
- Doppler assessment of the uterine artery can show absent or reversed end-diastolic blood flow in pre-eclampsia.
- Reduced liquor volume can also indicate placental insufficiency.

Diagnosis
By definition: pregnancy-induced hypertension measured on 2 separate occasions at least 4 hours apart, accompanied by significant proteinuria.

Method of BP measurement
- The woman should be seated at 45° degrees with the arm at the level of the heart.
- An appropriate sized cuff should be used. If the mid-arm circumference is >33cm, a large cuff should be used.
- Korotkoff phase 1 should be used for systolic BP, and Korortkoff phase 5 should be used for diastolic BP.
- Automated cuff measurements regularly underestimate systolic BP.

Definition of significant proteinuria
- Spot urinary protein:creatinine ratio (PCR) >30mg/mmol.
- 24 hour urine collection >300mg protein.
- An automated reagant strip test of 1+ should prompt a PCR or 24 hour collection.

Clinical features supportive of the diagnosis
- Headache.
- Visual disturbance.
- Epigastric pain.
- Vomiting.
- Liver tenderness.
- 3 beats of clonus.
- Papilloedema.

Blood investigations supportive of the diagnosis
- Platelet count< 100×10^6/l.
- Abnormal liver enzymes (ALT/AST>70 IU).
- Uric acid or urate is a marker of oxidative stress and associated with poorer maternal and neonatal outcomes—0.33 at 38 weeks is the upper limit of normal.

Additional considerations
- Clinical symptoms and signs may precede measurable rises in blood pressure and detectable proteinuria, therefore a high level of clinical suspicion is required in order to avoid missing cases.
- IUGR may be the presenting feature.
- Severe PET can be diagnosed with mild or moderate hypertension if complicated by HELLP (haemolysis, elevated liver enzymes, low platelets), renal dysfunction, or eclampsia.
- The diagnosis of HELLP, which is part of the spectrum of pre-eclampsia, can be made with normal blood pressure and no proteinurea,
- The mother can deteriorate rapidly without warning, therefore clinical vigilance is necessary in all cases of pre-eclampsia.

Pathophysiology of pre-eclampsia

The exact cause and mechanism of pre-eclampsia is unknown, but a two-stage pathological process is widely supported:

- Impaired placentation is the 1st stage, leading to maternal endothelial changes in the 2nd stage, resulting in the systemic clinical manifestations. Impaired trophoblast invasion of the myometrial arteries leads to failure of spiral artery remodelling.
- This results in an unusually high resistance in the spiral arteries due to lack of breakdown of the muscular walls. Irregular perfusion then leads to placental hypoxia and reperfusion, which results in oxidative stress. It is hypothesized that the cause of the placental stage of pre-eclampsia is an atypical maternal immune response to trophoblasts.
- The 2nd systemic maternal phase of the disease is thought to be an exaggerated endothelial activation and generalized hyper-inflammatory state.
- Placental oxidative stress results in the release of inflammatory cytokines into the maternal circulation. This leads to maternal endothelial dysfunction and associated increased vascular reactivity resulting in the onset of the clinical disease.
- The overall effect is a low output, high resistance cardiovascular state.
- The linking mechanism between stage 1 and 2 of the disease may differ and thus explain different manifestations of the spectrum of clinical presentations associated with pre-eclampsia, such as HELLP and acute fatty liver of pregnancy (AFLP) syndromes.
- Early onset disease is associated with a much more aggressive placental phase, leading to a small placenta and IUGR. This disease process may account for early miscarriages.
- In late onset disease, placental size and villous morphology is often normal, and predisposing factors may play a greater role in initiating the placental and systemic inflammatory response.
- Pre-eclampsia is now known to be linked to an increased risk of developing cardiovascular and metabolic diseases in later life.

Cardiovascular changes

In a recent study, hypertension is thought to be primarily due to increased cardiac output, due to both an increased inotropic effect and impaired diastolic function. In addition, generalized vasoconstriction leads to increased SVR and contributes to the hypertension.

Capillary permeability leads to redistribution of fluid into the interstitial space. Intravascular depletion and hypovolaemia occur as a consequence of the above.

Peripheral oedema is seen due to:
- Increased capillary permeability.
- Hypoalbuminaemia, therefore reducing colloid oncotic pressure.
- Increased capillary hydrostatic pressure due to increased SVR and the effects of the gravid uterus.

Pulmonary and cerebral oedema may occur in severe cases and can be life-threatening. Modest administration of IV fluids, fluid shifts at delivery, and

LV dysfunction contribute to their severity. Pulmonary oedema can be secondary to marked diastolic dysfunction, where the mechanism is in part due to oedema within the myocardial muscle.

Respiratory changes

- Increased lung water causes reduced lung compliance and increased work of breathing. Therefore, an increase in respiratory rate and falling oxygen saturations, especially on air, are early signs of impending pulmonary oedema.
- Upper airway oedema of face, neck, tongue, and larynx. Voice changes and difficult intubation are early changes, with stridor occurring late. The cricoid cartilage may be difficult to palpate.

Renal changes

- Endothelial damage leads to protein loss and decreased albumin/colloid oncotic pressure.
- Decreased glomerular filtration leads to increased serum uric acid, which is an indicator of disease severity.
- Tubular ischaemia secondary to vasoconstriction and hypovolaemia.
- Acute kidney injury (AKI) requiring dialysis is rare but is a serious prognostic indicator due to its association with severe disease.

Hepatic changes

- Oedema, haemorrhage, and ischaemic necrosis of the liver can occur.
- Raised aspartate aminotransferase (AST), and alanine aminotransferase (ALT) are a poor prognostic sign (see HELLP syndrome).
- AFLP may also be part of the pre-eclamptic spectrum, with hypoglycaemia being a marker of deteriorating hepatic function. Urgent delivery is indicated if diagnosed.
- Liver capsule distension—may present with epigastric pain. This may cause a subcapsular hepatic haematoma or even hepatic rupture.

CNS changes

- Risk of cerebral haemorrhage secondary to hypertension.
- Cerebral vasoconstriction, cerebral oedema, and raised intracranial pressure leads to cerebral ischaemia and may precipitate eclamptic seizures.
- Variable neurological symptoms and signs—headache, vomiting, visual disturbance, confusion, decreased Glasgow Coma Score (GCS), hyper-reflexia, and clonus.

Haematological changes

- Thrombocytopaenia.
- Haemolysis and anaemia.
- Coagulopathy—in severe disease with hepatic dysfunction. DIC is rare and associated with haemorrhage or placental abruption.

Feto-placental unit

- IUGR is often seen.
- There is a significant risk of placental abruption.

Antenatal management of pre-eclampsia

Primary prevention

Low dose aspirin has been shown to reduce the overall risk of PET by ~19%. The number needed to treat (NNT) varies depending on the baseline risk, from 69 in low risk women to 18 in those 'at high risk' of PET. There is also an associated reduction in fetal mortality. Women at risk of developing PET should take 75mg of aspirin daily from 12 weeks until the birth of the baby. Those at high risk include those with:

• Hypertension during a previous pregnancy.
• Chronic renal disease.
• Autoimmune disease, e.g. SLE.
• Type 1 and 2 diabetes mellitus.
• Pre-existing hypertension.

In addition, women with more than one moderate risk factor should take low dose aspirin from 12 weeks:

• >40 years old.
• Pregnancy interval >10 years.
• Multiple pregnancy.
• Family history of PET.

Management of gestational hypertension and pre-eclampsia

• Admission to hospital is necessary if hypertension is severe, i.e. >160/110mmHg for monitoring, investigation and treatment.
• Investigations will include assessment of proteinuria, blood tests for FBC, renal function, electrolytes, and liver function tests.
• Oral labetalol is usually the first line antihypertensive treatment of choice, with a target BP of <140–149/90–99mmHg. The BP needs to be checked regularly in order to ensure effectiveness of treatment.
• Alternative anti-hypertensives include nifedipine and methyldopa.
• There is no current evidence to suggest that any of these agents is superior to any other. However, labetalol should be avoided in asthmatics. Following delivery neonates of mothers taking labetalol are at increased risk of hypoglycaemia and will require blood sugar monitoring.
• If a woman has pre-eclampsia, repeated quantification of proteinuria does not need to be assessed, as it is not been proven to be an effective prognostic tool for decision-making regarding delivery timing.
• Fetal monitoring will include CTG, ultrasound for assessment of growth, amniotic fluid, and Doppler assessment of the uterine artery flow.
• Timing of delivery and requirement for antenatal steroids will need to be considered.
• Mother and fetus require frequent monitoring to assess disease progression.
• Early management of BP may extend the pregnancy to allow better fetal maturity.
• The CHIPS study found that tight blood pressure control in non-proteinuric, non-severe hypertension conveyed no benefit over less tight control in terms of maternal and fetal outcomes. This finding may lead to future modification of the NICE guidelines for the management of mild to moderate hypertension in pregnancy.

Mild/moderate pre-eclampsia management plan

Definition
- **Mild**—BP 140–149 systolic and/or diastolic 90–99.
- **Moderate**—BP 150–159 systolic and/or diastolic 100–109.
- Proteinuria >300mg in 24h **or** PCR >30mg/mmol.

Management
- Admit to hospital.
- Measure BP 4 times a day.
- Monitor/manage BP to maintain systolic BP between 140–149mmHg, and diastolic BP between 90–99mmHg.
- Assess fetal size, and monitor growth.
- Assess/monitor uterine artery blood flow.
- **Mild**—check FBC, U&Es, LFTs 2 times/week.
- **Moderate**—check FBC, U&Es, LFTs 3 times/week.
- Consider steroids to improve fetal lung maturity.
- Monitor for symptoms/signs of development of severe pre-eclampsia.

Further reading

Magee L.A. et al. Chronic Hypertension in Pregnancy Study (CHIPS) *Hypertension* 2016; 68: 1153–1159.

Severe pre-eclampsia

Definitions vary, but ~5 per 1000 maternities have 'severe' pre-eclampsia in developed countries. It should be noted that no criteria detects all women with severe pre-eclampsia, as some women present with eclampsia and no prodromal symptoms. It is also possible to have severe pre-eclampsia with normal BP measurements, although in such cases the BP usually subsequently rises. In these cases, the diagnosis should be made on grounds of clinical suspicion and probability.

Definition

BP >160 systolic and/or >110 diastolic (confirmed on repeat measurement 4 hourslater), associated with proteinuria>300mg/24hrs or PCR 30mg/mmol

OR

Mild/moderate pre-eclampsia (BP >140 systolic and/or >90 diastolic confirmed on repeat measurement and proteinuria (>300mg in 24h **or** PCR >30mg/mmol) with ≥2 of the symptoms/signs or haemotological/biochemical changes listed below:

- Severe headache.
- Visual disturbance.
- Clonus (three or more beats).
- Papilloedema.
- Epigastric pain and/or vomiting.
- Liver tenderness.
- Platelet count <100×10^9/L.
- Abnormal LFTs (ALT/AST >70IU/L).
- Features of HELLP syndrome (see below).

Eclampsia

- Eclampsia is defined as one or more convulsions superimposed on any degree of pre-eclampsia.
- Diagnosis is sometimes only possible retrospectively, when manifestations of pre-eclampsia become apparent after the convulsion.
- It affects 5 per 10,000 maternities in the UK.

HELLP syndrome

- This is a rare, severe form of PET characterized by rapid deterioration and the following features: **H**aemolysis—detected on a blood film, **E**levated **L**iver enzymes, and **L**ow **P**latelets.
- It is more common for women to present with 1 or 2 features rather than all 3, or the features develop at different times.

General management

- Multidisciplinary management—senior obstetric, anaesthetic, midwifery, and critical care staff, either managed in a high dependency area of delivery suite or in a critical care unit facility.
- Maintain patent IV access at all times.
- BP should be measured every 15–30min or continuously by invasive arterial monitoring if BP is difficult to control.

- Hourly oxygen saturations, HR and respiratory rate, and 4 hourly temperature should be recorded and documented.
- Accurate fluid balance recording is essential. Catheterization for accurate hourly urine measurement.
- Daily blood tests should include U&E, LFTs, serum calcium, phosphate, and magnesium, serum uric acid, FBC, and coagulation profile. Blood bank should hold a 'group and save' sample if delivery is imminent or blood made available by electronic issue.
- More severe cases may require monitoring of blood tests more frequently than daily and may also require regular analysis of arterial blood samples. Placement of an arterial cannula should be considered to facilitate this sampling.
- Regular assessment of fetal well-being should be according to local protocols, i.e. CTG, Doppler studies.
- Administer oral omeprazole 20–40mg 12 hourly if delivery imminent or there is risk of eclampsia.

Control of blood pressure

The mode and agents used will depend on the severity of hypertension and the response to various treatment modalities. Frequently patients are managed initially with oral therapy, but as the disease process becomes more severe, intravenous agents may be required.

- Acute antihypertensive treatment should be started in all women with BP >160 systolic, >125 mean, or >110 diastolic to reduce the incidence of cerebral haemorrhage.
- Target BP should be ideally 140–149mmHg systolic, <125mmHg mean, and 90–99mmHg diastolic BP.
- Treatment may also be considered for women with lesser degrees of hypertension if there are other markers of severe PET.
- Non-invasive automatic BP monitoring should be compared periodically with a manual sphygmomanometer measurement to assess its accuracy.

Oral treatment regimens

Labetalol
- 100–400mg tds, maximum dose 1200mg over 24 hours.
- Beware of neonatal hypoglycaemia.

Nifedipine
- Intermediate acting 10–20mg bd/tds, maximum dose 60mg/24h.
- Long acting 20–90mg once daily.

Therapy with labetalol and nifedipine may be combined.

Methyldopa
- 250mg–1g tds, up to a maximum dose of 3g/24h.
- Takes effect over several days and is best used to maintain out-patient therapy.

Contra-indicated anti-hypertensives
- ACE inhibitors and angiotensin receptor blockers are contraindicated for fear of teratogenicity.
- Diuretics are contraindicated to avoid limiting the desired expansion of circulating volume, although would be indicated in pulmonary oedema.

Intravenous treatment regimens
When intravenous therapy is necessary, the blood pressure can be extremely labile and should therefore be monitored every 15–30mins non-invasively, or alternatively, continuously, via an arterial line. The requirement for intravenous therapy should necessitate senior obstetric and anaesthetic involvement. A careful fluid pre-load (500ml crystalloid) should be given prior to commencing intravenous agents, particularly hydralazine. IV fluid should not be given if there are signs of pulmonary oedema and treatment requires close monitoring with an arterial line.

Labetalol
- Initially 50mg slow IV bolus, then start infusion at 20mg/hr.
- Double infusion each 15mins until BP controlled.
- Maximum infusion 160mg/hr.

Hydralazine
- Initially 5mg over 20min.
- Repeat at 30min intervals to maximum 4 boluses.
- Infusion 1–5mg/hr.

Treatment and prevention of seizures
- Magnesium sulphate has been shown to be beneficial in preventing seizures in the most severe cases of pre-eclampsia.
- Magnesium sulphate should be used as first-line management if an eclamptic fit occurs. Dosing regime is set out in eclampsia sub-section.
- Care is required with its administration in the face of renal impairment.

Fluid balance
General principles
- Excessive fluid administration is harmful in severe pre-eclampsia, and can cause pulmonary and cerebral oedema.
- Fluid restriction has been shown to be safe in severe pre-eclampsia, and fluid intake should generally be limited to 1mL/kg/h, administered through an infusion pump to avoid accidental over infusion.
- Post-delivery oral fluids can be commenced but total fluids (oral + IV) should be monitored and restricted.
- Fluid restriction should be continued until resolution of the illness causes a spontaneous diuresis.
- Fluid intake and output must be carefully recorded and, for this purpose, an indwelling urinary catheter is required. In general, a urine output (UO) >0.5mL/kg/h is satisfactory.

- Oxygen saturations should be monitored regularly for the onset of pulmonary oedema, i.e, SpO2 <94% on air is a worrying sign, and any changes in neurological state should raise the suspicion of cerebral oedema.
- AKI requiring renal replacement therapy (RRT) is an uncommon complication of pre-eclampsia alone but confers a high mortality due to its association with severe disease and haemorrhage. Most cases of AKI in pre-eclampsia are associated with placental abruption or haemorrhage.
- The risk of AKI is higher if there is pre-existing chronic renal impairment or if NSAIDs are used.
- Fluid balance is particularly difficult in a patient who has concurrent blood loss.
- Volume replacement without excess should be aimed for, but this is often easier said than done—particularly if the haemorrhage is severe.
- Good clinical judgement by an experienced team, possibly supplemented by invasive monitoring, is important.
- There is growing evidence that careful fluid boluses directed by echo CO monitoring by those expert in the technique is helpful in complex cases.

CVP measurement
- Measuring CVP can aid fluid balance management in severe disease associated with oliguria.
- It is most helpful when pre-eclampsia is complicated by haemorrhage.
- However, CVP may be unreliable, and pre-eclamptic patients can develop pulmonary oedema with a normal or low CVP measurement.
- Trends in CVP readings, rather than absolute values, are more important and useful to monitor.
- Any consideration of insertion of CVP line should trigger a senior anaesthetic review.

Diuretic administration
- Does not alter the outcome or progression of the disease.
- Many pre-eclamptic patients will produce a diuresis after IV furosemide 20mg.
- Diuretics can therefore be useful in the overall management of fluid balance.
- A progressively positive fluid balance is associated with pulmonary oedema, and diuretic administration when the mother is in 1500–2000mL positive balance can prevent this complication.

Intensive care management of severe pre-eclampsia

- Although level 3 critical care (ICU) will be required for some pre-eclamptic patients, the majority of patients will only require level 2 critical care (HDU).
- The latter would include patients who require invasive BP monitoring via an arterial line, and occasionally a central venous line in place.
- Whilst patients requiring level 3 care will need to be managed in a general ICU environment, the situation for patients only requiring level 2 care is less clear.
- In many obstetric units such patients can be managed within a high dependency area on the delivery suite, although it is important

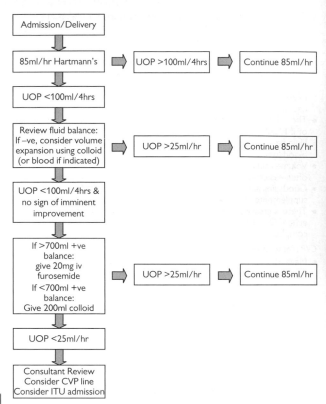

Fig. 19.1 Fluid balance in severe pre-eclampsia/eclampsia. UOP = urinary output.

that midwives or obstetric nursing staff are trained and supported
appropriately in managing such patients.
- Continuing the management of level 2 patients on the delivery suite
allows easier access to a senior obstetric anaesthetist and obstetricians,
who are more experienced in managing pre-eclampsia.
- However, it is important that an intensivist is readily accessible for
advice if there is any deterioration in the mothers' condition and
particularly to discuss the management of those cases where the
boundary between level 2 and 3 care is blurred.

Indications for level 3 care would include:
- Decreased level of consciousness requiring airway protection, e.g.
cerebral oedema/haemorrhage.
- Recurrent convulsions requiring general anaesthesia for airway and
seizure control.
- Ventilatory support, e.g. for pulmonary oedema.
- Renal support for AKI, usually triggered by hyperkalaemia, acidosis, or
fluid overload.

While many aspects of the care of a pre-eclamptic patient requiring level
3 care would be along general ICU principles, it remains important that
ongoing obstetric and obstetric anaesthesia input is available to advise
on issues specific to pre-eclampsia.

Further reading

Royal College of Obstetricians and Gynaecologists Green Top Guideline 10(A) The Management of
Severe Pre-Eclampsia and Eclampsia 2006

Dennis AT et al. Haemodynamics of women with untreated pre-eclampsia. *Anaesthesia* 2012;
67: 1105–1118.

Chen SSM et al. Myocardial tissue characterisation and detection of myocardial oedema by cardiovascular magnetic resonance in women with pre-eclampsia: a pilot study. *International Journal of
Obstetric Anesthia*. 2018;36: 56–65.

Dennis AT Transthoracic echocardiography in women with preeclampsia. *Current Opinion in
Anaesthesiology* 2015;28:254–260.

Eclampsia

Prevention

- The MAGPIE trial showed that women with severe pre-eclampsia had a 58% lower risk of eclampsia when given magnesium.
- Magnesium should be commenced once severe PET has been diagnosed. The patient does not necessarily have to have severe hypertension. This usually coincides when a decision to deliver is made, and should be continued for 24 hours after delivery or last convulsion.
- It is thought to reverse the cerebral vasoconstriction and ischaemia that leads to eclampsia, and is indicated in all patients who fulfill the criteria for severe pre-eclampsia.

Treatment of eclampsia

- The patient should be turned into the left lateral position.
- **A**irway, **B**reathing, and **C**irculation should be assessed and supported as per advanced life support (ALS) protocol.
- High flow oxygen by face mask should be given.
- Venous access should be secured (any size initially, but will require large bore if going for CS).
- ECG/oxygen saturation/BP monitoring should be commenced.
- The drug of choice for eclampsia is magnesium sulphate.
- Most eclamptic fits are short lived, and magnesium therapy is given to prevent a second fit.
- Blood sugar should be checked by finger prick and 25–50mL of 50% glucose given if <5mmol/L.
- Fetal well-being should be assessed as soon as practical as this may influence the timing of delivery. In the short term, however, appropriate treatment of the mother will have the most beneficial effect on the fetus, rather than rushing to a precipitant delivery.
- Second fits can be treated with another dose of magnesium if renal function is not impaired or IV lorazepam 4mg.

Magnesium therapy

Magnesium loading dose

For those women not on magnesium already:

- Give 4g IV over 5–10min—Draw up 10mL of 50% magnesium sulphate = 5g, with 40mL of normal saline to give a total volume of 50mL. Infuse 40mL over 5–10min.

For those women on a magnesium infusion:

- Take blood for urgent Mg^{2+} level then give extra 2g IV (20mL of above mixture) over 10min.

Continue magnesium infusion at 1g per hour for 24 hours.

Relative contraindications to magnesium include:

- Hypersensitivity to magnesium.
- Hepatic coma.
- Severe renal failure.

- Myasthenia gravis.
- Absent/diminished tendon reflexes.
- Caution with concurrent use of nifedipine or muscle relaxants.

The usual doses of Mg^{2+} should be reduced (typically halved) in the presence of significant renal dysfunction, e.g. urinary output <100mL/4h or abnormal urea/creatinine.

Signs of magnesium toxicity
- Muscle weakness/respiratory depression.
- Absent tendon reflexes.
- Severe toxicity may cause:
  - Muscle paralysis/respiratory arrest.
  - Heart block/cardiac arrest.
- Regular checking of respiratory rate and maternal reflexes reliably detects toxicity in the majority of cases.
- Routine checking of serum magnesium level is no longer considered necessary, but serum magnesium should be checked if there are concerns regarding toxicity, in the presence of renal disease or if there are recurrent convulsions (when it may be sub-therapeutic).
- Absent tendon reflexes and respiratory rate <14/min are indications to stop the infusion and check serum magnesium level.

Treatment of suspected magnesium toxicity
- Support respiratory/cardiovascular systems as per ALS algorithm.
- Calcium gluconate 1g (10mL) over 10min should be given for signs of significant toxicity.
- The infusion should be restarted at half the previous rate once respiratory depression has resolved.

Side effects of magnesium
- May potentiate the effects of depolarizing muscle relaxants.
- May prevent the appearance of fasciculation with suxamethonium (but no effect on subsequent myalgia).
- Magnesium may lower BP by vasodilation. Although sometimes useful, it is not routinely given for this purpose.
- Inhibition of uterine contraction.

Complications of eclampsia
- Failure to recover consciousness rapidly, recurrent convulsions, evidence of significant aspiration or the need for immediate CS are indications for intubation.
- Rapid sequence induction with thiopental and suxamethonium should be performed. Long-acting muscle relaxants may make diagnosis of recurrent seizures more difficult and should be used sparingly.
- If convulsions are not recurrent, it is usually best to control the seizures with magnesium and achieve cardiovascular stability before proceeding to delivery of the baby.

Liver disease and pre-eclampsia

PET /eclampsia

- Liver involvement is not common with PET but signifies severe disease. Increases in AST and ALP enzymes are the most usual change; bilirubin often remains relatively normal.
- Clinical signs include right upper quadrant pain and epigastric pain.
- The pathological process involves vasoconstriction of the hepatic vasculature and deposition of fibrin.
- Liver involvement is an indication for delivery.
- Biochemical changes usually resolve within 2 weeks of delivery.

HELLP syndrome

- **H**aemolytic anaemia, **E**levated **L**iver enzymes, and **L**ow **P**latelets are the features of HELLP, and lactate dehydrogenase >600IU/L, AST, and ALT >70IU/L and platelets <100×10^9/L are significant in the diagnosis of HELLP.
- It complicates 10–20% of severe PET and 0.2–0.6% of all pregnancies.
- 20% of patients can develop HELLP without hypertension or pre-eclampsia.
- Usual presentation is 28–36 weeks gestation, but 30% can present up to 7 days postpartum.
- 5% will have jaundice.
- Its pathology is similar to PET, including intravascular fibrin deposition and raised sinusoidal pressures.
- Platelet consumption is due to aggregation of platelets at sites of endothelial inflammation.
- Diagnosis should be established as both maternal and fetal morbidity and mortality are significant.
- Progression is usually rapid with platelets dropping at a rate of 35–50% every 24 hours.
- Sub-capsular liver haematoma and liver rupture can occur.
- Treatment includes anti-hypertensives and magnesium as prophylaxis against seizures.
- Vaginal delivery can be considered in uncomplicated cases but CS is usual.
- Liver enzymes often remain elevated until at least 48 hours postpartum.
- Haemolysis and thrombocytopenia may persist for 72 hours post partum.

Acute fatty liver of pregnancy

- A rare disease that presents in late pregnancy with clinical and histological manifestations similar to those of PET.
- Incidence is approximately 5/100,000 pregnancies, but accounted for 3 maternal deaths in the 2009–2012 CEMACE report.
- Presents in late pregnancy as the mother becomes increasingly reliant on fatty acid oxidation as a source of energy.
- The disease is thought to originate in defective mitochondrial dysfunction in the placenta leading to increased oxidative stress.

- The release of fatty acids and metabolites in the maternal blood leads to microvesicular steatosis and hepatocyte apoptosis.
- Diagnosis can be made with a liver biopsy showing typical features including fatty deposits around nuclei giving the cytoplasm a foamy appearance. However, a liver biopsy is not often practical, in part due to the associated coagulopathy.
- The 'Swansea' criteria, based on clinical and biochemical results, have been validated as a suitable alternative, to make a presumptive diagnosis in the absence of an alternative. AFLP is likely if a patient in late pregnancy has 6 out of 14 of the following in the absence of an alternative explanation:
  - Vomiting.
  - Abdominal pain.
  - Polydipsia /polyuria.
  - Encephalopathy.
  - Elevated bilirubin >14mmol/l.
  - Hypoglycaemia <4mmol/l.
  - Uric acid >340mmol/l.
  - Leucocytosis >11×10^9/L.
  - Ascites or bright liver on ultrasound.
  - Elevated transaminases >42IU/L.
  - Elevated ammonia >47mmol/l.
  - Creatinine >150mmol/l.
  - Prothrombin time >14 seconds or APPT>34 seconds.
  - Microvesicular steatosis on liver biopsy.

Management
- Immediate delivery is indicated.
- Coagulopathy and hypoglycaemia should be anticipated.
- Broad spectrum antibiotic cover particularly against gram-negative bacteria.
- Critical care for monitoring post delivery.
- Complications include encephalopathy, renal failure, and haemorrhage.
- Most patients improve within days of delivery. Occasionally prolonged supportive management is required, although the need for a transplant is extremely rare.

Further reading

Joshi D et al. Liver disease in pregnancy. *Lancet* 2010; 375: 594–605.

Morton A, Laurie J. Physiological changes of pregnancy and the Swansea criteria in diagnosing acute fatty liver of pregnancy. *Obstetric Medicine* 2018; 11: 126–131.

Timing and mode of delivery

In all but the most urgent cases, the timing and mode of delivery should be carefully considered. The woman should be stable, fluid status should be optimized, and hypertension and seizures should be treated. The most senior staff available should be present in unstable cases, and neonatal specialist care provision should be available for the baby.

MBRRACE emphasizes the importance of controlling maternal blood pressure, even if this results in a delay in delivery with a consequent adverse fetal outcome. Failure to control maternal blood pressure at the time of delivery, particularly at laryngoscopy has resulted in fatal maternal cerebral haemorrhage.

Before 34 weeks gestation

- Women should receive corticosteroids to aid fetal lung maturity if delivery is anticipated before 34 weeks gestation. Where possible, delivery should be delayed for 24 hours after administration of corticosteroids. It may be necessary to re-assess the risks/benefits of delivering the baby after this period.
- Women should be offered delivery before 34 weeks gestation, if hypertension becomes refractory to treatment, or if other maternal or fetal disease markers rapidly deteriorate.
- Examples of maternal indications include rapidly falling platelets <100×10⁹/L, elevated liver enzymes, and deteriorating renal function.
- Examples of fetal indications include absent or reversed end-diastolic flow using Doppler assessment of the uterine artery.
- Where possible, the mother should receive an infusion of magnesium sulphate (if not already receiving magnesium) to reduce the risk of cerebral hypoxic injury to the neonate, if birth is anticipated within the next 24 hours.
- Before 24 weeks gestation, survival of the baby is unlikely, and delivery is considered only if necessary to save the mother's life.
- Between 24 and 34 weeks, the chances of survival increase steadily, although there is a significant risk of disability before 28 weeks.
- Delivery before 34 weeks would usually be by CS.

After 34 weeks gestation

- Survival of the baby approaches 100% and delivery stops the pre-eclampsia process, although it may take several days to fully resolve and symptoms may worsen immediately after delivery.
- Most women with severe PET after 34 weeks gestation should therefore be delivered as soon as their clinical condition allows.
- Induction of labour may be warranted if the condition of the cervix is favourable, provided the fetal condition and presentation are satisfactory.
- A CS will be otherwise required.

Anaesthetic management

Labour

Women may present in labour and subsequently be found to have signs of pre-eclampsia—usually proteinuria and mild hypertension. Alternatively, some women diagnosed with pre-eclampsia may be assessed as suitable for induction of labour. In these women, treatment of hypertension and anaesthetic review should be undertaken prior to attempted induction of labour as their risk of CS is higher.

- All women with pre-eclampsia in labour should have antacid prophylaxis.
- Continuous CTG monitoring in labour is required.

Epidural analgesia

- Early epidural analgesia is recommended for most women with pre-eclampsia during labour to reduce surges in BP due to pain.
- Prior to insertion of epidural analgesia, thrombocytopenia and coagulopathy should be excluded.
- A recent platelet count i.e. <2h should be available. If this is >100, there is no need to carry out further coagulation studies unless there is some other indication, e.g. cholestasis of pregnancy.
- A platelet count <100 is relative contraindication to epidural placement and a 'risk/benefit' assessment and discussion with a senior anaesthetist. Formal coagulation tests should be checked as part of this assessment. Alternative analgesia may be offered, e.g. Entonox® or IV PCA opioids.
- Trends in platelet count are more important than absolute figures, as they indicate disease progression.
- Technique of insertion should be as usual, without fluid preloading. It may be wise for the epidural to be sited by the most experienced person available.
- A poorly functioning epidural should not be accepted. The epidural should be working well enough such that the anaesthetist is confident to use it for either instrumental delivery or CS.

Post-delivery

Before removing the epidural catheter:

- Re-check the platelet count if a significant period of time has elapsed since the last count. This is especially important if the platelet count was low, or if it was falling rapidly pre-insertion.
- The same acceptable platelet counts should be applied to catheter removal as to epidural insertion.
- If the platelet count is too low for safe removal, options are either to wait until recovery of the platelet count or give platelet transfusion if removal is urgent.

Caesarean section

- Ideally the patient should be fully pre-assessed, fasted, and have received antacid prophylaxis.
- The BP should be controlled, and up to date blood tests should be available.
- Magnesium prophylaxis should be started if necessary.
- Blood bank should have a recent blood sample. Cross-match may be indicated. A pre CS platelet transfusion is occasionally required.
- In the urgent situation, some or all of this preparation may not be possible.
- Large-bore venous access is mandatory, but excess fluid administration should be carefully avoided.
- The need for invasive haemodynamic monitoring should be assessed on a 'case by case' basis, but an arterial line can be very useful and there should be a low threshold for its insertion.
- NSAIDs for postoperative analgesia should be avoided in any women with moderate/severe PET or a creatinine >70, to avoid oliguria and may increase the risk of AKI. Hyperkalaemia, leading to a maternal death has been linked to the use of NSAIDs for post-operative analgesia in PET.
- Standard DVT prophylaxis should be provided postoperatively unless contraindicated, e.g. ongoing bleeding, platelet count <70×10^9/L.

Regional anaesthesia

- Regional anaesthesia is preferable to GA if it can be safely performed.
- Regional anaesthesia is NOT contraindicated after an eclamptic fit if the mother has fully regained consciousness.
- As well as the usual contraindications, a recent platelet count should be available. If this is >100×10^9/L, there is no need to carry out further coagulation studies unless there is some other indication, e.g. cholestasis of pregnancy.
- A platelet count <70×10^9/L is a contraindication to a spinal blockade and a GA will usually be required. A platelet count between 60 and 70 should involve a 'risk/benefit' assessment for each individual patient by the most senior anaesthetist available. Formal coagulation tests should be checked as part of this assessment if time allows.
- Fluid preloading should be minimized.
- 'Prophylactic' vasopressors should be used with extreme caution.

Spinal anaesthesia

- Spinal anaesthesia has the advantage of simplicity and familiarity, and usually gives a better quality of block than epidural anaesthesia.
- There has been concern that a sudden vasodilation due to spinal anaesthesia might cause significant hypotension in some patients. In practice this is rarely seen, and most patients with pre-eclampsia tend to have less hypotension than other patients. Where seen, hypotension must be carefully treated—restoring similar BP to pre-spinal levels whilst avoiding hypertension.
- Response to vasopressors may be exaggerated in patients with pre-eclampsia, so they should be used sparingly.
- The usual doses of LAs/opiates should be used for spinal anaesthesia in pre-eclampsia. However in pre-term deliveries, e.g. <30 weeks gestation, an increased dose of LA is advised as reduced cephalad spread is often seen with a smaller uterine size.

Epidural anaesthesia
- For many years epidural anaesthesia was the traditional, preferred technique for CS in pre-eclampsia. However, spinal anaesthesia or a CSE technique have been proven to be safe for the last 2 decades.
- If an epidural catheter is *in situ* for labour, the block can be extended for a CS.
- 'Top-ups' should be with the usual agents with which the user is familiar, but they should be given cautiously with full monitoring (including CTG) in theatre.
- Any BP changes are likely to be more gradual if an epidural is topped-up compared to spinal anaesthesia.
- Continuation of epidural analgesia into the postoperative period may aid analgesia and BP control.
- Drawbacks of epidural anaesthesia include greater technical difficulty, slower onset of block and sometimes a less satisfactory block. Poor blocks arise from severe peripheral oedema or interstitial fluid in the epidural space.

Combined spinal–epidural
- The CSE technique confers the advantage of a lower dose spinal anaesthetic, 'topped-up' with subsequent epidural injections.
- It potentially combines a relatively rapid, predictable block with minimal cardiovascular derangement and the ability to extend the block if required, including use for postoperative analgesia.

General anaesthesia
GA for CS in pre-eclampsia may be required if:
- Immediate delivery is required—life of mother or fetus at risk. Control of maternal systolic hypertension is required and should be prioritized over immediate concerns for the fetus.
- There is thrombocytopenia/abnormal coagulation (or need for urgent CS before blood test results available).
- Poorly controlled convulsions.
- Severe haemorrhage/high risk of haemorrhage.
- Patient refuses regional anaesthesia.
- Technical failure of regional anaesthesia.
- Other regional contraindication, e.g. severe aortic stenosis or sepsis.

Management of general anaesthesia
- A senior anaesthetist should be available.
- BP and convulsions should be as well controlled.
- Large-bore venous access is mandatory and invasive monitoring may be required.
- Careful airway assessment is mandatory—voice changes/hoarseness/stridor should alert to the possibility of laryngeal oedema.
- If present, stridor should be treated with 0.2mg/kg dexamethasone IV and 5mg nebulized adrenaline prior to intubation. Fibreoptic intubation equipment or videolaryngoscopy should be considered.
- A smaller tracheal tube than usual may be necessary. It may be wise to keep the patient intubated at the end of the procedure until the swelling subsides and there is a 'leak' around the endotracheal tube.

- Lesser degrees of pharyngeal oedema may still increase the risks of failed intubation.
- Careful pre-oxygenation followed by a modified rapid sequence induction is the most common technique.
- A short-acting opiate (e.g. alfentanil 10–20 micrograms/kg or remifentanil 0.2 micrograms /kg/min infusion for approximately 2 minutes) is recommended before induction to reduce the hypertensive response or tachycardia related to laryngoscopy and intubation. If opiates are used prior to delivery of the baby, the neonatal team should be informed.
- Other agents that have been used to control BP during induction are labetalol (50mg) and magnesium sulphate (2g).
- Induction with thiopental 5mg/kg and suxamethonium 1–1.5mg/kg.
- It should be noted that muscle fasciculation may not be seen following suxamethonium, especially if the patient is on magnesium. Magnesium may also prolong the effects of non-depolarizing muscle relaxants.
- Cardiovascular system stability should be maintained and paO_2 and $paCO_2$ kept within the normal range.
- Intraoperative control of BP may be achieved with volatile anaesthetics and/or IV labetalol/hydralazine.
- Any concurrent pulmonary oedema may make ventilation/oxygenation more difficult. PEEP/high FiO_2 may be required.
- Control of convulsions, level of consciousness, condition of the airway, FiO_2 requirement, and concurrent factors, e.g. haemorrhage, will dictate whether the patient is extubated at the end of the procedure or transferred to ITU.
- Where possible, the patient should be extubated at the end of surgery. It is equally important to control blood pressure during extubation.

Further reading

Dennis AT. Management of Pre-eclampsia: issues for anaesthetists. *Anaesthesia* 2012; 67:1009–1020.

Embolic disease

Abrie Theron

Venous thromboembolism

Pregnancy is a pro-thrombotic state, therefore the incidence of deep vein thrombosis (DVT) and pulmonary embolism (PE) is increased during both the antenatal and postnatal periods.

- The MBRRACE 2012–2014 report confirms that PE is still the leading cause of direct maternal deaths.
- There were 20 deaths reported in 2012–2014, giving a calculated incidence of 0.85 per 100,000 maternities in the UK.
- PE can occur during the antenatal, peripartum, or postpartum period.
- There is a higher incidence of PE and consequently death following an untreated DVT than a treated DVT.

Risk factors

In the 19th century, Virchow identified a triad of risk factors for venous thromboembolism (VTE):

- Venous stasis.
- Injury to the blood vessel intima.
- Changes in the coagulation properties of blood.

> **Many of the important risk factors related to pregnancy are based on this triad**
> - Pregnancy itself increases the risk 5-fold.
> - Mothers aged >40yrs are at very high risk.
> - Increasing parity.
> - Caesarean section.
> - Family history.
> - Obesity.
> - Hypertensive disease of pregnancy.
> - Immobility.
> - Dehydration.
> - Haematological conditions, e.g. antithrombin deficiency, protein C, and S deficiency.
> - Long-distance travel.

The RCOG guidelines for LMWH dosage for thrombo-prophylaxis based on early pregnancy/booking weight are outlined in Table 20.1

Table 20.1 RCOG Thrombo-prophylactic doses for LMWH

Body Weight	Enoxaparin	Dalteparin	Tinzaparin
<50kg	20mg daily	2500U daily	3500U daily
50–90kg	40mg daily	5000U daily	4500U daily
91–130kg	60mg daily	7500U daily	7000U daily
131–170kg	80mg daily	10000U daily	9000U daily
>170kg	0.6mg/kg/day	75U/kg/day	75U/kg/day
High prophylactic dose for women 50–90kg	40mg 12hrly	5000U 12hrly	4500U 12hrly

Pulmonary embolism

The clinical presentation of PE varies from progressive dyspnoea to sudden cardiovascular collapse. Symptoms can be non-specific, so a high index of suspicion is required, particularly when a patient has risk factors.

Symptoms

- The most common symptoms are dyspnoea, pleuritic chest pain, and haemoptysis.
- Patients can be asymptomatic or have an atypical presentation.
- Other symptoms are cough, leg pain, and back pain.
- In massive PE, central chest pain, convulsions, and cardiac arrest can occur.

Signs

- Tachycardia and crepitations on chest auscultation may be the only findings.
- Look for signs of a DVT (more commonly in the right leg).
- In a massive PE, evidence of right heart failure can occur. Look for features such as jugular venous distension, an enlarged liver, and parasternal heave.

Differential diagnosis

- Differential diagnoses are extensive.
- Consider all the causes for chest pain and dyspnoea, including myocardial infarction, myocarditis, pericarditis, pneumonia, pleuritic, and musculoskeletal pain.

Investigations for pulmonary embolism

- Investigations in PE are crucial, because clinical assessment alone is unreliable.
- Failure to diagnose PE is associated with high mortality, but incorrect diagnosis of the condition unnecessarily exposes the patient to the risks of anticoagulant therapy.
- A combination of tests according to the clinical features will increase the sensitivity and specificity.
- Unless contraindicated, women should be treated with LMWH until PE is excluded.

Blood tests

- Blood should be taken and sent to the lab for a FBC, coagulation study, U&E, and LFT prior to starting anticoagulation therapy.
- A thrombophilia screen prior to commencement of anticoagulation is not recommended.

Arterial blood gas

- Hypoxaemia with normal or low PaCO2 may occur.
- Normal blood gases do not exclude even a major PE.

ECG

- May be normal, but sinus tachycardia and non-specific ST segment and T wave changes are the most common findings.
- Right axis deviation, right bundle branch block, or S1 Q3 T3 pattern are rare.

Chest X-ray
- Findings are often non-specific.
- Atelectasis, collapse, consolidation, focal infiltrates, and raised hemi-diaphragm may occur. Wedge-shaped infarction is rare.
- The radiation risk to the fetus from a chest X-ray is minimal.
- If the chest X-ray is abnormal a CT pulmonary angiogram should be performed rather than a V/Q scan.

Bilateral duplex Doppler ultrasonography of legs
- Should be done in all suspected cases of DVT or confirmed PE, including calf, thigh, and groin regions.
- If the ultrasound is negative and there is little clinical suspicion, anticoagulation should be stopped. If negative with a high level of clinical suspicion, anticoagulation can also be stopped but arrangement should be made for a repeat scan on day 3 and 7.
- In women with a suspected PE where ultrasonography confirms a DVT, further investigation is not indicated and treatment for VTE should be continued.

Echocardiogram
- Echocardiogram is a very useful non-invasive bedside test, which may reveal a large PE demonstrated by RV dysfunction.

Ventilation/perfusion (V/Q) scan
- This is a useful test with minimal radiation exposure risk, but compared with CTPA carries a slightly higher risk of childhood cancer.
- V/Q scans detect areas of lung that are ventilated but not perfused, as occurs in PE.
- The results are reported as normal, low, intermediate, or high probability of PE based on patterns of V/Q mismatch. A completely normal scan can essentially exclude PE. A high probability scan provides enough evidence of PE in those patients with a high clinical suspicion.
- Perfusion deficits may occur in many other lung conditions such as pleural effusion, chest mass, pulmonary hypertension, pneumonia, and chronic obstructive pulmonary disease (COPD).

CT pulmonary angiography (CTPA)
- CT with radiocontrast is effectively a pulmonary angiogram imaged by CT. It is increasingly used as the mainstay in diagnosis.
- Whereas the V/Q scan displays the secondary effect of the PE on the pulmonary vasculature, CTPA actually visualizes the clot.
- Other advantages include better availability, cost-effectiveness, identification of alternative diagnoses, and the ability to image pelvic and lower extremity veins in the same study.
- The disadvantages are a large contrast load and a high radiation dose, which slightly increases the risk of breast cancer compared with a V/Q scan.

Management

Supportive therapy

- Ensure adequate Airway (100% oxygen), Breathing, Circulation.

Anticoagulation

Low molecular weight heparins (LMWH)

- Anticoagulation should start until the diagnosis is excluded, unless there is a strong contraindication.
- LMWH should be started using the woman's early pregnancy/ booking weight. See Table 20.2 for LMWH therapeutic dosing.
- If the patient is near term consideration should be given to using unfractionated heparin for easier manipulation of anticoagulation.
- DO NOT START LMWH if there is a possibility of early delivery as the effects of a treatment dose is long lasting (24h) and difficult to reverse.
- LMWH should be discontinued 24 hours before a planned delivery. Woman should be told not to inject any further doses of LMWH when she thinks she is going into labour. Regional anaesthesia should not be undertaken within 24 hours of the last therapeutic dose.
- Anti-Xa activity should only be monitored in patients at extreme weight (<50kg/> 90kg) and with complicating factors like renal impairment and recurrent VTE.
- LMWH has advantages over UFH; it has a high bioavailability, is longer acting, needs less monitoring, and has fewer side effects.

Table 20.2 RCOG Therapeutic doses for LMWH

Body Weight	Enoxaparin	Dalteparin
<50kg	40mg bd / 60mg od	5000IU bd / 10000IU od
50–69kg	60mg bd / 90mg od	6000IU bd / 12000IU od
70–89kg	80mg bd / 120mg od	8000IU bd / 16000IU od
90–109kg	100mg bd / 150mg od	10000IU bd / 20000IU od
110–125kg	120mg bd / 180mg od	12000IU bd / 24000 IU od
>125kg	Discuss with haematology	Discuss with haematology

Tinzaparin 175 units/kg once daily (Early pregnancy/booking weight).

Adapted from: Royal College of Obstetricians and Gynaecologists table 1a, 1b, and 1c of Green top Guideline 37b "Thromboembolic Disease in Pregnancy and the Puerperium: Acute Management London: RCOG; April 2015, with the permission of the Royal College of Obstetricians and Gynaecologists.

Unfractionated heparin

- Unfractionated heparin (UFH) is the drug of choice in massive PE, with cardiovascular compromise and when a patient is near term.
- Units should have their own guidelines on IV UFH administration, e.g. commence infusion at 1000U/h, then aim for a dose to ensure APTT 1.5–2.5 times normal. Patients can be changed to LMWH later.
- Platelet counts should not be monitored routinely, except in patients who have had surgery. In this group, a platelet count should be performed every 2–3 days from days 4 to 14 post-op or until heparin is stopped.
- Specialist advice should be sought regarding alternative anticoagulation in women who develop heparin induced thrombocytopenia or allergy. Consideration should then be given to the newer anticoagulants (argatroban, fondaparinux, r-hirudin).

Warfarin

- Warfarin is rarely used antenatally for venous thromboembolism because of its unacceptable side effects for mother and fetus. It is useful in the postpartum period after initial heparin therapy.
- Warfarin should be avoided until 5 days postpartum, and even longer in women with a persistent risk of postpartum haemorrhage.
- The need for frequent blood tests to monitor warfarin dosing should be explained to the mother and she should be offered a choice between LMWH and warfarin postnatally.

Postnatal instructions

- Therapeutic anticoagulation therapy should be continued for at least 3 months; throughout pregnancy and for a minimum of 6 weeks postnatally.
- The continuing risk of thrombosis should be assessed before anticoagulation is stopped. Once anticoagulation is stopped thrombophilia testing could be performed, but this should only be done if the results would guide the patient's future management.
- Woman should be informed that there is no contraindication to breast feeding while on heparin, LMWH, or warfarin.

Treatment options for life-threatening PE

- A shocked, collapsed woman should be assessed by an experienced multidisciplinary team. A bedside echocardiogram or CTPA should be performed as soon as possible.
- Intravenous UFH is the treatment of choice in woman with cardiovascular compromise due to a massive PE.
- The decision to use thrombolysis or embolectomy will depend on patient assessment and multidisciplinary team discussion.

Thrombolysis therapy
- Has been described in pregnancy.
- Is not recommended except in extreme life-threatening collapse.
- Is associated with a very high risk of antepartum and postpartum haemorrhage, which can cause fetal demise and may significantly complicate the management of the collapsed parturient.

Pulmonary embolectomy
- Has been described as an open and percutaneous procedure.
- May be lifesaving in the severely compromised parturient.
- Open procedures, especially associated with cardiac bypass, are associated with a very high incidence of fetal demise.

Other treatment
- If a DVT is present, leg elevation and graduated elastic compression stockings should be used to reduce oedema and mobilization should be encouraged.
- Vena cava filters should be considered in patients with iliac vein VTE and for patients with recurrent PE despite adequate anticoagulation.

Further reading
Knight M et al (Eds.) on behalf of MBRRACE-UK. Saving Lives, Improving Mothers' Care—Surveillance of maternal deaths in the UK 2012–14 and lessons learned to inform maternity care from the UK and Ireland Confidential Enquiries into Maternal Deaths and Morbidity 2009-14. Oxford: National Perinatal Epidemiology Unit, University of Oxford 2016.

Thomson A, Greer I on behalf of the Royal College of Obstetricians and Gynaecologists. Thromboembolic Disease in Pregnancy and the Puerperium: Acute Management. Green-top Guideline No. 37b: www.rcog.org.uk.

Nelson-Piercy C, MacCallum P, Mackillop L on behalf of the Royal College of Obstetricians and Gynaecologists. Reducing the Risk of Venous Thromboembolism during Pregnancy and the Puerperium. Green-top Guideline No. 37a: www.rcog.org.uk.

Amniotic fluid embolus

Description

- Amniotic fluid embolus (AFE) is a rare but devastating condition, responsible for 16 maternal deaths in the MBRRACE 2012–2014 report, with an estimated incidence in the UK of 2 cases per 100,000 maternities.
- Entry of amniotic fluid into the maternal pulmonary circulation causes profound effects upon gas exchange and haemodynamic status, frequently leading to cardiorespiratory arrest.
- Coagulopathy occurs within 30min, if the patient survives that long.
- Deterioration is rapid, with up to half of deaths within 1 hour of presentation.
- Early recognition is associated with improved survival.
- Mortality may be as high as 80%.

Aetiology

- May occur at any time during pregnancy, and has been described after termination of pregnancy, amniocentesis, and immediately post delivery.
- Risk factors include induction of labour, advanced maternal age, multiple pregnancies, trauma, precipitant labour or delivery of a large baby, obstructed labour, placental abruption, placenta previa, and CS.
- The role of uterine stimulation as a cause or effect of AFE is uncertain; however, they appear to be associated with one another.
- Ethnic minority is also associated with increased risk of AFE and these women tend to have a worse outcome.

Pathophysiology

- An underlying mechanism of anaphylaxis has been proposed since fetal tissue can be found in the maternal circulation in asymptomatic individuals.
- Right heart failure occurs due to intense pulmonary vasoconstriction.
- LVF ensues, with pulmonary oedema, hypoxia, and cardiorespiratory arrest.

Clinical features

- Presentation may be subtle in the first instance with premonitory symptoms, e.g. restlessness or altered behaviour followed by:
  - Dyspnoea.
  - Seizures.
  - Cardiovascular collapse.
  - Coagulopathy.
- Coagulopathy is severe with marked features of DIC. Severe haemorrhage is associated with the condition, and frequently is a major factor in maternal collapse and death.

Diagnosis

- Clinical: usually by exclusion.
- High index of suspicion in patients with:
  - Severe hypoxia.
  - Collapse.
  - Coagulopathy (DIC).
- Point of caretesting: the increasing availability of near-side automated machines to measure fibrinogen on delivery suites can be used to rapidly identify coagulation failure, suggestive of AFE.
- Laboratory: fetal squames may be aspirated from the pulmonary vasculature using a pulmonary artery flotation catheter, but this is not diagnostic of AFE.
- At postmortem: fetal elements (squames and lanugo hair) should be looked for in the pulmonary vasculature.

Differential diagnosis

Other causes of cardiorespiratory arrest
- Major haemorrhage.
- Pulmonary thromboembolism.
- Air embolus.
- Acute anaphylaxis.

Other causes of cardiac failure
- Acute coronary syndrome.
- Cardiomyopathy.

Other causes of altered neurological status
- Eclampsia.
- Local anaesthetic toxicity.
- Intracranial haemorrhage.

Management

- No specific therapy exists, with supportive care being the mainstay of treatment.
- Multidisciplinary involvement (senior obstetrician, anaesthetist, intensivist, haematologist).
- Supportive treatment: Airway, Breathing, Circulation.
- Cardiopulmonary resuscitation if required.
- Expedite delivery of the baby if appropriate.
- Invasive cardiovascular monitoring (arterial line, CVP monitoring).
- Treatment of cardiac failure.
- Treat haemorrhage and correct coagulopathy.
- Transfer to ICU for ongoing critical care.

Long-term sequelae

If the patient survives the insult of emboli and coagulopathy, long-term recovery may be complicated by neurological deficits. Women who died or have permanent neurological injury were more likely to suffer cardiac arrest and to have had a hysterectomy. They were also less likely to have received cryoprecipitate.

AFE register

UK Obstetric Surveillance System (http://www.npeu.ox.ac.uk/UKOSS) has established a voluntary database for all cases of suspected AFE. It aims to gather more information on the epidemiology of the disease. Due to the extreme rarity and significant mortality associated with AFE surveillance is still ongoing. By comparing outcomes of different cases, it is hoped advances in management can be achieved.

Intraoperative blood cell salvage

Specific concerns regarding AFE have meant that blood cell salvage has traditionally not been used in obstetric practice. From the clinical trials to date, it appears the risk remains theoretical since no cases of AFE or DIC have been associated with cell salvage when used with the appropriate filter.

Further reading

Knight M et al. Amniotic fluid embolism incidence, risk factors and outcomes: a review and recommendations. *BMC Pregnancy and Childbirth* 2012;12:7.

Knight M et al. Incidence and risk factors for amniotic-fluid embolism. *Obstetrics and Gynecology* 2010; 115: 910–917.

NHS National Institute for Health and Clinical Excellence. Intraoperative cell salvage in obstetrics. November 2005, updated / minor maintenance 22 January 2012. http://www.nice.org.uk/guidance/IPG144.

Vascular air embolism

Description

- Massive air embolus is a rare phenomenon in obstetrics, but is potentially lethal.
- It has been described during CS, manual removal of placenta, and termination of pregnancy.
- Air may be entrained into the utero-placental veins, which form an open plexus during removal of the placenta.
- Minor air embolus is probably very common during CS, especially when the uterus is exteriorized, and showers of small bubbles can be seen using Doppler ultrasound in the vena cava during routine surgery.
- This observation is a possible explanation for the frequent maternal complaint of heaviness or tightness in the chest around the time of placental removal.
- Fluid administration sets provide a route for air to enter the circulation. Epidural insertion, especially with loss of resistance to air, also provide a route.
- Symptoms may manifest after 0.5mL/kg/min of air has entered the circulation.

Pathophysiology

- A large bolus of air enters the RV and obstructs outflow into the pulmonary circulation.
- Smaller amounts of air can enter the pulmonary vasculature, with the development of bronchospasm, pulmonary hypertension and subsequent RVF.

Clinical features

- Presentation will vary according to the rate and volume of air that enters the circulation.
- Clinical signs may appear late in vascular air embolism (VAE).
- Fluctuating symptoms of restlessness and dyspnoea are frequently seen as a prequel to a major collapse.
- In the awake patient, air embolism may present as severe chest pain, dyspnoea, haemoptysis, or altered mental status.
- Clinical signs include cyanosis, tachypnoea, tachycardia, raised jugular venous pressure, hypotension, and a 'millwheel' murmur on auscultation of the heart.
- In patients with unexplained persistent hypotension and hypoxia during CS, VAE should be considered.
- If the patient is under GA, consider the diagnosis if there is a sudden fall in end-tidal CO_2, accompanied by hypoxia and ECG abnormalities (e.g. tachyarrhythmias, AV block, acute ischaemic changes).
- Massive air embolism can present with cardiorespiratory arrest, usually in pulseless electrical activity (PEA).
- Paradoxical emboli can occur in patients with a patent foramen ovale (PFO), causing neurological signs and cardiac symptoms.

Differential diagnosis

Respiratory distress
- Bronchospasm.
- Pneumothorax.
- Pulmonary oedema.

Other embolic phenomena
- Thromboebolism.
- AFE.

Primary cardiac event
- Acute coronary syndrome.
- Cardiomyopathy.

Other causes of PEA
- Consider the 4 Hs (Hypoxia, Hypovolaemia, Hyper/hypokalaemia, Hyperthermia) and 4Ts (Tension pneumothorax, Tamponade—cardiac, Toxins, Thrombosis—coronary or pulmonary).

Diagnosis
- Initially difficult as it is a rare cause of collapse in obstetrics. A high index of suspicion is required.
- Special monitoring to detect VAE, e.g. transoesophageal echo, precordial Doppler, and oesophageal stethoscope are not routinely used in obstetric anaesthesia.
- If GA is employed, capnography will detect most clinically significant emboli.
- The final diagnosis is usually one of exclusion after the other two causes of embolic collapse have been investigated:
  - High right-sided pressures on echo and CVP.
  - Cardiovascular collapse.
  - No evidence of coagulopathy.
  - No evidence of thrombolic event from duplex Doppler scans, V/Q, and CTPA.

Management
- Airway: check for a patent airway.
- Breathing:
  - Stop nitrous oxide if administered (as this can expand intravascular gas) and administer 100% oxygen.
  - If the capnograph trace has suddenly changed, check for leaks or disconnection.
  - CPAP or PEEP has been proposed since the rise in mean intrathoracic pressure will elevate CVP, in turn limiting the extent and progression of an air embolus, but it may increase paradoxical air embolism.
  - Hyperbaric oxygen therapy could be considered if available.
- Circulation:
  - Avoid further air entering the circulation: Flood the wound with saline and compress the open veins of the uterus. Tilting of the operating table to lower the uterus and limiting the negative pressure gradient, should be considered.
  - Check all lines for the presence of air.
  - Give an IV fluid bolus and use vasopressor agents to raise the CVP.
  - The classical description is to aspirate air from the right ventricle using a CVP line with the patient in the left lateral position in a head-down tilt. This should only be performed if central access is in place.
  - Cardiopulmonary resuscitation if there is cardiopulmonary arrest. The act of chest compression may help break up the bubbles of air, dispersing them into the pulmonary vasculature where they are absorbed.

Prevention
- Prevention is key to the management of VAE.
- Exteriorization of the uterus while suturing during CS is associated with an increased incidence.
- Avoid all air in IV lines and syringes. This is essential if patients are known to have a PFO.

Further reading
Mirski M et al. Diagnosis and treatment of vascular air embolism. *Anesthesiology* 2007; 106: 164–77.
Webber S et al. Gas embolism in anaesthesia. *British Journal of Anaesthesia CEPD Reviews* 2002: 2: 53–57.

The collapsed parturient

Rachel Collis

Cardiac arrest

Introduction

- Cardiac arrest at term is a rare but serious event.
- A recent survey based in the UK found an incidence of 2.78 per 100,000 maternities (1:36,000; 95% confidence interval 2.2–3.6). There was a case fatality rate of 42%.
- 24% of cardiac arrests occurred as a direct result of anaesthesia due to high blocks, local anaesthetic toxicity, and airway problems.
- 75% of women who arrested solely as a consequence of obstetric anaesthesia were obese.
- Those who died were more likely to have collapsed at home and peri-mortem CS (PMCS) was performed in 74%, and 22% had the PMCS in the emergency department.
- The time from collapse to PMCS was significantly shorter in women who survived (median interval 3 vs 12 minutes, P = 0.001).
- 80% of babies were born alive; 55% to surviving mothers and 24% to women who had died.
- It is essential to diagnose the cause of the arrest as soon as possible as the fatality rate is highly dependent on the cause, and the treatments are significantly different.
- Although not as common as anaesthesia related arrest, cardiac disease is the number one cause of maternal arrest and seems to be especially associated with sudden arrhythmic death syndrome.
- As maternal cardiac arrest is a rare event, it should be part of regular 'skills and drills' up-date.
- For an over-view of the management of CPR algorithm: see Fig. 21.3

Immediate resuscitative measures

- Position the patient in full left lateral, if patient has a CO.
- If NO cardiac output—Place supine, use left manual displacement of uterus demonstrated in Figs 21.1–2.
- Commence standard basic life support/advanced life support protocols.
- Administer 100% oxygen using a tight-fitting mask.
- Establish IV access above the diaphragm and administer a fluid bolus.
- Ascertain if there are any pre-existing medical conditions, e.g. cardiac disease or pregnancy related conditions e.g. pre-eclampsia.
- If on magnesium infusion—STOP and administer calcium chloride 10ml in 10% solution OR calcium gluconate 10ml in 10% solution.

Immediate response

- The latest basic and advanced life support algorithms from the Resuscitation Council UK should be used at a maternal cardiac arrest, see Fig. 21.4.
- External automated defibrillators can be used if necessary.
- There should be a specific maternal cardiac arrest call. This will include an obstetrician, paediatrician, and equipment brought to the arrest to perform an immediate peri-mortem CS.

- Ideally there should be three team leaders:
  - Medical care.
  - Obstetric care.
  - Paediatric care.
- Do not delay usual measures such as defibrillation and the administration of IV medication.
- Aorto-caval decompression manoeuvers are essential, preferably manual left uterine displacement (Figs 21.1–2).
- Consider airway difficulties. The most experienced provider should manage the airway.
- Intravenous access should be placed above the diaphragm.
- There should be a dedicated timer to document when 4 minutes after the onset of a maternal cardiac arrest has elapsed, in order to make a decision on the need for a PMCS.
- PMCS should be performed by 5 minutes after the onset of a maternal cardiac arrest if there is no return of spontaneous circulation. Therefore it should be considered by 4 minutes with the usual resuscitation measures.
- Consider an expanded aetiology list for the cause of the cardiac arrest in a pregnant woman.
- Disconnect the fetal heart rate monitor. Prioritize the mother.

Factors impeding resuscitation in pregnancy

Airway
- In pregnancy there is an increased risk of failed intubation due to poor positioning, airway oedema, and enlarged breasts impeding intubation.
- The most experienced team member who is present should intubate with a size 7 endotracheal tube.
- Management of the airway and managing difficulties with the airway should follow the last recommendations.

Breathing
- Ventilation is more difficult due to reduced chest compliance.
- Mothers are less tolerant of apnoea, due to decreased FRC, and increased metabolic demands, leading to rapid desaturation, with the risk of hypoxic brain damage.
  - Oxygenate well, monitor, and avoid desaturation.
  - Avoid respiratory alkalosis.
  - Consider reducing the ventilatory volumes.
  - Be aware of the risk of aspiration.

Circulation
- Aorto-caval compression dramatically reduces VR and CO from 20 weeks gestation, i.e. uterus palpable above the umbilicus.
- The ideal position of the mother should be supine with manual left uterine displacement.
- Allowing the patient to remain supine improves:
  - Airway access.
  - Ease of defibrillation.
  - IV access is easier to achieve.
  - Enables simultaneous high quality chest compressions.

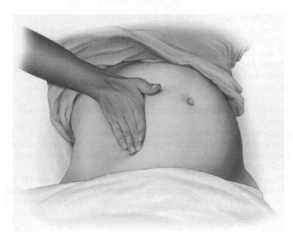

Fig. 21.1 Left manual uterine replacement one hand.

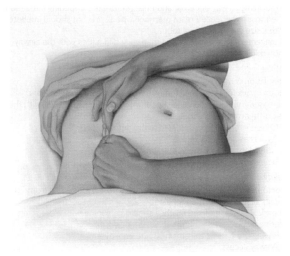

Fig. 21.2 Left manual uterine replacement two hand.

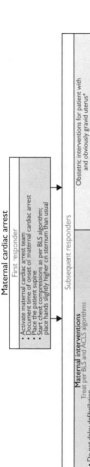

Maternal cardiac arrest

First responder
- Activate maternal cardiac arrest team
- Document time of onset of maternal cardiac arrest
- Place the patient supine
- Start chest compressions as per BLS algorithm;
  place hands slightly higher on sternum than usual

Subsequent responders

Maternal interventions
Treat per BLS and ACLS algorithms
- Do not delay defibrillation
- Give typical ACLS drugs and doses
- Ventilate with 100% oxygen
- Monitor waveform capnography and CPR quality
- Provide postcardiac arrest care as appropriate

Maternal modifications
- Start IV above the diaphragm
- Assess for hypovolemia and give fluid bolus when required
- Anticipate difficult airways; experienced provider is preferred for advanced airway
  placement
- If patient is receiving IV/IO magnesium prearrest, stop magnesium and give IV/IO
  calcium chloride 10 mL in 10% solution, or calcium gluconate 30 mL in 10% solution
- Continue all maternal resuscitative interventions (CPR, positioning, defibrillation,
  drugs, and fluids) during and after cesarean section

Search for and treat possible contributing factors (BEAU-CHOPS)
Bleeding/DIC
Embolism: coronary/pulmonary/amniotic fluid embolism
Anesthetic complications
Uterine atony
Cardiac disease (MI/ischemia/aortic dissection/cardiomyopathy)
Hypertension/preeclampsia/eclampsia
Other: differential diagnosis of standard ACLS guidelines
Placenta abruptio/previa
Sepsis

**Obstetric interventions for patient with
and obviously gravid uterus***
- Perform manual left uterine displacement (LUD); displace uterus
  to the patient's left to relieve aortocaval compression
- Remove both internal and external fetal monitors if present

  Obstetric and neonatal teams should immediately
  prepare for possible emergency cesarean section

- If there is no ROSC by 4 minutes of resuscitative efforts, consider
  performing immediate emergency cesarean section
- Aim for delivery within 5 minutes of onset of resuscitative efforts
- An obviously gravid uterus is a uterus that is deemed clinically to
  be sufficiently large to cause aortocaval compression

Fig. 21.3 Over-view of management of cardiac arrest in pregnancy.

Maternal Cardiac Arrest algorithm.

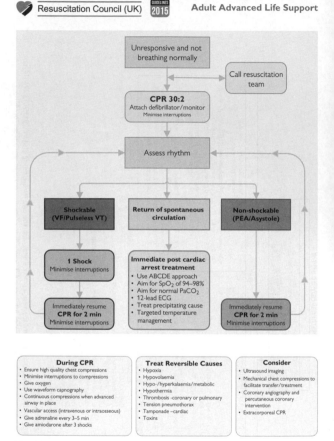

Fig. 21.4 Adult Advanced Life Support Algorithm.

Reproduced with the kind permission of the Resuscitation Council (UK) 2015: Adult advanced life support algorithm. Resuscitation Council (UK).

- Previously, left lateral tilt had been recommended to reduce aortocaval decompression, but evidence now shows that that:
  - Tilt will reduce the forcefulness of the chest compression.
  - It affects quality of chest compression.
- It negatively impacts on survival.

Establish cause of cardiac arrest

The well-known general mnemonics should be considered.
- 4Ts: tension pneumothorax, tamponade, thromboembolism, toxic/therapeutic disturbances.
- 4Hs: hypoxaemia, hypovolaemia, hypo/hyperkalaemia, hypothermia.

Causes specific or more common in pregnancy

Haemorrhage
- Obstetric haemorrhage can often be concealed, and usually young, fit parturients can appear to have cardiovascular stability despite excessive ongoing bleeding. They then decompensate rapidly.
- Commence fluid resuscitation, using blood (O-negative or group-specific if necessary) and blood products early to prevent a significant coagulopathy developing.
- For further management of obstetric haemorrhage, see Chapter 18.

Thromboembolic disease
- PE is more common in pregnancy due to the hypercoaguable pregnancy state.
- Anticoagulate if history and examination suggestive of diagnosis. CTPA is the diagnostic test of choice.

Amniotic fluid embolism
- Presents with acute hypotension proceeding to circulatory collapse, hypoxia, convulsions, and coagulopathy, either during labour or at time of delivery.
- A sudden onset severe DIC is characteristic and clotting studies should always be taken immediately. Point of care VHA can rapidly confirm the diagnosis with characteristic severe hypofibrinogenaemia.
- Bleeding associated with this coagulopathy should be treated with high doses of fibrinogen (cryoprecipitate or fibrinogen concentrate and plasma).

Severe pre-eclampsia or eclampsia
- Cardiac arrest can occur from sudden decompensated heart failure associated with severe diastolic dysfunction.
- Treat with standard heart failure regimes.
- Hypoxia and an obstructed airway can occur from an eclamptic fit. Treat with 4G IV magnesium and support airway.
- For further management, see Chapter 19.

Magnesium toxicity
- Should be considered in patients receiving magnesium therapy. It may be secondary to an accidental over-dosage (concentration/infusion rate/pump error) or reduced excretion resulting from renal impairment.
- Treatment: stop magnesium infusion, give 10mL IV calcium gluconate 10% or 10mL IV calcium chloride 10%.

Anaesthesia related
- This is a leading cause of cardiac arrest, severe hypoxaemia resulting from a failed intubation or difficult airway.
- Always confirm endotracheal tube placement with end-tidal CO_2 monitoring. If in doubt, replace the endotracheal tube.
- Failed intubation and failed ventilation—commence failed intubation drill. See Chapter 12 p. 337.
- Total or high spinal anaesthesia—high sensory block, profound hypotension, bradycardia may lead to reduced conscious level.
- For causes and advice on early identification and treatment see p. 550.

Systemic local anaesthetic toxicity
- Prodromal symptoms, e.g. perioral tingling, dizziness, tinnitus, followed by convulsions ± cardiovascular collapse.
- IV lipid treatment for bupivacaine toxicity: 100mL of 20% Intralipid® is recommended.

Cardiac disease
- Patients with adult congenital heart disease, ischaemic heart disease, or peripartum cardiomyopathy can decompensate rapidly.
- Consider any past medical history, older mothers, smokers, or presence of chest scars.
- Consider dissection of the aorta in high risk mothers, e.g. previous aortic surgery, bicuspid aortic valve, Marfan's syndrome.
- An echocardiogram should be considered an early investigation, e.g. to confirm a cardiac cause of pulmonary oedema.

Further management
- If the mother responds quickly to resuscitation, the viability of the fetus needs to be assessed by an ultrasound scan.
- A management plan for delivery should made in conjunction with the ongoing investigation and treatment of the mother.
- Transfer the mother to an appropriate place depending on the cause of the collapse, e.g. theatre or intensive care for ongoing management.

Investigations

All parturients
- FBC, U&E, blood glucose, LFTs, clotting studies.
- Point of care viscoelastography if available.
- Blood group and save ± cross-match blood.
- Arterial blood gas with special attention to lactate.

As indicated
- Magnesium level
- Chest X-ray.
- ECG.
- Echocardiogram.
- V/Q scan, spiral CT scan, or CTPA if a PE is suspected.
- CT head.

Peri-mortem caesarean section

If vaginal delivery is imminent, then an assisted vaginal delivery is acceptable

- An emergency CS needs to be considered as soon as a pregnant mother has a cardiopulmonary arrest.
- It should be performed if resuscitation is not successful at 4min and delivery completed by 5min, to improve the chance of both maternal and fetal survival and outcome.
- Emptying the gravid uterus significantly improves maternal outcome with complete aorto-caval decompression after 20 weeks gestation, i.e. uterus felt above the umbilicus.
- Case reports have shown a dramatic return of maternal pulse and BP once the uterus is emptied.
- Precious minutes should not be wasted moving the mother to theatre or preparing a sterile field. This may mean performing the CS in a less than ideal environment, e.g. in the emergency department or antenatal clinic. In reality, minimal equipment is likely to be needed, e.g. a scalpel and a pair of artery forceps.
- Bleeding at the time of peri-mortem CS is not usually problematic because of a low CO.
- A classical uterine incision may allow quickest delivery of the baby.
- Continue CPR throughout and afterwards.
- Consider transabdominal open cardiac massage.
- Fetal prognosis is poor, becoming worse with prolonged time to delivery. The paediatrician should be part of the arrest team, therefore immediately available as the baby is delivered.
- Transfer the mother and baby to the appropriate place, e.g. theatre or ICU once stable, for ongoing treatment.
- A peri-mortem cardiac arrest 'drill' should be practiced in different in-hospital locations to assess readiness, i.e. emergency department, postnatal ward, and antenatal clinic.

Further reading

For up to date resuscitation guidance see: https://www.resus.org.uk/resuscitation-guidelines/

Jeejeebhoy FM et al Cardiac arrest in pregnancy: A scientific statement from the American Heart Association. *Circulation* 2015; 132: 1747–1773.

Jeejeebhoy FM, Morrison LJ. Maternal cardiac arrest: a practical and comprehensive review. *Emergency Medicine International* 2013; 2013: 274814. doi: 10.1155/2013/274814.

Beckett VA et al. The CAPS Study: incidence, management and outcomes of cardiac arrest in pregnancy in the UK: a prospective, descriptive study. *British Journal of Obstetrics and Gynaecology* 2017; 124:1374–1381.

Bonnet MP et al. Maternal death due to amniotic fluid embolism: A National Study in France. *Anesthia and Analgesia* 2018; 126: 175–182.

Adams J et al. Management of maternal cardiac arrest in the third trimester of pregnancy: A simulation-based pilot study. *Critical Care Research and Practice.* 2016; 2016: 5283765.

Eldridge AJ, Ford R. Perimortem caesarean deliveries. *International Journal of Obstetric Anesthia* 2016; 27: 46–54.

High regional blocks: Causes

This is a term used to describe a central neuroaxial block that rises to the upper thoracic level and above, with associated cardiorespiratory symptoms.

Definition

- **High block** that extends to the upper thoracic or lower cervical dermatomes which can cause some cardiorespiratory compromise and maternal anxiety, but does not cause diaphragmatic paralysis.
- **Total spinal** where the block extends to the upper cervical dermatomes and brainstem, which leads to complete paralysis and respiratory failure, followed rapidly by desaturation, airway compromise, and cardiac arrest if not dealt with appropriately.

It is important to recognize the two situations, because the management, although overlapping, is different.

Mechanism of high blocks/total spinal

Spinal
- Excessive dose.
- Patient position.
- Spinal injection after an epidural.

Epidural
- As a result of excessive dosage into epidural space.
- Unintentional injection of LA into the subarachnoid space.
- Subdural catheter placement.

CSE
- Epidural top-up after a recent spinal injection.

Spinal anaesthetic

Excessive dosage
- It is common in non-obstetric practice to use 3–4mL 0.5% heavy bupivacaine for lower limb orthopaedic and lower abdominal surgery. These doses may lead to excessive blocks in the pregnant woman, who can have an acceptable intra-abdominal block with doses from 1.5 to 2.5mL 0.5% bupivacaine.
- Experience with the 'usual' non-obstetric spinal doses of LA in pregnant women has shown that there can be significant variability in the extent of block achieved.
- Increased intra-abdominal pressure from the pregnancy causing epidural venous engorgement, and a reduction in volume of both epidural and subarachnoid space is thought to be a major factor.
- The reduced LA requirements are seen as early as 8–12 weeks of pregnancy, well before the mechanical effects of gravid uterus are present. The explanation is that either pregnant nerve fibres are more sensitive to LAs or there is enhanced diffusion of LA across the nerve membrane.

- High progesterone levels in CSF and/or blood during pregnancy may be the cause of the different response to subarachnoid injection of LA during late pregnancy.
- The dose of LA during pregnancy should be reduced by at least 25% compared with similar non-pregnant patients, and tailored to the individual parturient depending on gestation i.e. smallest dose in the full-term parturient.
- Occasionally a woman with a very short stature (<152cm) can get an excessive block from <2.5mL of bupivacaine.

Position
- This may also play a part in the aetiology.
- High intra-abdominal pressure and engorged epidural veins may make the pregnant woman more vulnerable to developing an excessive block, in a flat or slightly head-down position, compared with a non-pregnant patient.

Spinal anaesthesia after an epidural
- May cause either a high block or a total spinal.
- The subarachnoid space is squeezed by the volume of LA already in the epidural space, facilitating cephalad spread of subarachnoid LA.
- If a spinal block is performed within 45min of an epidural top-up the dose should be reduced by ~25%.
- Drug flux is the movement of drug from the epidural space to the subarachnoid space via the dural hole made by the spinal needle. Some of the LA from the epidural space can pass through the dural hole and enter the subarachnoid space, further extending the block.

Excessive epidural doses
- Most likely to cause a high block rather than a total spinal.
- Large doses of epidural LA can give rise to a high block associated with cardiorespiratory features.
- This is usually seen when one is faced with a block, which after top-up for operative delivery, is unequal. When the final block height is achieved, it may lead to a high block especially on one side.
- This is more likely to happen after a single bolus volume >20mL or divided boluses >30mL total volume.
- An early presentation of high block is a unilateral Horner's syndrome. However, the appearance of Horner's syndrome does not predict cardiorespiratory compromise and the mother should be reassured.

Subdural block
- Can cause a high block or a modified type of total spinal.
- Incidence is quoted to be 0.82%.
- Results from unintentional catheterization of the subdural space at insertion, as well as delayed migration of the epidural catheter.
- The block behaves more like an epidural than a subarachnoid block.
- Time to maximal block ranges from 20 to 30min, but the extent produced by a given volume of LA is greater.
- Subdural block is often patchy, asymmetric, with minimal motor block and hypotension.

- Retention of sacral sensation distinguishes it from spinal block.
- As it extends intracranially, a subdural block can involve the cranial nerves and can cause unconsciousness.
- A subdural block can unexpectedly lead to a sudden subarachnoid block. A sudden increase in pressure generated in the subdural space by the injection of LA may rupture the arachnoid.
- The onset of a subarachnoid block in the absence of CSF during placement of the catheter, inability to aspirate fluid through the catheter before injection and free flow of CSF after injection confirms this.

Unintentional subarachnoid block

Accidental dural puncture during epidural placement
- This may cause a high block or a total spinal.
  - 65% of the time this is recognized at the time of epidural needle insertion by the free flow of CSF.
  - 35% of the time it is due to the catheter puncture. It may not be as obvious, and a negative aspiration of CSF via the catheter does not guarantee that it is not placed in the subarachnoid space.
- Administration of a test dose should help identify subarachnoid placement of a catheter.
- If unrecognized, injection of a large volume of LA may rapidly lead to a high/total spinal.
- A high block may result from an epidural injection of LA given into the intervertebral space adjacent to an inadvertent dural perforation with a 16 or 18G Tuohy needle.
- It is suggested that the frequent uterine contractions of labour can result in some of the LA solution being forced through the puncture hole into the subarachnoid space.
- If an epidural catheter is resited after an inadvertent dural puncture this should be performed above and well away from the original interspace to minimize this risk.
- A multi-holed catheter may be placed partly in the epidural and partly in the subarachnoid space. With initial slow injection, the LA emerges from the proximal holes. With a subsequent rapid injection LA will emerge from the distal holes, resulting in a subarachnoid block. The block may have features of an epidural, subdural, and subarachnoid block.

Catheter migration from the epidural into the subarachnoid space
- This may cause a high block or a total spinal.
- High blocks occurring on second or subsequent top-ups may be due to migration of an originally correctly placed epidural catheter into the subarachnoid space.
- However, a postmortem study has shown that the epidural catheter is unable to puncture the dura.
- It is likely that the epidural catheter in this circumstance was originally in the subdural space and, because it provided some analgesia, was not recognized.
- Sudden disruption of arachnoid mater results in a sudden, late, high block.

Combined–spinal epidural

- This can cause a high block or total spinal, and can follow an epidural top-up administered to augment the initial spinal injection.
- The volume effect and mechanical compression of the dural sac by the epidural fluid displacing the CSF in the cephalad direction. This is supported by studies demonstrating the increase in LA block even when saline is injected into the epidural space.
- To minimize this risk there should be a 10 minute time gap between the spinal injection and the first epidural top-up.
- The epidural top-up volume should not exceed 5mL of saline or LA solution at a time.
- Drug flux is movement of drug from the epidural space to the subarachnoid space via the dural hole made by the spinal needle. The clinical effect of such drug flux is thought to be affected by the size of the dural hole. It is probably minimal with the conventional use of 24–27G spinal needles during this technique, although deliberate use of this technique has been described.
- The epidural catheter may be accidentally placed in the subarachnoid space and, because of the initial intended spinal block, a test dose through the epidural catheter can be difficult to interpret.
- It is therefore suggested that a low concentration of LA be used and each subsequent bolus should be treated as a test dose.

High regional blocks: presentation

High block

Nausea and vomiting

- Is common and may be due to hypotension or cerebral hypoxia.

Hypotension

- Although common in obstetric spinal anaesthesia, the rapidity and severity with which it occurs during high blocks can put the patients' life and the fetus at risk if treatment is delayed.
- The major factor in the development of hypotension is the height of the block. The sympathetic outflow from the spinal cord is between T1 and L2. A block below that level has little effect on the BP. The sympathetic supply to the adrenal medulla is from T8 to L1, and a block to T8 will affect the BP by inhibition of systemic release of catecholamines, in addition to venous pooling of blood in the lower half of the body secondary to vasodilatation.
- All these effects are compounded by any degree of aorto-caval compression, resulting in a severe fall in venous return, CO, and BP.

Bradycardia

- Is usually secondary to blockade of T1–T4 cardio-acceleratory fibres.
- Decreased right atrial filling from aorto-caval compression may be a contributing factor, i.e. Bezold–Jarisch reflex, where the onset of bradycardia can be very sudden and severe, e.g. HR <20/min or asystole.

Respiratory difficulty

- This is due to paralysis of the intercostal muscles.
- During pregnancy, the intercostal muscles contribute more than normal during quiet respiration due to diaphragmatic splinting.
- Patients may complain of difficulty especially in taking a deep breath or coughing, but will usually be able to speak normally.
- Patients may complain they cannot speak normally, only whisper. This is an important sign and can signify impending unconsciousness.

Tingling in the hands and fingers

- Indicates a sensory block at T1, although beware of the anxious hyperventilating patient who may develop similar symptoms.

Somnolence

- This is a very important sign of an impending total spinal.
- It can be a difficult sign to interpret, as excessive fatigue and the effect of opioids can have a similar effect.
- When associated with a high block, it is caused by the sensory component spreading several dermatomes above the motor block to the brainstem.
- Motor function may be surprisingly unaffected; however, beware, as the patient may not complain of any difficulties before a respiratory arrest occurs.

Total spinal

Loss of consciousness
- Due to spread of LA into the brainstem.
- Loss of airway reflexes due to involvement of cranial nerves.

Respiratory arrest
- May occur without warning.
- Due to phrenic nerve paralysis, which may be preceded by difficulty in coughing and phonation.
- The medullary respiratory centre may also be affected.

Cardiovascular collapse
- Profound hypotension and severe bradycardia due to total block of sympathetic nervous system.
- Cardiac arrest may occur.
- All cardiovascular problems are compounded by aorto-caval compression.

High regional blocks: assessment and management

High block

- The mainstay of treatment includes prompt recognition and early treatment aimed at providing adequate oxygenation and correcting hypotension and bradycardia. Senior anaesthetic and ODP help should be sought early if simple measures are unsuccessful in stabilizing the mother.
- It is common for a mother with a block required for a CS to complain of some breathing difficulty. This is caused by the paralysis of intercostal muscles and the supine position required for surgery. The extent of the block should be quickly ascertained.
- It is common for the mother to complain of some numbness to cold in the high thoracic T1 and lower cervical C7-8 dermatomes, i.e. inner border of arm and little finger.
- If the numbness involves the whole hand, this indicates an abnormally high block.
- The sensory block extends above the motor block and, even if there is a significant sensory block, the ability to squeeze her hand closed is a reassuring sign for the mother and anaesthetist.
- Place a firm additional pillow or wedge under the mid thoracic curve to prevent a block that has reached the lower cervical dermatomes from rising further.
- This manoeuvre will in addition allow the descent of the diaphragm and improve respiratory function. This will make the mother feel less breathless and reduce her associated anxiety.
- Administer high flow oxygen via a face mask.
- If there is doubt about respiratory effort, tidal volume can easily be assessed through most modern anaesthetic machines using a tight-fitting anaesthetic face mask.
- The additional value of this approach is that 100% oxygen can be administered, and pre-oxygenation has taken place if intubation is rapidly required.
- The anaesthetist must stay in close contact with the mother, both to reassure her and to assess her respiratory status.
- Ensure adequate lateral tilt to prevent aorto-caval compression. If possible, a full lateral position may be more effective.
- Lifting the legs above the level of the heart increases the VR. The patient must not be placed in a head-down position as this may extend the block and increase respiratory difficulty because of reduced pulmonary volume. Raising the knees flattens the lumbar curve and raises intra-abdominal pressure; both manoeuvres may also extend the block further.
- Atropine boluses of 300–600 micrograms may be needed to treat bradycardia.
- Boluses of ephedrine 6–9mg or phenylephrine 25 micrograms as required, or by increasing the IV phenylephrine infusion, to restore and maintain the systolic BP. Phenylephrine may be a more useful drug, although there is frequent anxiety about its use in a patient who is

bradycardic. It is a more potent drug than ephedrine, has a more direct alpha action, and is therefore effective against an excessive sympathetic block and improves venous return.
- IV fluids should be administered, e.g. 1000mL crystalloid and/or 500mL colloid. Fluid therapy should not be used alone and, if it is not rapidly effective, the early use of other manoeuvres, i.e. change of position and vasopressors should be adopted.
- Reassurance is extremely useful to calm the anxious mother.
- Sometimes it is not possible to achieve good haemodynamic stability with a high block, even if the mother remains conscious. Delivery of the baby will improve this and may be indicated. Further anaesthesia is not usually necessary unless the block progresses and respiratory function declines.
- Depending on the circumstances, the block may progress to a total spinal, and preparation should be made to protect and secure the airway as appropriate. The operating theatre on a maternity unit is usually the safest place.

Total spinal

The complaining agitated patient may have a high block BUT beware of the silent non-complaining somnolent patient.

- Hypotension can be of sudden onset if it is secondary to an extensive subarachnoid block, when it presents as sudden loss of consciousness and collapse. However, it can be of slower onset if due to subdural or extensive epidural block. Hypotension may be severe enough to impair cerebral perfusion and cause loss of consciousness.
- The associated loss of airway reflexes as the cranial nerves are affected may lead to aspiration of gastric contents.
- Weakness of arm and hand indicates blockade of cervico-thoracic nerves.
- Once the phrenic nerve fibres (C3, 4, 5) start to be affected, difficulty in coughing and phonation develops. Respiratory arrest ensues as a result of complete respiratory muscle paralysis.
- LA action on the medullary respiratory centre will cause a direct cessation of respiration, and its effect on other brainstem functions will directly cause unconsciousness.
- Finally, fixed and dilated pupils are seen.
- Early recognition and treatment is of utmost importance for successful outcome, and every anaesthetist working on the maternity ward should be able to recognize this complication and treat.
- Treatment is aimed at protecting and securing the airway with restoration of ventilation and circulation.
- Endotracheal intubation is required in almost all the cases. A small dose of an anaesthetic, sedative agent, and an intubating dose of a muscle relaxant may need to be used to facilitate intubation.
- Controlled ventilation of the lungs with 100% oxygen should be instituted.
- Ensure adequate uterine displacement to prevent aorto-caval compression.

- Further management involves administration of fluids, atropine, and vasopressors to support the BP. An adrenaline infusion may be required to maintain a satisfactory level of BP and HR.
- The duration of the block depends on the type and dose of the LA injected into the subarachnoid space and usually starts to recede after 1–2h.
- The patient will not require further anaesthetic/sedative agents initially as her unconsciousness is caused by the LA action on the brainstem. Additional agents will only impair the anaesthetist's ability to assess the level of consciousness and cause unnecessary additional cardiovascular compromise. Additional sedation may be needed later if she is able to respond and open her eyes before the return of adequate respiratory function.

If the cardiovascular and respiratory features are recognized early and treated effectively, the outcomes of a total spinal for mother and baby are good.

Further reading

D'Angelo R et al. Serious complications related to obstetric anesthesia: the serious complication repository project of the Society for Obstetric Anesthesia and Perinatology. Anesthesiology. 2014; 120: 1505–1512.

Jenkins JG. Some immediate serious complications of obstetric epidural analgesia and anaesthesia: A prospective study of 145,550 epidurals. International Journal of Obstetric Anesthia 2005; 14: 37–42.

Chau A et al. Dural puncture epidural technique improves labor analgesia quality with fewer side effects compared with epidural and combined spinal epidural techniques: A randomized clinical trial. Anesthesia and Analgesia 2017; 124: 560–569.

Local anaesthetic toxicity

Obstetric anaesthesia practice frequently involves the use of regional techniques, using large amounts of LA agents to establish effective analgesia and anaesthesia. Consequently, obstetric patients are at risk of developing systemic toxicity of LA drugs.

Systemic LA toxicity depends on a number of factors

- Site of injection, e.g. epidural space, pudendal block infiltration.
- Total dose in milligrams.
- Intravascular injection—this is the most common reason for systemic toxicity and is often unrecognized. The epidural veins in the obstetric patient are congested, and cannulation with the epidural catheter is common. Aspiration may not reliably reveal blood, as epidural veins are thin walled and may collapse.
- Speed of injection—slow injection of the LA drug will allow detection of toxicity earlier and is an important safety measure.
- The degree of protein binding and the presence of acidosis.
- The agent being used—levobupivacaine is recognized for its enhanced cardiovascular safety profile over bupivacaine.
- The British National Formulary guidelines recommend a total maximum dose (in mg) of bupivacaine or levobupivacaine of 150mg over a 4h period.
- Although a guide, the clinical manifestation of LA toxicity will depend on all the factors above, but in particular accidental intravascular injection.
- In the event of IV injection, a much smaller total dose of LA would be required to cause life-threatening complications.

Presentation

The manifestation of systemic toxicity may present acutely following accidental IV administration, or insidiously through systemic absorption. LAs act as membrane stabilizers within the heart and brain, leading to the following symptoms:

CNS complications
- Early excitation followed by CNS depression.
- Anxiety; light headed or drowsy.
- Facial paraesthesia, especially around the lips and tongue because of increased blood flow.
- Tinnitus.
- Loss of consciousness.
- Convulsions.
- Coma and apnoea.

Cardiovascular system complications
- Arrhythmias including VF/VT.
- Bradycardia and eventually asystole.
- Hypotension.
- Cardiac arrest.

Prevention

- Careful aspiration and observation of epidural catheters.
- Slow administration of increased concentration doses.

- If the patient has the first signs of LA toxicity, usually perioral tingling, stop injection and re-aspirate gently via the catheter.
- The use of adrenaline in LA administration is well known as a mechanism for the detection of inadvertent IV injection. Its use in obstetric patients is controversial as many patients are tachycardic and hypertensive, therefore the sensitivity and specificity are low.

Management

- STOP injection
- **A and B.** Maintain airway and give 100% O_2. Intubate and ventilate if indicated, e.g. patient obtunded/cardiovascular system collapse.
- Treat convulsions with IV diazepam 5–10mg or IV lorazepam 4mg.
- **C.** Left lateral tilt or wedge to reduce aorto-caval compression. Treat bradycardia with atropine and hypotension with appropriate vasopressors, e.g. ephedrine, phenylephrine, or adrenaline. Continue until clinical improvement. Consider IV vasopressor infusion for inotropic support. In event of cardiac arrest—Resuscitation Council ALS algorithm applies with emphasis on early delivery and avoidance of aorto-caval compression.
- CPR may have to be sustained for a considerable time, as cardiac arrest secondary to LA toxicity is very resistant to normal resuscitation practices (see below).
- Reduce individual adrenaline boluses to ≤ 1 microgram/kg.
- Vasopressin is not recommended.
- Avoid calcium channel blockers and beta-blockers.
- If ventricular arrhythmias develop, amiodarone is preferable.

The use of Intralipid for LA-associated cardiac arrest

Strong evidence now suggests that the use of a lipid emulsion, Intralipid® 20%, markedly improves outcome in cardiac arrest secondary to bupivacaine systemic toxicity.

Cardiac arrest secondary to LA toxicity
- Give 1.5mL/kg Intralipid® (20%) over 1 minute.
- Then immediately start infusion of Intralipid® at 0.25mL/kg/min.
- Repeat the bolus dose at 3–5 minute intervals until 3mL/kg total dose given.
- Continue the infusion until cardiovascular system stability is restored. Increase the infusion rate to 5mL/kg/min if BP decreases again.
- Maximum recommended dose is 8mL/kg.

Further reading

Neal JM et al. The American Society of Regional Anesthesia and Pain Medicine Checklist for Managing Local Anesthetic Systemic Toxicity: 2017 Version. *Regional Anesthesia and Pain Medicine..* 2018; 43: 150–153.

Mayr VD et al. A comparison of the combination of epinephrine and vasopressin with lipid emulsion in a porcine model of asphyxial cardiac arrest after intravenous injection of bupivacaine. *Anesthia and Analgesia* 2008; 106: 1566–1571.

Rothschild L et al. Intravenous lipid emulsion in clinical toxicology. *Scandinavian Journal of Trauma, Resuscitation and Emergency Medicine* 2010; 18: 51.

Magnesium toxicity

Magnesium is used in the treatment of severe pre-eclampsia and the prevention and treatment of eclampsia.

Side effects
- Flushing: if given too rapidly.
- Hypotension.
- Shortness of breath.
- Muscle weakness/paralysis, if given in an excessive dose especially in the presence of renal impairment. The patient on a magnesium infusion should have regular assessment of reflexes, and a serum magnesium level measured 4h after establishing the treatment.

Special consideration for the obstetric anaesthetist
- Suxamethonium neuromuscular blockade is not affected by magnesium but the muscle fasiculations are suppressed, making the timing of intubation difficult. A standard dose of suxamethonium 1–1.5mg/kg should be used. Its duration of action is unchanged.
- Magnesium will prolong and enhance non-deporalizing neuromuscular blockade. The dose of non-depolarizing muscle relaxant should be reduced, and attempts at reversal and extubation made only after assessment with a peripheral nerve stimulator.
- Care must be taken well into the postoperative period as recurarization has been described, which may lead to aspiration in the high risk obstetric patient and respiratory failure. The mother must have her respiratory rate and oxygen saturation monitored in a high dependency area on the maternity unit.
- IV calcium gluconate or chloride (10mL of 10% solution as a bolus) may be used if severe magnesium toxicity is present. Further management may include additional IV calcium and supportive care, often requiring critical care input.

Anaphylaxis

- This is an IgE-mediated type B, non-dose related hypersensitivity reaction. The causative antigen combines with IgE on mast cells and basophils, leading to the mass release of histamine and seretonin.
- Presentation includes any variation of; facial swelling, airway obstruction, bronchospasm, rash, oedema, erythema, profound hypotension, and shock. This condition is of major concern in the parturient and is associated with poor fetal outcome.
- Presentation may be within seconds of drug administration or over minutes.
- Common triggers in anaesthetic practice include muscle relaxants, latex, antibiotics, NSAIDs, colloids, hypnotics, and opioids—in decreasing order of frequency.
- A history of prior exposure is not required as cross-sensitivity is possible.

Immediate management
- Call for help (remember obstetric team).
- Remove suspected trigger.

Airway and breathing
- Maintain airway and give 100% O_2.
- Intubate and ventilate if significant upper airway obstruction.

Circulation
- Left lateral tilt or wedge to minimize aorto-caval compression.
- Adrenaline 50 micrograms IV increments (0.5mL 1:10,000 solution) or 0.5–1mg. IM. Repeat as necessary to support BP and continue until clinical improvement.
- Elevate legs and commence rapid IV fluid resuscitation.
- Expedite early delivery and paediatric support if situation is not rapidly improving.

Further management
- Chlorphenamine 10–20mg by slow IV injection for less severe reactions.
- Hydrocortisone 100–300mg IV.
- Consider continued inotropic support with adrenaline (0.05–0.1 micrograms/kg/min) or noradrenaline (0.05–0.1 micrograms/kg/min), and critical care transfer. Noradrenaline can be particularly useful if the hypotensive pressure is resistant to treatment with adrenaline.
- Consider nebulized bronchodilators, salbutamol 2.5–5mg, if continuing bronchospasm.
- Leak test endotracheal tube before extubation to exclude possible airway oedema.

Differential diagnosis

- Amniotic fluid embolus (AFE) has a very similar presentation; however, profound DIC is common with an AFE.
- Latex sensitivity. Risk factors include healthcare workers, spina bifida, need for recurrent bladder catheterization, and some fruit allergies (including banana, kiwi, and tomato).
- Cardiac disease of pregnancy, which is the most common indirect cause of maternal death. Can present with cardiogenic shock and wheeze secondary to cardiac failure.

Investigation/follow-up

- Plasma tryptase. Take 10mL blood after resuscitation and up to 1h following the reaction. Store at −20°C and inform biochemistry. Note down time of sample on form and in the patient notes. A further sample should be taken at 6 and 24h post reaction.
- Arrange anaesthetic follow-up and immunology referral for further investigation.
- Suspected drug reactions require CSM reporting via a yellow card— https://yellowcard.mhra.gov.uk
- A clear record of the allergy must be made in the notes, a full explanation given to the patient, and a MedicAlert® bracelet issued.

Further reading

Nel L, Eren E Peri-operative anaphylaxis. *British Journal of Clinical Pharmacology* 2011; 71: 647–658.
Rutkowski K et al. Anaphylaxis: current state of knowledge for the modern physician. *Postgrad Medical Journal* 2012; 88: 458–464. https://www.resus.org.uk/anaphylaxis/emergency-treatment-of-anaphylactic-reactions/
Harper NJN et al. Anaesthesia, surgery, and life-threatening allergic reactions: management and outcomes in the 6th National Audit Project (NAP6). *British Journal of Anaesthesia* 2018; 121: 172–188.

Uterotonic effects

Oxytocin

- Oxytocin is normally produced by the posterior pituitary and is structurally very similar to vasopressin.
- May cause hyper-stimulation of the uterus, uterine dysfunction, and fetal distress when used to promote or induce labour.
- It has some antidiuretic activity and can contribute to oliguria and fluid overload.
- This is especially likely in the context of PPH where a large amount of fluid/blood will be required in conjunction with an oxytocin infusion.
- Rapid bolus causes flushing, peripheral vasodilatation, and hypotension with occasional cardiac arrest.
- Give a bolus of 5U IV slowly, followed by a second dose only if required. Follow by an infusion 10U/h post delivery to avoid complications.

Ergot alkaloids

- Ergometrine is the classic example of this group; however, Syntometrine® (a combination of ergometrine and oxytocin) is also frequently used. It is administered IM postpartum to promote tetanic uterine contraction and decrease blood losses.
- May be given IV, IM, or intramyometrially to treat large blood losses.
- The IV route is associated with marked hypertension, nausea, and vomiting.
- A slow IV injection (dilute in 20mL of normal saline) will decrease the incidence and magnitude of these side effects. An anti-emetic, e.g. ondansetron 4mg IV is recommended pre-emptively.
- Avoid in pre-eclampsia/severe essential hypertension.

Prostaglandins

- Synthetic prostaglandins (analogues of E_2 and $F_2\alpha$) are used for the induction of labour and in the treatment of PPH.
- Carboprost is an example of this group used in the treatment of PPH.
- Most frequently given by the IM and intramyometrial route.
- May cause severe:
  - Bronchospasm—it contraindicated in asthmatics.
  - Cyanosis.
  - Systemic hypertension.
  - Diarrhoea—20–30% incidence.
  - Pulmonary hypertension.
  - Pulmonary oedema.
  - Arrhythmias, including VF.
  - Anaphylaxis.
- It is important to realize that these drugs may convert one life-threatening situation, e.g. uterine atony and PPH, to another!
- Beta-agonist treatment may be required to treat bronchospasm and may increase uterine atony.

Trauma in the obstetric patient

The principles of trauma resuscitation are the same for pregnant and non-pregnant patients. Pregnancy causes major physiological changes and altered anatomical relationships involving almost every organ system. These changes may alter the response to injury. Trauma is the major cause of death in young people, and the pattern of death demonstrates a trimodal distribution:

- Instantaneous—within seconds to minutes of the injury.
- Early—from a few minutes to a few hours.
- Late—hours to weeks.

When attending a pregnant trauma victim, it must be remembered that there are two patients; a successful outcome for the fetus relies on prompt resuscitation of the mother and early consultation with other specialties.

A systematic approach to resuscitation with the appropriate team can prevent deaths especially during 'the golden hour'.

Anatomical alterations of pregnancy relating to trauma

First trimester
- The uterus lies within the pelvis and it and the fetus are therefore well protected from traumatic damage.

Second trimester
- The uterus expands into the abdomen but the fetus remains somewhat protected, now by the proportionally large volume of amniotic fluid.

Third trimester
- The uterus is now large and increasingly thin walled, which makes the fetus more vulnerable; the fetal head lying within the pelvis is at danger in the event of maternal pelvic fracture.
- The lack of elasticity of the placenta when compared with that of the uterus exposes it to shearing forces, thus causing placental abruption.
- The bowel is pushed to the upper part of the abdomen posteriorly and is therefore relatively protected.

Physiological changes of pregnancy relating to trauma

- There can be initial haemodynamic stability, despite blood loss of up to 1500mL (Grade 3–4 shock), due to the expansion of plasma volume by 50%, which is normally seen in pregnancy.
- The CO is increased and SVR decreased, resulting in an overall decrease in BP during second trimester. The BP returns nearly to normal values at term.
- The supine position can reduce CO by 30% from the second trimester because of aorto-caval obstruction.
- The haematocrit is reduced.
- Vasoconstriction in placental vasculature occurs easily in response to hypotension and circulating catecholamines during trauma causing increased vascular resistance, reduced blood flow, and fetal hypoxaemia.
- Increased oxygen consumption and lowered arterial carbon dioxide can make interpretation of arterial blood gases difficult.

Assessment and treatment

- Ideally any injured pregnant woman needs to be seen and treated as early as possible after injury by a multidisciplinary team including anaesthetist, surgeon, obstetrician, paediatrician, and midwife.
- During the primary survey, life-threatening injuries are identified and treated using the **ABCDE** sequence of resuscitation.
- During the secondary survey, other important injuries which might not be life threatening are identified and treated during a head to toe, back to front examination.

Special measures for mother and fetus are required

- Injured mother must be resuscitated in a position that minimizes aorto-caval obstruction.
- If a spinal injury is suspected, a lateral tilt on a spinal board or lateral displacement of the uterus may be needed.
- Fetal monitoring is required for at least 4h, even after trivial trauma, using a CTG.

Maternal monitoring should continue for 24h with specific attention to the following

- Uterus—fundal height, position of fetus, contractions, irritability.
- Vagina—evidence of blood, amniotic fluid.
- Cervix—effacement suggesting preterm labour.

If a patient has multiple injuries

- X-rays of chest and pelvis are mandatory at some stage when the patient is stable. This MUST NOT be deferred because of the pregnancy.
- Cervical spine X-ray including the C7/T1 junction can be difficult to achieve and time should not be wasted; if there is any doubt in a critical situation, assume the neck is unstable and treat other life-threatening injuries.
- Nominate a team leader to ensure a systematic approach to resuscitation and reassessment of the multiply injured patient.

Airway

Acute airway obstruction may result from:

- Anatomical distortion from trauma.
- Debris such as blood or vomit.
- Oedema from inhalation injury and head injury.

Immediate recognition and resolution is vital

- Basic and advanced airway manoeuvres with cervical spine control and oxygenation.
- Immobilization of the neck is achieved with a correct sized stiff collar, tapes, and sand bag.

If considering endotracheal intubation, expect a difficult airway

- Term pregnancy and associated laryngeal oedema.
- Head not in the 'sniffing the morning air' position.
- Increased risk of regurgitation.
- Collar impedes movement of jaw and mouth.
- A rapid sequence induction is required using thiopental and suxamethonium.
- Nasogastric and nasotracheal tubes are contraindicated if a base of skull fracture suspected.

Breathing

- Inspection—respiratory rate, depth, symmetry, bleeding, wounds.
- Palpation—tenderness, asymmetry, crepitus, midline trachea.
- Percussion—hyper-resonance or dullness.
- Auscultation—loss of air entry.

Clinical examination should identify these life-threatening injuries

- Tension pneumothorax—treat with needle thoracocentesis in the second intercostal space, mid-clavicular line with a 16G needle.
- Open pneumothorax—use a three-sided occlusive dressing.
- Flail chest—consider lung contusion and need for ventilation.
- Massive haemothorax—chest drain losses of 1500mL of blood or continued loss of 200mL in 1h needs a thoracotomy.
- Cardiac tamponade—difficult to diagnose; Becks triad of muffled heart sounds, raised jugular venous pressure, and reduced arterial pressure. Aspiration of pericardial blood required with ECG monitoring.

Circulation

- Site two 14/16G cannulae in the antecubital fossae.
- Blood should be sent for FBC, cross-match, U&E, and glucose.
- Rapidly infuse 2L of warmed Hartmann's solution and check response.
- Apply compression to any external source of bleeding, e.g. open femoral fracture and obvious vascular injuries.
- Avoid aorto-caval obstruction in any shocked pregnant patient.

- Remember that in the third trimester the mother will be hypercoagulable and blood products should be used with a pregnancy specific protocol (see Chapter 18 MOH)

During fluid therapy, patients may be classified as follows:

- Stable.
- Responding to fluid therapy.
- Transient responders.
- Non-responders.

Fetal compromise demonstrated with the CTG may the first sign of maternal haemorrhage.

Further monitoring, fluid and surgery may be required.

Any suspected source of bleeding must be identified

- Intrathoracic—CXR, Echo, or CT Thorax.
- Abdomen—CT abdomen or diagnostic peritoneal lavage has been used to detect free blood in the abdominal cavity. Ultrasound, i.e. focused abdominal sonography for trauma (FAST) may be preferred to detect haemorrhage.
- Retroperitoneal space—large engorged pelvic vessels that surround the gravid uterus can contribute to massive retroperitoneal bleeding after blunt trauma.
- Pelvis—sacroiliac joints and symphysis pubis widen in pregnancy.
- Extensive placental separation or AFE can cause DIC with depletion of fibrinogen, clotting factors, and platelets. If this occurs, appropriate therapy should be given in liaison with the consultant haematologist.

- As little as 0.01mL of fetal blood can cause iso-immunization of Rhesus-negative mothers. Ig therapy should be considered in all Rhesus-negative mothers, irrespective of the extent and site of trauma, within 72h.
- A Kleihauer–Betke test to assess iso-immunization should be performed. A maternal blood smear allows detection of fetal RBCs in the maternal circulation. A positive test is also an accurate predictor of premature labour.

Disability

Non-pregnant and pregnant patients are assessed alike with the AVPU score: A fall in the level of consciousness is always serious.

- A—awake and orientated.
- V—responds to voice.
- P—responds to pain.
- U—unresponsive.

Eclampsia is a complication of pregnancy that may mimic head injury. The diagnosis needs to be considered if a patient has a head injury. Look for evidence of hyper-reflexia, peripheral oedema, and proteinuria.

Environment

- The patient needs to be completely exposed to assess for injury. The ambient temperature needs to be increased to prevent hypothermia and further clotting abnormalities.
- Domestic violence is rapidly becoming a major cause of injury to women during cohabitation, marriage, and pregnancy—17% of injured patients experience trauma as a result of another person. This needs to be considered.

Some indicators of domestic violence include

- If the partner insists on being present for interview and examination and monopolizes discussion.
- Diminishing self-image, depression, history of suicide attempts.
- Self-blame.

Secondary survey

This does not begin until the primary survey has been completed and the immediate life-threatening injuries identified and treated.
Other important potential injuries include:

- Simple pneumothorax.
- Haemothorax.
- Aortic disruption.
- Diaphragmatic injury.
- Blunt cardiac injury.
- Fetal survival is completely dependent on adequate resuscitation of mother. Fetal survival does not necessarily equate with the injury severity score, and fetal demise can occur with trivial maternal trauma and at any gestational age.
- Vigilant monitoring of mother and fetus is needed.

Specific maternal and fetal injury

Blunt injury
- The abdominal wall, uterine myometrium, and amniotic fluid act as buffers to direct fetal injury from blunt trauma.
- Direct injuries to fetus and uterus causing rupture can occur during motor vehicle accidents and indirect ones from shearing forces resulting in placental abruption.

Penetrating Injury
- As the gravid uterus increases in size, the remainder of the viscera are relatively protected from penetrating injury, while the risk of uterine injury increases.
- Energy is absorbed by the uterus from any penetrating injury, resulting in good maternal survival and poor fetal survival.
- Maternal volume status should be monitored with early placement of a CVP line.
- An abnormality of fetal heart baseline, repetitive decelerations, absence of acceleration, or beat-to-beat variability may indicate fetal compromise.
- A vaginal examination is mandatory to assess cervical effacement and dilatation, fetal presentation, and relationship of fetal presenting part to ischial spines.

Uterine rupture
- If this has occurred, peritoneal signs may be difficult as usual peritoneal signs are attenuated.
- Abdominal guarding and tenderness may be present.
- Odd lie of uterus with an inability to feel fundus or fetal presentation.
- Suspicion of uterine rupture requires surgical exploration.
- Placental abruption is a leading cause of death after blunt trauma and occurs after relatively minor trauma in late pregnancy.
- Vaginal bleeding can be occult (30%).
- Uterine tenderness, premature contractions, irritability, or tetany may occur.
- The fundal height may increase.
- Maternal shock is very likely.

Amniotic fluid embolism
- If bleeding vaginally after rupture of membranes, there is a possibility of a life-threatening AFE and a consumptive coagulopathy.
- Early monitoring of coagulation preferably with VHA is essential.

Outcome
- Pregnancy is likely to end unsuccessfully with placental, uterine, or direct fetal injury.
- Fetal death occurs in 80% of cases where there has been maternal haemorrhagic shock.
- Maternal survival may depend on surgical evacuation of uterus and fetus.
- Post-mortem CS is advised in the event of fatal maternal trauma, since it may result in fetal salvage despite prolonged hypoxaemia.

Further reading
Jain V et al. Guidelines for the management of a pregnant trauma patient. *Journal of Obstetrics and Gynaecology: Canada* 2015; 37:553–574.

Anaesthesia for non-obstetric surgery

Martin Garry

General principles

Up to 2% of pregnant women undergo surgery unrelated to pregnancy each year. The most common procedure during the first trimester is laparoscopy. Appendicectomy and cholecystectomy are the most commonly performed open abdominal procedures. Surgery during pregnancy can be associated with premature labour and fetal loss. Lower abdominal and pelvic surgery carries a higher risk.

Anaesthetic concerns

A thorough knowledge of physiological changes of pregnancy and of placental transfer of drugs is essential.

Major anaesthetic concerns are:

- Maternal risk resulting from anatomical and physiological changes of pregnancy.
- Maintenance of adequate uteroplacental blood flow.
- Teratogenic effects on the fetus of drugs administered to the mother.

Surgical concerns

- The changes of pregnancy can often modify the disease process and make initial diagnosis difficult.
- Patients may therefore present late with advanced or complicated disease.
- Surgical management is also more complicated than in non-pregnant patients.

Timing

- Whenever possible, elective surgery should be delayed until 6 weeks postpartum.
- More urgent surgery should be delayed until after the period of organogenesis of the first trimester, unless there is an immediate threat to the mother.
- If emergency surgery is necessary, ensure the obstetric team are informed.

Preparation

- Thorough preoperative evaluation including airway assessment should be performed and gestational age noted.
- The mother should be counselled about the relative risks of surgery to the pregnancy.
- Premedication may be necessary to allay maternal anxiety, as excess maternal catecholamines are harmful to fetal well-being.
- All women >14 weeks pregnant should have antacid prophylaxis, as hormonal changes at the lower oesophageal sphincter increase the risk of regurgitation and aspiration.

Anaesthetic principles

- Where possible, a regional technique should be used. It has the benefits of the woman maintaining her own airway and providing good analgesia. However, hypotension should be aggressively treated to maintain uteroplacental circulation.

- Ensure correct positioning for all women >20 weeks gestation whatever surgery is being performed. Aorto-caval compression must be avoided by placing a wedge under the right hip and manual uterine displacement. Even when aorto-caval compression does not cause maternal hypotension, it can reduce placental perfusion and cause fetal compromise.
- It is usually not necessary to monitor the fetal heart rate (FHR) during surgery as the effects of general anaesthesia (GA) drugs make interpretation difficult.
- If the mother is near term, especially if the surgery is abdominal, then there should be careful consideration around delivery of the baby by caesarean section (CS).
- Maternal FRC is reduced and oxygen requirement increases in pregnancy. Pre-oxygenate for at least 3 mins prior to GA.
- Avoid hypoxia, hypotension, hypercarbia, and hyperventilation regardless of the anaesthetic technique used.
- If a GA is used, adequate depth of anaesthesia should be maintained. Consider a depth of anaesthesia monitor. Light anaesthesia increases maternal catecholamine release and reduces uteroplacental perfusion. In addition, the tocolytic effect of volatile anaesthetics is beneficial.
- During laparoscopic surgery, minimize pneumoperitoneum to 8–12mmHg.
- Treat blood loss early and vigorously. Physiological changes of pregnancy mask early signs of blood loss, and subclinical hypovolaemia will compromise placental perfusion. Hypotension from hypovolaemia in a pregnant woman may not be evident until 25–30% of blood volume is lost.

Fetal monitoring

- Continuous FHR monitoring using transabdominal Doppler is possible from 16 weeks of gestation. However fetal monitoring is controversial, especially if the fetus is very premature.
- Prior to 24 weeks gestation, the fetus is generally not usually considered viable, and confirmation of fetal well-being should be performed at an appropriate time in the postoperative period.

If urgent surgery is required after the fetus is viable at 22–24 weeks:

- The neonatology team should be informed.
- External tocodynamometry should be applied in recovery during the early postoperative period. It can detect the onset of preterm labour, so that tocolysis can be started early. Prophylactic tocolysis is controversial.
- Tocolysis can be administered in the post-operative period if there are signs of labour either from the use of tocodynomometry or the onset of regular painful contractions.
- The CTG can be difficult to interpret in the presence of GA or opioid drugs.
- Acute fetal distress is uncommon unless the surgery is complicated by hypotension. The cause should be aggressively treated.

Effect of anaesthetic drugs on fetus

Teratogenicity has been defined as any significant postnatal change in function or form in an offspring after prenatal treatment.

- Causes of teratogenicity are diverse, and include infection, pyrexia, hypoxia, and acidosis as well as the better recognized hazards of drugs and radiation.
- It is estimated that drug/chemical exposure is the cause of 2–3% of birth defects.
- Ionizing radiation is a known human teratogen. Exposure below 5–10rads is safe. Fetal exposure from a chest radiograph is ~8mrads.
- The teratogenic potential of drugs is influenced by genetic predisposition, dose, duration, and timing of exposure.
- The fetus can be affected at three stages:
  - During the first 2 weeks of intrauterine life, the teratogens have either a lethal effect or none at all on the fetus.
  - The 3rd to 8th week is the most vital period for organogenesis. Drug exposure during this period would cause most teratogenic effects and subsequent organ abnormalities.
  - From the 8th week onwards, the organ formation is completed and then organ growth takes place. Drug exposure after 8 weeks gestation should not cause major organ abnormalities, but can cause fetal growth retardation.

Premedication

Antacids
- Sodium citrate is safe.
- Omeprazole is not known to be harmful in pregnancy.

Anxiolytics

Although animal studies have shown an association of benzodiazepines with cleft lip and cleft palate, effects on humans are still controversial. A single dose has not been shown to be teratogenic. Long-term exposure should be avoided, as it can cause neonatal withdrawal symptoms following delivery; exposure just before delivery can cause neonatal drowsiness and hypotonia.

Anticholinergics
- Glycopyrronium bromide is preferred to atropine if an anticholinergic is required. It does not readily cross the placenta and is a better antisialogogue.
- Atropine crosses the placenta and can cause fetal tachycardia and loss of FHR variability when given in large doses.

IV induction agents

It should be remembered that opioids and IV induction agents decrease FHR variability, and this should not be a cause of concern.

Thiopental
- Clinical experience shows that this is a very safe drug to use, although formal studies have not been conducted.
- Ideal if rapid sequence induction is planned.

Propofol
- It is not teratogenic in animal studies.
- Its use in early human pregnancy has not been formally investigated. However, it is safe to use during CS at term.

Etomidate
- Is a potent corticosteroid inhibitor and, when used during CS, neonates have reduced cortisol levels.
- Its use in early pregnancy has not been formally investigated.

Ketamine
- Should be avoided during early pregnancy, as it increases intrauterine pressure and can cause fetal asphyxia. This effect is not seen in the third trimester of pregnancy.

Inhalational anaesthetic agents

All volatile anaesthetic agents decrease the uterine tone, dilate uterine arteries, and increase uterine blood flow up to a MAC of 1.5. However, at higher concentrations, the uterine blood flow decreases secondary to falls in maternal BP and CO.

- Halothane and isoflurane have been used extensively in pregnancy and are safe. The halogenated vapours also cause uterine relaxation, which may be beneficial for surgery during pregnancy.
- Since nitrous oxide inhibits methionine synthetase, there is a concern that it can affect DNA synthesis in a developing fetus. It has been shown to be consistently teratogenic during the peak organogenic period in animal studies, but there is no evidence of such an effect in humans. However, given that anaesthesia can be safely delivered without nitrous oxide, it is sensible to avoid this agent.

Analgesics

- Opioids are highly fat-soluble and readily cross the placenta. Although brief exposure is safe, long-term exposure will cause symptoms of withdrawal when the fetus is delivered. Animal studies show possible fetal teratogenicity if prolonged hypercapnia or impaired feeding develop as side effects of opioid exposure.
- Paracetamol and codeine are the safest analgesics for minor surgery during pregnancy.
- NSAIDs are contraindicated in the first and third trimester and especially shortly before delivery as they may prevent closure of the neonate's ductus arteriosis at delivery.

No anaesthetic drugs, with the exception of cocaine, have been associated with proven teratogenic effects.

Anaesthetic management

General principles

- The mother should be counselled and reassured whenever possible about the risks to the pregnancy.
- The obstetric team should be involved.

Regional is preferable to general anaesthesia.

Meticulous anaesthesia is required with attention to:
- Good oxygenation.
- Normal CO_2 (for pregnancy).
- Normotension and normovolaemia.

First trimester

- Ideally avoid surgery or at least delay to second trimester if possible.
- Care with potential teratogenic drugs.
- Avoid N_2O.
- Consider the possibility of undiagnosed pregnancy in all women of reproductive age.

Second trimester

- This is the optimum time for surgery.
- Care with positioning to avoid/minimize aorto-caval compression.

In order to minimize risk of aspiration:
- Pre-medicate with omeprazole 20–40mg 1h before surgery.
- Sodium citrate 20mL immediately before induction.
- Rapid sequence induction with cricoid pressure.
- Monitor uterine activity and FHR post surgery. Treat with tocolytic agents if necessary.

Third trimester

As for second trimester regarding:
- Positioning.
- Risk of aspiration.
- Fetal and uterine monitoring.
- At particular risk of premature induction of labour, so that postoperative uterine monitoring is essential.

Anaesthetic drugs

During pregnancy, the response to anaesthetic drugs is altered:
- MAC for inhalational anaesthetics is decreased.
- Neuronal block from spinal and epidural anaesthesia is more extensive.
- Enhanced block from peripheral nerve blocks.
- Plasma cholinesterase levels decrease by >25% and the effect of suxamethonium may be prolonged.
- Albumin concentration is reduced and thus plasma binding of drugs decreases, resulting in a greater fraction of unbound drug. This explains the increased toxicity of bupivacaine during pregnancy.

Postoperative considerations

- Venous thrombo-embolic prophylaxis is mandatory for all pregnant women, i.e. anti-embolic stockings and LMWH, e.g. enoxaparin 40mg SC. Pregnant women are hypercoaguable with a high risk of post-operative DVT.
- Give adequate postoperative analgesia. The sympathetic response from pain and stress increases maternal catecholamine levels, which causes vasoconstriction of all blood vessels, including those of the uteroplacental circulation.

Further reading

Goodman S. Anesthesia for nonobstetric surgery in the pregnant patient. *Seminars in Perinatology* 2002; 26: 136–145.

Kuczkowski KM. Nonobstetric surgery during pregnancy: what are the risks of anaesthesia. *Obstetrical and Gynecological Survey* 2004; 59: 52–56.

Rosen MA. Management of anesthesia for the pregnant surgical patient. *Anesthesiology* 1999; 179: 1643–1653.

The fetus

Christine Conner

Fetal circulation *in utero*

Oxygen and nutrients are brought to the placenta by the maternal uteroplacental circulation, with delivery to the fetus by the separate fetoplacental circulation.

Uteroplacental circulation

- Maternal CO together with the spiral arteries within the uterine myometrium and decidua determine blood flow to the intervillous space and fetus.
- Physiological adaptations in pregnancy increase the maternal CO by 40%.
- Oxygen-carrying capacity is increased up to 28% by an increase in the red cell mass.
- Spiral arteries become more tortuous and lose elasticity through placental trophoblast invasion to adapt to the increasing demand of blood supply to the placenta.
- Trophoblast erosion of the spiral arteries occurs in two phases to produce a low pressure, high blood flow system within the placenta.

  - Phase 1 occurs in the first trimester and involves trophoblast erosion of the decidual portions of the spiral arteries.
  - Phase 2 in the second trimester involves trophoblast erosion into the myometrial portion of the spiral arteries.

- The loss of elasticity within the spiral arteries removes vasoregulation. Therefore, blood flow to the placenta is directly proportional to the maternal CO.
- Oxygenated blood enters the intervillous space from the spiral arteries as jets of blood directed towards the chorionic plate of the placenta.
- Transplacental gas exchange occurs by simple diffusion.
- Blood then flows towards the basal placental plate, aided by uterine contractions and movement of the chorionic villi.
- Deoxygenated blood drains into the uterine veins.

Umbilical circulation

- In the fetus, the placenta performs the functions of the lungs and kidneys.
- Two umbilical arteries (UAs) carry 50% of the fetal CO to the placenta.
- One UA arises from each fetal internal iliac artery and leaves the fetus through the umbilical cord to the placenta.
- In the placenta, the arteries divide into small branches, which enter the chorionic villi where further subdivision into arterioles and capillaries and transplacental gas exchange occur.
- Fetal blood then flows through corresponding venous systems, which drain into a single umbilical vein carrying oxygenated blood back to the fetus through the umbilical cord.
- Approximately 50% of the blood from the umbilical vein passes into the ductus venosus, which enters the inferior vena cava (IVC), bypassing the fetal liver.

- On reaching the heart, a large proportion of blood within the IVC is directed by the crista dividens through the foramen ovale into the left atrium, avoiding entry into the right heart channel.
- This oxygenated blood passes into the left ventricle from where it is pumped into the aorta.
- From the aorta, two large carotid arteries distribute a large share of the oxygenated blood to the cerebral circulation.
- The smaller portion of blood in the IVC that does not pass through the foramen ovale mixes in the right atrium with deoxygenated blood carried by the superior vena cava (SVC) and the coronary sinus.
- This blood passes to the right ventricle from where it is pumped into the pulmonary circulation.
- Pressure within the pulmonary circulation is much higher than in the aorta, resulting in most of the blood being diverted along the ductus arteriosus, which joins the aorta below the origins of the carotid arteries.
- Less than 10% of the fetal CO enters the pulmonary circulation.
- The blood which passes down the fetal aorta to supply the viscera contains mainly blood that has circulated through the head and arms together with a lesser amount from the LV.
- Two-thirds of the blood from the aorta is pumped along the umbilical arteries to the placenta, with a small amount entering the femoral arteries to the legs.

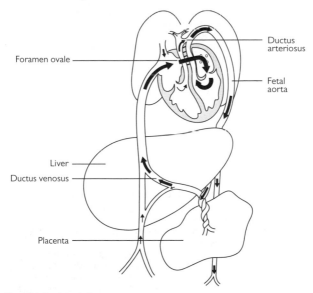

Ductus arteriosus

Foramen ovale

Fetal aorta

Liver

Ductus venosus

Placenta

Fig. 23.1 Fetal circulation.

Physiological changes to fetal circulation at delivery

At birth, a rapid sequence of cardiovascular and respiratory events occur to enable the newborn to switch from placenta to lungs for effective gaseous exchange. This sequence results in the transition from a fetal to an adult pattern of circulation.

• Labour-induced stresses stimulate catecholamine and steroid responses within the fetus, which prepare the lungs for air breathing by reducing the amount of lung fluid secretion and increasing the release of lung surfactant.
• Uterine contractions reduce the flow of blood into the intervillous space, resulting in deterioration in the fetal blood gas status.
• Compression of the fetal thorax as it descends through the birth canal at delivery helps expel some of the fetal lung fluid. Fluid within the alveolar spaces and tracheobronchial tree is absorbed into pulmonary lymphatics.
• Expansion of the fetal thorax as it emerges from the vagina at delivery enables the proximal airways to fill with air.
• Clamping of the umbilical cord results in a deterioration of blood gases and low arterial pO_2.
• This change is detected by the carotid and aortic body chemoreceptors and provides a very powerful stimulus to initiate breathing.
• Exposure to other sensory stimuli with delivery (temperature, pain, pressure, tactile stimuli) helps to initiate breathing.
• Entry of air into the lungs raises the interstitial pO_2, resulting in a reduction in PVR, an increase in pulmonary blood flow, a rise in the pO_2 and increased filling of the left atria.
• Clamping of the cord removes the low resistance placental circulation, with a resulting increase in SVR and reduced VR to the right atrium.
• The pressure gradient within the atrial chambers reverses with the increased pressure in the left atrium, resulting in a functional closure of the foramen ovale.
• This separates the circulatory system into two halves—the right and left.
• The fall in the PVR causes a reversal of blood flow within the ductus arteriosus shunt.
• The perfusion of the ductus arteriosus with oxygen-rich blood together with locally produced vasoactive substances results in its closure.

Physiological remnants of the fetal circulation

• The foramen ovale becomes the adult fosse ovalis.
• The ductus arteriosus becomes the adult ligamentum arteriosum.
• The extrahepatic portion of the umbilical vein becomes the adult ligamentum teres hepatis.
• The ductus venosus becomes the adult ligamentum venosum.
• The proximal portions of the fetal right and left umbilical arteries become the adult umbilical branches of the internal iliac arteries.
• The distal portions of the umbilical arteries become the adult medial umbilical ligaments.

Fetal haemoglobin

The partial pressure of oxygen within the umbilical vein at term is between 30 and 40mmHg. To meet its tissue oxygen requirements at this relatively low pO_2, the fetus has made adaptations to hypoxia.
- At term, the fetal haemoglobin concentration is high, between 160 and 180g/L, which increases the oxygen-carrying capacity of the blood.
- Fetal haemoglobin is predominantly (60–80%) HbF, which has a higher affinity for O_2 than adult haemoglobin (HbA).
- This enables fetal blood to take up oxygen more readily from maternal blood.
- The O_2 dissociation curve for HbF is steeper than that for HbA over the range of pO_2 found in fetal tissues, allowing better delivery of oxygen to these tissues.
- The anatomy of the fetal circulation ensures that the pO_2 within the ascending aorta is 30% higher than in the descending portion, providing more oxygenated blood to the developing brain and heart muscle than to the other fetal organs.

Assessment of fetal well-being during pregnancy

Obstetric patients are risk stratified at booking into two main groups:
- Low risk: no identifiable risk factors. They will have the majority of their care in community-based midwifery-led antenatal clinics.
- High risk: identified by either their past obstetric or medical history. Their care in pregnancy will be co-ordinated through hospital obstetrician-run antenatal clinics.
- All obstetric patients require antenatal fetal assessment, but the frequency and forms of assessment will vary according to risk.
- Patients who initially start as low risk may, during the course of either their pregnancy or labour, develop obstetric complications necessitating additional fetal assessment.

Fetal growth

- Normal fetal growth is dependent on an adequate supply of oxygen and nutrients to and across the placenta with sufficient fetal uptake, together with overall regulation of the growth process.
- Any factor which interferes with these processes can result in IUGR.
- The severity of the IUGR will depend on the gestational age at onset, the magnitude of the injury, and the success of adaptive mechanisms.
- Factors affecting fetal growth can be broadly subdivided into maternal, uterine, placental, and fetal categories.

  - **Maternal factors** include:
    - Any chronic medical condition.
    - Smoking.
    - Alcohol and drug addiction.
    - Maternal age <16 and >35 years.
    - Low BMI.
  - **Uterine abnormalities** include:
    - Congenital uterine malformation.
    - Uterine fibroids.
  - **Placental factors** include:
    - Impaired trophoblast invasion as seen with pre-eclampsia.
    - Placental abruption.
    - Placental infarction.
    - Chorio-amnionitis.
    - Placenta praevia.
  - **Fetal factors** include:
    - Chromosomal abnormalities.
    - Structural abnormalities.
    - Congenital infection.
    - Inborn errors of metabolism.
    - Multiple pregnancy.

- All obstetric patients require assessment of fetal growth.
- Any method employed to assess fetal growth requires an accurate knowledge of gestational age.
- Most of the tests currently used detect the small for gestational age (SFG) fetus rather than the fetus with IUGR.

- The IUGR fetus is one who has failed to reach its own growth potential. Not all SFG fetuses will be suffering from IUGR, as many will be healthy constitutionally small babies.
- Differentiating the pathological IUGR fetus from the healthy SFG fetus is clinically important as IUGR is associated with an increased risk of:
  - Stillbirth.
  - Prematurity.
  - Intrapartum fetal distress.
  - Perinatal morbidity.
- Tests used to assess fetal growth are more sensitive and specific when applied to high risk pregnancies compared to the low risk population.

Symphyseal fundal height

- A useful screening test for all obstetric patients.
- The measurement is taken from the top of the maternal symphysis pubis to the top of the uterine fundus and is measured in centimetres.
- Between 20 and 35 weeks gestation, the normal symphyseal fundal height (SFH) should approximate the number of weeks of gestation with an acceptable variation of ±2cm.
- After 35 weeks gestation, the margin of error is ±3cm.
- It does not differentiate between SFG and IUGR and is subject to significant intra- and inter-observer error.
- Serial SFH measurements increase its sensitivity as a screening test.
- Sensitivity is further limited by factors including:
  - Maternal obesity.
  - Uterine fibroids.
  - Abnormal amniotic fluid volume.
  - Abnormal fetal lie.
  - Multiple pregnancies.
- Customized charts which adjust for maternal factors, including BMI, parity, and ethnicity, improve the sensitivity and increase the antenatal detection of SFG babies.
- Further investigation, in the form of an ultrasound examination, is required if the SFH measurement differs by more than the expected for gestation.

Ultrasound biometry

- Ultrasound is the best available method for detecting a SFG fetus and in monitoring growth.
- Any fetus thought to be at risk of IUGR, from either the maternal obstetric or medical history, should be assessed with serial ultrasound biometry.
- The fetal biparietal diameter, head circumference (HC), abdominal circumference (AC), and femur length are the measurements obtained at ultrasound examinations.
- Growth charts are available for each of these measurements, and most are based on cross-sectional rather than longitudinal population studies.
- An estimated fetal weight (EFW) can be calculated from these fetal measurements using various formulae and plotted according to gestational age.
- On most charts, the 5th, 50th, and 95th centiles are plotted.
- The AC, which includes the fetal liver, the size of which is dependent on stored glycogen and hence fetal nutrition, is the best measurement for detecting IUGR.
- The EFW is becoming more widely used to assess fetal growth. A SFG fetus is defined as a weight below the 10th percentile for the gestational age.

Two patterns of growth restriction exist
- **Symmetric IUGR** where both head size and AC are simultaneously reduced, with a HC/AC within normal limits.
  - Constitutionally small babies at the lower end of the normal range.
  - Pathological due to an insult early in pregnancy at the time of general organ growth. This includes congenital abnormalities, chromosomal abnormalities, and congenital infections.
- **Asymmetric IUGR** is the result of fetal adaptation to an inadequate supply of nutrition in order to protect the developing brain.
  - AC is reduced more than the head measurements, giving an increased HC/AC ratio.
  - Usually seen in conditions with a later pathological onset, e.g. pre-eclampsia, placental abruption, or infarction.
- Ultrasound scanning also enables assessment of the amniotic fluid volume (AFV) and the UA Doppler status, which are both useful in distinguishing the healthy SFG fetus from the one with IUGR.

Amniotic fluid volume
- After 16 weeks gestation, the fetal kidneys produce most of the AFV.
- If the supply of oxygen and nutrients to the growing fetus is insufficient, adaptations occur, with redistribution of fetal blood away from the kidneys in favour of the brain and the myocardium.
- The reduced blood flow to the kidneys results in an overall reduction in the AFV.
- Ultrasound provides the most reliable method of assessment of AFV, which is expressed as the amniotic fluid index (AFI).
- Oligohydramnios is defined as either an AFI of <5cm or a single maximum pocket of <2cm.
- The perinatal mortality is increased in pregnancies with reduced AFV on ultrasound scanning compared with those where the AFV is normal.

Umbilical artery Doppler
- Assessment of the UA Doppler waveform is widely used in the antenatal surveillance of pregnancies with IUGR.
- The UA Doppler waveform is affected by the resistance of blood flow within the placenta and the degree of villous formation.
- Normal placental villous formation produces a low resistance system facilitating forward flow of blood within the UA throughout the fetal cardiac cycle, described as positive end-diastolic flow (EDF) (Fig. 23.2a).
- Various parameters including the resistance index can be calculated from the UA Doppler waveform and are used to assess the degree of resistance within the UA (Fig. 23.2a).
- Conditions such as IUGR and pre-eclampsia are associated with an inadequate maternal vascular response to placentation and result in increased resistance in the placental circulation.
- With increasing placental resistance, the EDF decreases (Fig. 23.2b).
- Further damage with increasing resistance will eventually lead to no forward flow, known as absent EDF (Fig. 23.2c) or, in extreme cases, to reversal of flow, known as reversed EDF (Fig. 23.2d).
- By this stage, ~60–70% of the villous vascular tree is damaged.
- Abnormal UA Doppler flow patterns indicate an increased risk of fetal hypoxia and acidaemia.

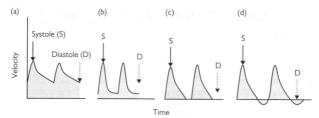

Fig. 23.2 Umbilical artery waveform patterns. (a) Normal UA Doppler with normal resistance index. (b) UA Doppler waveform showing increased resistance index. (c) UA Doppler waveform showing absent end-diastolic flow. (d) UA Doppler waveform showing reversed end-diastolic flow.

- Both perinatal mortality and morbidity rates increase with the degree of abnormality within the UA Doppler recording.

Management of IUGR

Once fetal IUGR has been confirmed by serial scanning, the subsequent management will depend on the gestation.

- With early-onset IUGR before 32 weeks gestation or symmetric IUGR, consider chromosomal abnormalities, congenital anomalies, and congenital infection.

  - Detailed anomaly scan to look for structural abnormalities.
  - Consider fetal karyotyping.
  - Maternal viral screen (TORCH screen for toxoplasmosis, rubella, cytomegalovirus, and herpes simplex).
  - Maternal corticosteroid administration, in case preterm delivery <36 weeks is required, to help fetal lung maturation.
  - Intensive fetal monitoring as for late-onset IUGR.

- Late-onset IUGR after 32 weeks gestation.

  - Regular fetal monitoring using ultrasound scanning assessment of the AFV, the UA Doppler status, serial biometry, and CTG.
  - Consider maternal steroid administration if delivery before 36 weeks is necessary.

- If the UA Doppler waveform and other tests remain normal, continue twice-weekly fetal monitoring. Some obstetricians may consider delivery at ~36 weeks whilst others may continue monitoring until term.
- If the UA Doppler shows absent EDF but other tests are normal, consider delivery if an adequate gestation has been reached. Otherwise, careful frequent monitoring at least twice weekly.
- If the UA Doppler shows reversed EDF or the CTG or other biophysical parameters suggest hypoxia, proceed to immediate delivery.

Assessment of fetal well-being during labour

Meconium

- Clear amniotic fluid drainage is a reassuring feature in labour.
- Meconium-stained liquor (MSL) is present in ~15% of all labours.
- The main factors influencing the passage of meconium are gestational age and possible fetal compromise. Therefore, the presence of MSL must be interpreted accordingly.
- Meconium is produced in the fetal gut from 10 weeks, but is rarely passed by the fetus before 34 weeks gestation. By term, MSL is present in ~30% of cases, increasing to 50% by 42 weeks.
- In preterm infants, MSL is very uncommon and is associated with infections such as listeriosis, which produce a fetal gut enteritis.
- Maternal obstetric cholestasis is associated with increased risk of MSL.
- Fresh thick meconium is frequently passed with a fetal breech presentation in the late first and second stage due to mechanical forces on the presenting part in labour.
- Acute and subacute fetal compromise can lead to the passage of meconium.
- In very acute situations such as cord prolapse or placental abruption, this may not occur.

Grading of meconium

- Meconium is often graded according to its appearance, which will be affected by the volume of amniotic fluid around the fetus and the temporal relationship between its passage and the timing of membrane rupture.
- Meconium consistency will be determined by the diluting influence of the AFV. With decreasing amounts of amniotic fluid, the thickness of meconium will increase.
- Meconium passed several days before rupture of the membranes is often brown and described as old.
- Recently passed meconium is green and often referred to as new or fresh.
- Significant meconium is defined as dark green or black amniotic fluid that is thick or tenacious or amniotic fluid containing lumps of meconium.

Management of meconium-stained liquor in labour

- Continuous fetal monitoring is recommended if there is significant meconium (see above).
- If the FHR is normal, no other specific action is required in labour.
- If the FHR is abnormal, consideration should be given either to performing a fetal blood sample or immediate delivery depending on the clinical setting.

Meconium aspiration syndrome

- Aspiration of meconium into the fetal or neonatal lungs can lead to meconium aspiration syndrome (MAS).
- Meconium aspiration, defined as the presence of meconium below the vocal cords, occurs in ~35% of fetuses with MSL.

- Clinically MAS can range from a mild transitory condition to severe respiratory compromise.
- Meconium aspiration can occur *in utero*, at delivery or after birth.
- *In utero* meconium aspiration is thought to occur as a result of fetal breathing movements.
- In an infant who has not been exposed to intrauterine hypoxia, meconium aspiration usually results in mild MAS, which is asymptomatic in 90% of cases.
- In severe cases, neonatal mortality can be as high as 40%.
- Meconium causes physical airway obstruction, displaces surfactant, resulting in atelectasis, and produces a local chemical pneumonitis.

Risk factors for severe MAS
- Fetal hypoxia.
- Presence of thick meconium, more common in post-term pregnancies and with oligohydramnios.

Management at delivery
- A paediatrician should be present for delivery in all labours where there is MSL.
- If the baby is vigorous and active following delivery, irrespective of grade of meconium, no further action should be taken.
- With a non-vigorous baby, the vocal cords should be visualized. If meconium is present on or below the cords, direct tracheal suction is required.
- Saline lavage is not recommended as it carries the risk of removing surfactant and it may facilitate further spread of meconium within the lung.
- There is no evidence to support the technique of clamping the chest to delay the first breath, nor is gastric suctioning recommended.

The cardiotocograph

The CTG is a continuous simultaneous recording of the FHR and uterine contractions, known as continuous electronic fetal monitoring (EFM).

- EFM can be performed with external transducers; Doppler ultrasound scanning to assess the FHR and a tocodynamometer, a strain gauge attached to a belt, to assess uterine contractions.
- Alternatively, internal devices such as an electrode applied directly to the presenting fetal part and a calibrated intrauterine pressure catheter can be used.
- External tocography assesses frequency and duration of contractions.
- An intrauterine pressure catheter is required to assess the intensity of contraction.

Fetal monitoring in labour

- In labour, uterine contractions restrict maternal blood supply to the placental bed, which is further compounded by the effects of pushing in the second stage.
- Each fetus has a different capacity to withstand the stress of labour.
- On admission in labour, an assessment is made to identify risk factors that may affect the fetal reserve.

Risk factors
- Maternal factors.
  - Medical problems: essential hypertension, IDDM (insulin-dependent diabetes mellitus).
  - Antenatal events: antepartum haemorrhage, pre-eclampsia.
  - Induced labour.
  - Prolonged pregnancy.
  - Past obstetric history: previous CS, previous stillbirth.
- Fetal factors.
  - Prematurity.
  - IUGR.
  - Oligohydramnios.
  - Abnormal UA Doppler studies.
  - Multiple pregnancy.
  - Breech presentation.
  - MSL.
- Intrapartum risk factors.
  - Augmentation with IV oxytocin.
  - Epidural anaesthesia.
  - Intrapartum bleeding.
  - Maternal pyrexia.
  - Development of fresh meconium in labour.
  - Abnormal FHR on intermittent auscultation.

Two options exist for fetal monitoring in labour:
- For low risk cases, intermittent FHR auscultation is acceptable.
- For high risk cases, continuous EFM is recommended.

External fetal monitoring

- EFM was introduced to try and reduce perinatal mortality and cerebral palsy (CP) rates.
- Only 10% of CP cases are thought to result from intrapartum events, the remainder being due to antenatal factors.
- EFM has failed to reduce CP rates but has led to an increase in instrumental-assisted vaginal delivery.
- EFM is very sensitive in detecting fetal hypoxia but lacks specificity.
- Fetal blood sampling has helped to improve overall specificity.

CTG interpretation in labour

Several CTG classification systems are in existence, e.g. NICE, FIGO (International Federation of Gynecology and Obstetrics). A systematic approach is required to ensure correct CTG interpretation.

- Any existing obstetric risk factors need to be considered and in particular the presence of meconium or fetal sepsis.
- Assessment of uterine contractions is required to allow their effect on the FHR to be established.
- A systematic assessment should be made hourly or more frequently if there are concerns.
- Do not make any decisions about a woman's care in labour on the basis of CTG findings alone.

Features of the FHR to be considered

Baseline rate

- The mean FHR when it is stable, over a 5–10min period with both accelerations and decelerations excluded.
- Normal baseline rates vary depending on which classification system is used.
- Normal baseline rate in labour is between 110 and 150bpm (Fig. 23.3).
- A change in baseline may indicate gradually developing hypoxia.

Baseline variability

- The degree to which the baseline varies, i.e. the width of the baseline, excluding accelerations and decelerations.
- Normal variability is between 5 and 25 beats (Fig. 23.3).
- Normal baseline variability is an indicator of adequate oxygenation of the autonomic system.
- Reduced variability <5bpm may represent a quiet sleep phase, may be secondary of medication or may be due to hypoxia to the CNS.
- Increased variability >25bpm is called salutatory and needs further consideration.

Presence or absence of accelerations

- Acceleration is a transient increase in the FHR of ≥15bpm lasting ≥15s.
- The presence of accelerations suggests the integrity of the somatic nervous system in a healthy fetus, that has sufficient reserve to supply non-essential somatic activity.
- Presence of accelerations is a marker of a healthy non-hypoxic fetus.

Presence and type of decelerations

- A deceleration is a transient decrease in the FHR of ≥15bpm lasting ≥15s.
- Decelerations have been traditionally described as early, variable and late; however beware that in labour, more than one pathophysiological process may arise simultaneously.

- **Early decelerations:**
  - These are due to compression of the fetal head causing stimulation of the vagus nerve producing a bradycardia.
  - Tend to appear in the late first and second stage of labour with descent of the head.
  - They are synchronous with contractions and tend to be uniform in shape (Fig. 23.4).
  - If isolated and other CTG parameters normal, they are usually benign.

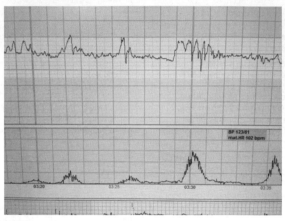

Fig. 23.3 A CTG trace showing a normal baseline and baseline variability with accelerations.

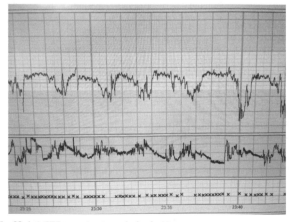

Fig. 23.4 A CTG trace showing early decelerations.

- **Late decelerations**:
  - These decelerations are late with respect to the uterine contractions and are associated with uteroplacental insufficiency.
  - The retroplacental space provides a variable-sized reservoir of oxygenated blood. In a fetus with IUGR, this reservoir will be small. At the start of a contraction, the fetus uses its reservoir of oxygen.
  - Due to restriction of uteroplacental blood supply during a contraction, a hypoxic deceleration begins and continues throughout the contraction.
  - Recovery occurs some time after the contraction when full oxygenation has been restored.
  - Late decelerations are associated with fetal hypoxaemia, hypercarbia, and developing acidosis.
  - Depending on the clinical scenario, interventions to increase the uteroplacental circulation should be considered, including changing maternal position, administering IV fluids, reducing oxytocin infusion or the use of tocolytics, e.g. terbutaline.
- Variable decelerations:
  - Most common type of FHR decelerations are a consequence of umbilical cord compression with contractions.
  - As the cord can be compressed in a different way with each contraction, their appearance can vary in shape, size, and timing.
  - In the cord, the umbilical vein is thinner and is compressed first before the arteries.
  - This results in loss of some of the fetal circulating volume, and autonomic responses result in an increased FHR to compensate, which is seen as an acceleration.
  - Further compression of the cord then occludes the thicker umbilical arteries with a relative restoration of the fetal circulation.
  - Stimulation of fetal baroreceptors leads to a precipitous fall in the FHR. The nadir of the deceleration occurs when both the umbilical vein and artery are compressed.

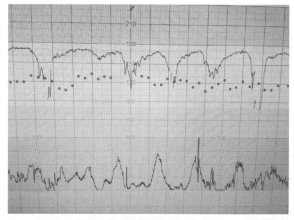

Fig. 23.5 A CTG trace showing late decelerations with reduced baseline variability.

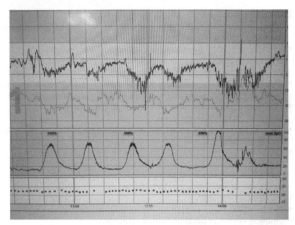

Fig. 23.6 A CTG trace showing typical variable decelerations.

- A normal well-grown fetus can tolerate cord compression for a considerable length of time before developing hypoxia. Small IUGR fetuses have less reserve.
- Variable decelerations can be sub-classified as typical and atypical.
- Typical variable decelerations characterized by a drop of <60bpm lasting for <60 seconds with the presence of shouldering and a slight increase in FHR before and after the contraction.
  - Suspicious features associated with atypical variable decelerations include reduced baseline variability, a rising baseline, late recovery, a combined variable, and a late deceleration component, and a duration of >60s with a loss of >60 beats from the baseline.
  - The presence of atypical variables makes progressive hypoxia more likely.

CTG classification

NICE classify the CTG as normal, suspicious or pathological.

- *Normal.* All four features are reassuring.
- *Suspicious.* No more than one non-reassuring feature and two reassuring features.
- *Pathological.* Two or more non-reassuring features or one or more abnormal features.
- Suspicious and pathological CTG traces are not always associated with acidosis.
- Special attention should be paid to fetuses susceptible to developing acidosis more quickly, including those with IUGR, preterm, post term, infected, where there is grade 3 meconium or minimal amniotic fluid draining.

Reassuring features on CTG

- Baseline FHR between 110 and 160bpm.
- Baseline variability between 5 and 25bpm.
- Decelerations—None or early or variable decelerations with no concerning characteristics for 90 minutes.

Non-reassuring or suspicious features on CTG
- Baseline FHR between 100 and 109bpm or 161 and 180bpm.
- Baseline variability <5 for 30–50min or >25 for 15–25min.
- Decelerations—variable with no concerning features for 90min or more, variable decelerations with any concerning characteristics in up to 50% of contractions for >30 minutes, or variable decelerations with any concerning features in over 50% of contractions for <30min or late decelerations in over 50% of contractions for <30min, with no maternal or fetal clinical risk factors or significant meconium.

Abnormal or pathological features on CTG
- Baseline FHR <100bpm or >180bpm.
- Baseline variability of <5bpm for >50min or >25bpm for more than 25min or sinusoidal pattern.
- Decelerations—variable decelerations with any concerning characteristics in over 50% contractions for 30min, late decelerations for 30min or less if any maternal or fetal clinical risk factors or significant meconium.
- Acute bradycardia or a single prolonged bradycardia lasting 3min or more.

Action with a normal CTG

Continue CTG monitoring

Action with a suspicious CTG

Correct any underlying cause:
- Uterine hyper-stimulation.
- Maternal hypotension from aorto-caval compression or epidural top-up.
- Maternal dehydration.
- Maternal pyrexia.
- Maternal need for analgesia.

Start one or more conservative measures—change position, administer IV fluids, reduce contraction frequency.

Action with a pathological CTG

- Exclude acute events—cord prolapse, placental abruption, uterine rupture.
- Correct any underlying cause—hypotension, uterine hyper-stimulation.
- Start conservative management—see above.
- Offer digital fetal scalp stimulations.
- If CTG continues to be pathological, consider fetal blood sampling or expedite birth.
- Take mother's preferences into account.

Need for urgent intervention

- Acute bradycardia or a single prolonged deceleration for 3min or more.
- Urgent obstetric review to exclude an acute event—expedite delivery if cord prolapse, placental abruption or uterine rupture.
- Correct any underlying causes such as hypotension or uterine hyperstimulation.
- Start 1 or more conservative measures.
- Make preparations for urgent delivery.
- Expedite birth if acute bradycardia persists for 9min.
- If FHR recovers at any point up to 9min, reassess any decision to expedite birth.

Fetal blood sample

Due to the high false-positive rate of CTG, peripheral tests of fetal well-being, including FBS, were developed to reduce intrapartum interventions. Any FBS result should be interpreted taking into account the clinical features of both the mother and baby, any previous FBS result and the progress of labour.

- An explanation should be given to the mother about the indication for the procedure and the planned action following the FBS.
- Verbal consent should be obtained.
- FBS is only technically possible once the cervix is dilated to 3cm or more.
- Occasionally, it may not be possible to obtain an adequate sample, therefore if the CTG abnormality persists, delivery is necessary.
- Midwifery and anaesthetic staff should be aware that the test is taking place in case urgent delivery is necessary.

Position
- Ideally, the mother should be in either the left or right lateral position.
- The lithotomy position should be avoided because of the risk of maternal hypotension from aorto-caval compression. This can produce an iatrogenic fetal hypoxia and acidosis, leading to an unnecessary operative delivery.

Procedure
- An aseptic technique is used and an amnioscope is passed through the vagina to reach the fetal scalp.
- The fetal scalp is dried using a dental swab and then sprayed with ethyl chloride to produce a hyperaemia, which aids bleeding.
- The fetal scalp is then smeared lightly with a water-repellent gel to help the blood form into a round drop.
- Under direct vision the fetal scalp is stabbed with a 2mm blade.
- The blood droplet is allowed to form and is then drawn up by capillary action into a pre-heparinized thin glass tube.
- A sufficiently sized sample is taken immediately to the blood gas analyser.

Analysis
- Measure the pH, the base deficit, the PO_2 and PCO_2.

FBS interpretation
As a general guide, Table 23.1 illustrates the subsequent action required following an FBS result according to published guidelines from the Royal College of Obstetricians and Gynaecologists and NICE.

Table 23.1 Fetal blood sample

Fetal blood sample result	Action
pH ≥7.25	Repeat FBS if the FHR abnormality persists
pH 7.21–7.24	Repeat FBS within 30min or consider delivery if rapid fall since last FBS sample
pH ≤7.20	Delivery indicated

Adapted from Fetal Blood Sampling: Clinical Guideline. Mid Essex Hospital Services NHS Trust.

CTG plus ST analysis of the fetal ECG (STAN)

- Although the use of intrapartum CTG has been shown to reduce the incidence of neonatal seizures, it has had little impact on long-term neonatal outcome. In addition, there is concern that its use has resulted in an increase in the CS rate.
- Whilst the use of FBS can help with CTG interpretation, there are situations where this may not be technically possible, e.g. in the early stages of labour.
- In an attempt to overcome some of these issues, newer methods of intrapartum fetal monitoring have been explored. These methods include CTG in conjunction with STAN (fetal ECG ST-analyser), the use of which is becoming more widespread.
- STAN monitoring assesses the oxygenation of the fetal heart.
- As part of the physiological response to *in utero* hypoxia, depression of the ST-segment of the fetal ECG has been observed and interpretation of such events with the CTG forms the basis of the STAN analysis.
- Application of a fetal scalp electrode (FSE) is necessary and therefore STAN can only be used in situations where this is technically possible, acceptable to the patient, and where no contraindications to the use of FSE exist (e.g. risk of bleeding disorder in the fetus, maternal HIV).
- The fetal ECG is monitored through the FSE. As soon as the FSE is applied, the machine calculates the normal T/QRS ratio for that particular fetus over the first 5min as a baseline. From this point, the machine analyses every 30 ECG complexes and compares them with the original baseline. If the analysed ECG differs significantly from the baseline, it will alert an ST event. It is critical that STAN monitoring is only commenced when the CTG is normal.
- In the presence of an ST event, it is necessary to classify the CTG trace using specific STAN criteria as normal, intermediate, or abnormal. This will determine whether the ST event is significant.
- There are three types of STAN events:
  - Episodic T/QRS rise—a response to a short lasting hypoxia <10min, significance depending on magnitude and classification of the CTG trace.
  - Baseline T/QRS rise—episode of hypoxia lasting >10min, significance depending on magnitude and classification of the CTG trace.
  - Biphasic events—a shift in the ST segment of which there are 3 degrees 1–3. Repetitive 2 and 3 biophysics are significant in the presence of an intermediate or abnormal trace.
- When interpreting any ST events/CTG changes, the whole clinical picture should be considered, including the presence of meconium, chorioamnionitis, IUGR, or vaginal bleeding. Immediate delivery may be indicated in the presence of any risk factors regardless of the significance of the ST event.
- In the presence of a normal CTG, any ST events can be managed expectantly.
- In the first stage of labour or passive second stage, a significant STAN event will require interventions to improve utero-placental oxygenation, e.g. IV fluids, change in maternal position, stop oxytocin infusion, or

acute tocolysis with 250 micrograms subcutaneous terbutaline. If the CTG changes improve and there are no further ST events, labour can be allowed to continue. If there are further significant ST events, the CTG should be reclassified and if no further conservative measure are possible, delivery within 20min is indicated.

• In the active second stage of labour, any significant ST events should be managed with immediate operative delivery by the safest and swiftest mode of delivery, unless an spontaneous vaginal delivery is expected within 5–10min. The anaesthetist must be kept fully informed of the situation to ensure the safest and most appropriate method of anaesthesia is employed.

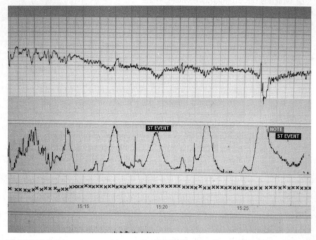

Fig. 23.7 A ST event on an intermediary CTG. The baseline rate has dropped very slightly and there are shallow decelerations. The CTG improved with simple measures of changing position and administering IV fluids.

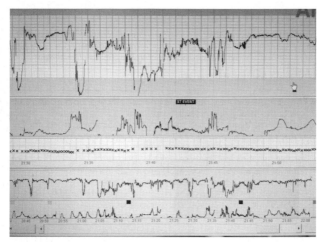

Fig. 23.8 A significant ST event on an abnormal CTG. IV oxytocin stopped and successful instrumental delivery performed within 15 mins.

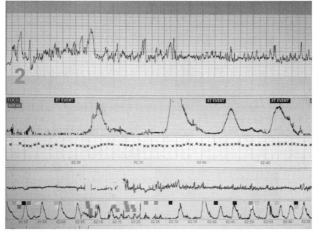

Fig. 23.9 A ST event on a normal CTG. No action was required.

Fetal acid–base

Normal functioning of the fetal enzyme systems depends on stability of the pH within the tissues. Derangements in pH may be primary due to respiratory or metabolic dysfunction, but the clinical picture is often mixed.

Normal gaseous exchange

- The placenta functions as the lung whilst the fetus is *in utero*.
- Free gaseous exchange depends upon normal flow of both maternal and fetal blood through the placental bed.
- High HbF concentration together with the higher affinity of HbF for O_2 ensures adequate amounts of O_2 are transferred to the fetus.
- Under normal conditions the fetus obtains the majority of energy by aerobic metabolism of glucose.
- Some of the waste product—CO_2—is carried in simple solution, but the vast majority is carried as dissociated hydrogen (H^+) and bicarbonate (HCO_3^-) ions. The H^+ ions are mainly buffered by Hb, and the HCO_3^- ions pass out into the extracellular fluid.
- At the placenta, the CO_2 in solution diffuses across to the maternal circulation. The CO_2 carried as H^+ and HCO_3^- ions is also released and transferred. Elimination of the CO_2 means the concentration of H^+ ions in the fetal blood is reduced.
- UA blood (from the fetus to the placenta) has a low pO_2, high CO_2, and a low pH (opposite of adult circulation).
- Umbilical venous blood (from the placenta to the fetus) has a high pO_2, low pCO_2, and a higher pH (opposite of adult circulation).

Disturbance of normal gaseous exchange

Various factors can disturb normal gaseous exchange at the placenta.

- *Maternal factors.* Hypotension from aorto-caval compression, regional analgesia, or anaesthesia. Uterine contractions may produce high pressure, reducing uterine blood flow. Chronic impairment of uteroplacental blood flow, e.g. pre-eclampsia.
- *Placental factors.* Placental abruption and abnormal placental circulation, e.g. pre-eclampsia.
- *Fetal factors.* Umbilical cord compression, fetal anaemia, and fetal arrhythmia.

Reduction of perfusion of the placenta from fetal vessels is manifest as variable decelerations, whilst a reduction in perfusion from the maternal circulation is manifest as late decelerations.

Consequences

Impaired gaseous exchange at the placenta has several consequences:

- *Respiratory acidosis.* During the early stages of reduced placental perfusion, CO_2 transfer across the placenta is reduced, leading to a high pCO_2 and a low pH. This may be transitory. If corrective measures are taken and the FHR improves, it may be treated conservatively. A degree of respiratory acidosis occurs in most uncomplicated labours.

- Further reduction in placental perfusion affects O_2 transfer, resulting in a low pO_2. Fetal adaptation occurs. Increased O_2 extraction with centralization of blood flow to brain and myocardium at the expense of other organs occurs. Physiological reserve of the fetus will determine how long this can be sustained, but will be reduced in high risk situations.

- *Metabolic acidosis.* If aerobic metabolism cannot be maintained because of reduced O_2 supply, anaerobic metabolism may supplement energy supplies, resulting in lactic acid formation. Lactic acid forms lactate and H^+ ions, some of which will be buffered by Hb and HCO_3^- ions. H^+ ions are not easily eliminated at the placenta and buffers have an finite capacity, and eventually the pH and bicarbonate levels will fall, producing a metabolic acidosis with a low pO_2, low pH, and low HCO_3^-. Metabolic acidosis is damaging to fetal tissues.

Base deficit

- Base deficit enables the physician to differentiate between a respiratory and a metabolic acidosis.
- Respiratory acidosis does not use up buffering capacity, whereas metabolic acidosis does.
- Base deficit measures how much available buffer has been used up, and is actually the amount of base (alkali) needed to add to the blood in order to restore the pH to normal.
- Base deficit is defined as the mmol/L of base required to titrate the blood back to a normal pH.
- A base deficit is negative and is calculated from the pH and the pCO_2.

Cord gas analysis

- Following delivery, cord gas analysis is useful in assessing the condition of the newborn and deciding subsequent neonatal management.
- The UA cord blood result better reflects the condition of the fetus.
- Sampling the smaller UA can be technically difficult compared with the vein. It is good practice to sample the UA and umbilical vein and compare results to ensure that the UA has indeed been analysed.
- Table 23.2 shows the mean blood gas results from both the UA and umbilical vein, with a mean difference in pH between the UA and UV of ~0.08 units.

Table 23.2 Mean blood gas results from umbilical artery and vein at delivery

Measurement	Umbilical artery	Umbilical vein
pH	7.26	7.35
pCO_2	7.3kPa	5.3kPa
Base deficit	2.3mmol/L	2.9mmol/L

Effect of analgesia and anaesthesia on the fetus

- The pain of labour causes hyperventilation, leading to respiratory alkalosis with resulting vasoconstriction and reduced placental blood flow and oxygen availability to the fetus.
- Many women request pharmacological methods of pain relief in labour, which may confer advantages to the fetus, but may also pose certain risks.
- Most systemic drugs given to the mother are transferred to the fetus. However, the amount transferred will depend on both maternal and fetal factors, as well as the characteristics of the drugs themselves.
- Blood levels of any transmitted drug are disproportionately higher in the fetal brain compared with other tissues.
- This is partly due to the high cerebral blood flow and relatively poor development of the blood–brain barrier in the fetus.
- Chronic fetal hypoxia further increases the levels in the fetal brain as a consequence of the redistribution of blood in favour of the cranial circulation.

Nitrous oxide

Nitrous oxide, in a 50:50 mixture with oxygen known as Entonox®, is the most widely available inhalational analgesic for labour.
- Entonox® rapidly crosses the placenta but is cleared quickly, resulting in minimal effect on the fetus or neonate.
- Neurobehavioural scores on babies exposed to *in utero* Entonox® have shown little effect at 2 and 24h.
- Maternal hyperventilation, to achieve adequate analgesia, can lead to respiratory alkalosis in the mother, displacing the oxygen dissociation curve to the left, resulting in reduced oxygen availability to the fetus.
- Prolonged use may cause vasoconstriction within the placental bed and reduce uteroplacental blood flow, reducing fetal oxygenation.
- Entonox® may reduce maternal respiratory drive, leading to periods of hypoventilation between contractions, with resulting hypoxia.

Systemic opioids

The opioids pethidine, diamorphine, and to a lesser extent morphine, are widely used to provide analgesia in labour.

Pethidine

- Rapidly crosses the placenta by passive diffusion, causing intrauterine sedation in the fetus.
- The effects are dependent on dose and timing, with maximal effects seen 2–3h after IM administration and with repeated doses. Fetal exposure can result in respiratory depression at birth, leading to lower Apgar scores, reduced oxygen saturations, and increased CO_2 tensions.
- If given within 1h of delivery, neonatal effects are minimal.
- Fetal sedation can result in CTG alterations.
- Reduction in baseline variability and accelerations are seen 25min after IV and 40min after IM administration.

- Reduced variability can last longer than the 40min normally associated with the quiet or sleep phase.
- CTG interpretation can be more difficult after administration, so it is important that the preceding CTG is normal and reactive.
- A reduction in fetal movements, altered fetal EEG activity, and reduced fetal scalp oxygen tensions have been observed, but these effects are of unknown clinical significance.
- Pethidine is a weak base, resulting in increased ionization and accumulation in the relatively more acidic fetal circulation.
- With fetal acidosis, this effect is further increased, making the pethidine less able to cross back into the maternal circulation (ion trapping).
- Norpethidine, the active metabolite of pethidine, compounds the neonatal effects and has proconvulsant properties.
- Neurobehavioural patterns are altered, with babies exposed to intrauterine pethidine tending to be sleepier, less attentive, and slower to establish breastfeeding.
- Administration of naloxone to the neonate can reverse the effects of opiates although it is increasingly controversial. The painful stimulus of an IM injection is thought to be largely responsible for 'waking the baby up'. The opioid effect outlasts the short-acting effect of naloxone.

Morphine and diamorphine
- The fetal side effects of morphine and diamorphine are very similar to those of pethidine.
- Equianalgesic doses of pethidine cause less neonatal respiratory depression than either morphine or diamorphine.
- The metabolite, morphine 3 glucuronide, does not have the side effects of norpethidine.

Regional analgesia and anaesthesia
- Maternal hypotension can occur as a result of either sympathetic blockade or aorto-caval compression, which can be detrimental to the fetus.
- If left untreated, this will cause fetal hypoxia with a fall in fetal pH.
- Continuous fetal monitoring is therefore mandatory following regional techniques.
- However, provided maternal hypotension is avoided and uteroplacental perfusion maintained, regional techniques are well tolerated by the fetus.
- Regional techniques do not influence the resistance in uterine vessels, intervillous blood flow or flow velocity in the UA.
- Relief of pain achieved with regional techniques, by reducing circulating maternal levels of catecholamines, increases placental blood flow.
- Maternal body temperature increases after epidural analgesia. The mechanism is unclear, but marked hyperthermia may result in a fetal tachycardia not associated with significant fetal hypoxia and fetal pH is not affected. This can give rise to an erroneous diagnosis of fetal distress or to a false diagnosis of intrauterine infection, increasing the number of newborns investigated and treated with antibiotics.
- Placental transfer of opioids occurs rapidly after epidural administration and should be considered when delivery is imminent.
- Epidural or intrathecal fentanyl doses >100 micrograms may cause neonatal respiratory depression and have an effect on establishing breastfeeding.

General anaesthesia
- If a GA is required for delivery, the ideal induction to delivery time is between 5 and 15min.
- Prolonged induction to delivery times increase the risk of fetal acidosis but can be minimized if both aorto-caval compression and hypotension are avoided.
- Lipid-soluble anaesthetic agents rapidly cross the placenta and a prolonged induction to delivery time allows progressive uptake by the fetus, resulting in neonatal sedation with low Apgar scores.

IV induction agents
- *Thiopental*: this remains the most commonly used induction agent and at 4mg/kg the baby is protected from excessive sedation because of the fetal circulation through the liver. At 8mg/kg neonatal depression will occur.
- *Propofol*: doses >2.5mg/kg can cause neonatal depression. Although associated with rapid wakening in the adult, this advantage has not been observed in the neonate.
- *Ketamine*: at doses of 1mg/kg, the neonatal condition is comparable with thiopental. At 2mg/kg, neonatal depression and low Apgar scores will result.
- *Benzodiazepines*: compared with thiopental induction doses, benzodiazepines double the time to sustained neonatal respiration. They can cause neonatal respiratory depression, lethargy, poor feeding, hypothermia, hypotonia, and jaundice; should be avoided.

Neuromuscular-blocking agents
- These agents are ionized compounds at normal physiological pH. Under normal circumstances, placental transfer is minimal with no effect on the fetus or neonate.
- There are case reports of suxamethonium apnoea in an affected neonate after suxamethonium was administered to an affected mother.

Inhalation anaesthesia
- *Nitrous oxide*: it freely crosses the placenta and if >50% is used, may cause neonatal depression with low Apgar scores. High concentrations of nitrous oxide can cause diffusion hypoxia and fetal acidosis. A 50:50 mixture with oxygen should be administered prior to delivery of the baby.
- *Volatile anaesthetic agents*: isoflurane, desflurane, and sevoflurane are widely used for CS.
  - These lipid-soluble drugs cross the placenta causing a dose- and time-dependent neonatal depression.
  - Using a 1 MAC equivalent with nitrous oxide and an induction–delivery interval of <11min, excessive neonatal depression is avoided.
  - Sevoflurane and desflurane are safe but have no benefits over isoflurane.
  - Sevoflurane metabolism is associated with fluoride ion production, causing an increase in neonatal serum fluoride 24h after delivery, the consequences of which are unknown.

Other medication

Magnesium sulphate

- Magnesium sulphate is the drug of choice for preventing and treating seizures in severe pre-eclampsia and eclampsia. Loading doses of 4g IV over 5min, followed by an infusion of 1g/hr for 24 hours after the last seizure. Recurrent seizures should be treated with a further dose of 2–4g given over 5min.
- Magnesium sulphate is also advised for mothers presenting in preterm labour before 30–32 weeks gestation, as a neuro-protective for those infants born pre-term. Loading and maintenance dosing regimes are as above. Can be given even if delivery is imminent but ideally within 4 hours of birth and for a maximum of 24 hours. If delivery is urgently mandated, do not delay delivery in order to administer magnesium sulphate. Stop treatment once the baby is delivered.
- It is widely regarded as a safe drug, however the mother should be monitored closely for signs of toxicity. See Chapter 21 p. 558 for further details.

Terbutaline

- The use of terbutaline is indicated to treat uterine hyperstimulation in the presence of CTG changes suggestive of acute or subacute fetal hypoxia.
- If removal of prostaglandin induction agents or cessation of an exogenous oxytocin infusion fail to reverse the hyperstimulation, acute tocolysis with 250 micrograms terbutaline administered subcutaneously may quickly restore utero-placental perfusion and reverse hypoxia.
- Signs of improvement in the CTG may be anticpated in 2–5min. A second dose may be appropriate in certain situations; however, the obstetric and anaesthetic team should be on standby to perform an emergency delivery unless the CTG normalizes.
- Terbutaline may cause maternal tachycardia and hypotension, and it may increase the risk of postpartum haemorrhage.

Further reading

NICE Guidelines Intrapartum Care 2017, www.nice.org.uk

Neonatal resuscitation

Angela Hayward

Overview

More than 90% of newborn infants will successfully make the transition from fetal to extra-uterine life. The remaining infants will require some assistance and fewer than 1% will need more extensive resuscitation efforts. Although the need for resuscitation can be predicted, there are occasions when a newborn is delivered in unexpectedly poor condition. It is vital that personnel who are present at delivery are able to provide prompt and effective basic newborn resuscitation, whilst additional help is summoned. Where the need for resuscitation has been predicted, the appropriately skilled teams should be in attendance at the delivery. Resuscitating a baby at birth is different from resuscitation of all other age groups, due to the unique physiological adaptations that occur around the time of birth.

Respiratory adaptation at birth

- During fetal life the lungs actively secrete lung liquid into the spaces that will contain air once air breathing commences after delivery.
- Lung liquid differs from amniotic fluid and plasma in that it has a high chloride and a low bicarbonate and protein concentration, which is essential to the growth and development of the normal lung structure before birth.
- If there is chronic drainage of the fluid, lung hypoplasia results, and if there is obstruction to the drainage of the fluid, lung hyperplasia results.
- To allow postnatal air breathing, the secretion of lung liquid has to be discontinued and the fluid must be absorbed.
- During labour, the fetus is stimulated to produce adrenaline, which results in active reabsorption of the lung fluid. Active contractions during labour also cause liquid to be expelled from the lungs.
- When delivery occurs prior to the onset of labour, e.g. pre-labour caesarean section, these processes are impaired resulting in increased respiratory morbidity.

Circulatory adaptation at birth

- The placenta is responsible for fetal gas exchange with just 10% of the right ventricular output entering the pulmonary circulation. This is due to the high pulmonary vascular resistance (PVR), the patent ductus arteriosus (PDA), and placental circulation.
- At birth, once the low resistance placental circulation is removed by clamping the umbilical cord, marked changes in the cardiovascular system occur to allow for gas exchange.
- The right atrial pressure decreases due to the loss of the placental bed circulation and the left atrial pressure increases due to the increased pulmonary venous return. This results in the foramen ovale closing and the ductus venosus closing because there is no longer any umbilical venous blood flow.
- The ductus arteriosus closes when the pressure in the aorta rises above that of the pulmonary artery and there is smooth muscle contraction in response to increased oxygen tension. The closure of the ductus arteriosus effectively separates the pulmonary and systemic circulations.

- The fall in PVR is mediated by ventilation of the lungs, increased oxygenation, and shear stresses. Prostaglandins, endothelial derived products, and nitric oxide all have a role in the regulation of PVR.
- Ventilation of the lungs and stretch forces result in the release of prostacyclins from the vessel walls causing an increase in pulmonary blood flow and hence a fall in PVR.
- Oxygen is a potent vasodilator. Nitric oxide is produced by vascular endothelial cells, it diffuses into smooth muscle cells where it increases guanosine monophosphate (GMP) production resulting in smooth muscle relaxation and a fall in PVR.
- During the early neonatal period, the pulmonary circulation remains fairly unstable, and in some disease conditions the PVR remains high resulting in persistent pulmonary hypertension.

Asphyxia during labour and delivery

- In everyday clinical practice, it is rare for a fetus to experience an event that causes acute asphyxia. More often, there is a more chronic process.
- During labour, uterine contractions will cause a transient hypoxaemia that the healthy fetus usually tolerates well.

Causes of asphyxia during labour and delivery
- Placental abruption: failure of gas exchange across the placenta.
- Cord compression/prolapse: interruption of umbilical blood flow.
- Severe maternal hypotension: inadequate perfusion of the placenta.
- Compromised fetus unable to tolerate labour, e.g. growth restricted fetus.
- Failure of lung inflation at birth: failure of the postnatal respiratory and circulatory adaptations.

Factors that may increase the risk of asphyxia

Maternal factors
- Pregnancy induced hypertension, anaemia, diabetes mellitus, prolonged rupture of membranes, haemorrhage, sepsis, and illicit drug or alcohol usage.

Labour and delivery factors
- Abnormal presentation, shoulder dystocia, instrumental delivery, uterine rupture, cord prolapse, opioid analgesia, general anaesthesia.

Fetal factors
- Preterm delivery, post term delivery, multiple delivery, meconium stained liquor, oligo/polyhydramnios, intrauterine growth restriction, macrosomia, congenital anomaly, hydrops fetalis, fetal anaemia.

Preparation and assessment

When there is a potential need for neonatal resuscitation, the neonatal team should be called in good time to allow for preparation. Not all resuscitations can be predicted, so it is vital that personnel trained in newborn resuscitation are available while additional help is summoned. The necessary equipment to institute resuscitation should have been pre-checked and in working order to avoid any delays.

Resuscitation equipment

The exact equipment and adjuncts to resuscitation will vary from institution to institution but would usually include as a minimum:

- Resuscitaire with radiant heater and a clock.
- Warm towels.
- Gas supply of air and oxygen and oxygen blender.
- Face mask appropriate to size of baby, bag-valve-mask apparatus.
- Pressure limited gas supply apparatus.
- Suction equipment and catheters.
- Airway adjuncts, intubation equipment, stethoscope.
- Portable saturation monitor.
- Resuscitation drugs, selection of needles and syringes.
- Equipment for umbilical vessel catheterization.

Environment and temperature control

- The delivery room and obstetric theatre should be kept warm and draught free to prevent the newborn being exposed to cold stress.
- Cold stress is known to lower arterial oxygen tension, increase metabolic acidosis, and inhibit surfactant production.
- All term babies should be dried and wrapped in a warm towel following delivery. Alternatively, they can be dried and placed skin to skin with their mother and covered in a dry towel.
- Preterm infants are at greater risk of cold stress and it is advised that their delivery room temperature is maintained at 26°C. Drying and wrapping alone may not be sufficient to maintain body temperature.

Assessment of the newborn and initial actions

- The initial assessment of the newborn consists of assessing colour, respiratory effort, heart rate, and tone.
- Whilst assessing the baby, ensure the clock has been started and that the baby is dried and wrapped in a warm towel.

At the first assessment, newborns will fit into the following groups

- Blue and becoming pink, with a healthy cry, heart rate >100, and good tone.
- Blue, good respiratory effort, heart rate >100, and good tone.
- Blue, minimal respiratory effort or gasping, heart rate 60–100, and poor/moderate tone.
- Pale, no respiratory effort, heart rate <60, and poor tone.
- Pale, no respiratory effort, heart rate undetectable, and poor tone.

- If the baby is pink with a healthy cry, it should remain in the care of its mother; all other babies will need additional assessment and intervention, usually on the resuscitaire.
- Resuscitation at birth follows a standard algorithm, see Fig. 24.1.

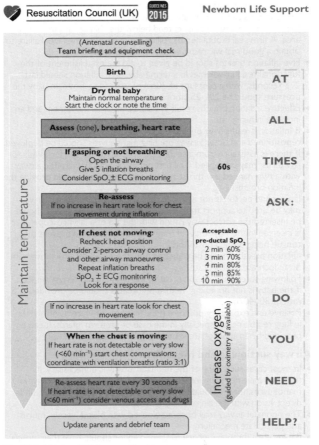

Fig. 24.1 Newborn Life Support Algorithm.

Reproduced with the kind permission of the Resuscitation Council (UK) Guidelines 2015: Newborn Life Support. Resuscitation Council (UK).

Airway and breathing support

Neutral head position and positive pressure ventilation

- Airway obstruction occurs if the neck is either flexed or hyperextended, the baby should be on a flat surface with the head in a neutral position. Applying a jaw thrust will assist with airway opening.
- The correct size face mask should be selected—the mask should cover the mouth and nose but not extend below the chin or into the orbital area. A firm seal is obtained by rolling the mask onto the face. Failure to obtain a good seal will result in failure to inflate the lungs.
- Five inflation breaths should be given to aid the establishment of the functional residual volume. In a term baby, each inflation should last 2–3 seconds, with a pressure of 30cm of water. In a preterm baby the pressure should be 20—25 cmof water.
- Effective inflation breaths result in visible chest wall movement and an increase in heart rate.
- If inflation breaths have been unsuccessful, the airway should be repositioned and other airway opening manoeuvres should be deployed.
- If there is assistance from a second person, a two-person technique for jaw thrust may be applied. The first person should stabilize the airway with a two-handed jaw thrust and the second person should provide the inflation breaths.
- If a second person is not available to assist, an oropharyngeal airway may be used to support the airway. The oropharyngeal airway should be inserted the correct way round with the aid of a laryngoscope. It is inserted in this way to avoid trauma to the palate and prevent the tongue being pushed posteriorly.
- Inflation breaths should be repeated until there is chest wall movement or an increase in heart rate.
- Following successful inflation breaths, the baby should be reassessed, if the baby is not breathing, ventilation breaths should be provided at a rate of 30–40/min.
- Positive end expiratory pressure (PEEP) at 5cm of water is of benefit in lung recruitment, especially in the case of preterm infants. It can be provided by an appropriate ventilation circuit.

Airway suctioning and meconium

- In most cases suctioning of the neonatal airway is unnecessary. If the lungs have not been inflated by inflation breaths or other airway manoeuvres, then it would be appropriate to inspect the airway, under direct vision with the aid of a laryngoscope.
- The neonatal airway may become blocked with blood, vernix, mucus, and particulate meconium.
- Babies born through meconium stained liquor should have their airway inspected and suctioned only if they are unconscious. It has been shown that there are no benefits in suctioning the airway of a vigorous baby.

Intubation

- In most newborn resuscitations, the airway can be managed without the need for intubation. Intubation may be helpful if there is a prolonged resuscitation, failed face-mask ventilation, or in special circumstances, e.g. congenital anomalies and administration of surfactant for preterm infants.
- Uncuffed straight endotracheal tubes with a diameter of 3.5–4mm for term infants and diameters of 2.5–3.0mm for preterm infants will be suitable. It is important to ensure a snug fit of the endotracheal tube at the laryngeal inlet. If there is a large leak, it may not be possible to achieve lung inflation. If there is a very tight fit, the tracheal wall and vocal cords may become damaged.
- Confirm the endotracheal tube position in the trachea by auscultation. End tidal carbon dioxide devices may also assist in confirmation of position in the delivery room.
- Secure the endotracheal tube at the correct length and obtain a chest X ray to confirm placement later. See Table 24.1 for endotracheal tube sizing.
- Laryngeal masks have been used successfully in infants greater than 2000g, when face mask ventilation has failed. They are not suitable for the smaller preterm infants.

Air verses oxygen at resuscitation

- Traditionally 100% oxygen has always been used in newborn resuscitations; however, more recently this has changed to 21% oxygen.
- Exposing hypoxic tissues to 100% oxygen may result in cellular damage by oxygen free radicals. It may also have adverse effects on breathing physiology and cerebral circulation.
- In term newborn infants, resuscitation in air has been shown to be as effective as resuscitation in oxygen.
- A healthy term newborn infant has preductal oxygen saturations of 60%; these will increase to 90% within the first 10min of life.
- If a newborn is receiving resuscitation, apply an oxygen saturation probe to the right wrist to record preductal pulse oximetry. The delivered oxygen can then be titrated to acceptable target oxygen saturations.

Table 24.1 Endotracheal tube (ETT) lengths by gestation and weight

ETT length at lips (cm)	Gestation (weeks)	Weight (kg)
5.5	23–24	0.5–0.6
6.0	25–26	0.7–0.8
6.5	27–29	0.9–1.0
7.0	30–32	1.1–1.4
7.5	33–34	1.5–1.8
8.0	35–37	1.9–2.4
8.5	38–40	2.5–3.1
9.0	41–43	3.2–4.2

Circulation support

It is vital to ensure that the lungs have been successfully inflated before moving on to support the circulation. In the event of circulatory failure, the best way to judge successful inflation of the chest is to see chest wall movement.

Chest compressions

- Chest compressions are delivered most effectively by encircling the chest with both hands, supporting the back with your fingers and compressing the sternum with your thumbs.
- The chest should be compressed one-third of the anterior posterior diameter just below the nipple line.
- Compressions should be at the rate of three compressions to one ventilation breath, aiming for 90 compressions and 30 breaths in 60 seconds.
- The baby should be reassessed every 30 seconds.

Drugs of resuscitation

- It is very rare for a newborn to require drugs of resuscitation.
- If a baby has failed to respond to effective ventilation and chest compressions, ideally drugs should be delivered via the umbilical vein.
- The umbilical cord should be cut down, the vein identified and an umbilical catheter inserted approximately 5cm until blood can be aspirated.
- Adrenaline is given for its β1 effects on the heart and peripheral α1 effects resulting in an increased blood flow to the heart and brain. The initial dose of adrenaline is 10 mg/kg intravenously; a larger dose of 30 milligram /kg may be given if the initial dose was not effective.
- Sodium bicarbonate is a controversial drug of resuscitation and should only be used when ventilation is effective, thus enabling the CO_2 produced during the buffering process to be eliminated. The dose of 4.2% sodium bicarbonate is 1–2 mmol/kg intravenously.
- Volume should be given in situations where there has been known or presumed blood loss to improve intravascular volume. In these situations the most appropriate volume is emergency blood. If there is a delay in obtaining emergency blood, isotonic crystalloid at 10mL/kg intravenously should be administered.
- Following insertion of the umbilical catheter, it is helpful to obtain a blood sugar. If the baby is hypoglycaemic, 2.5ml/kg of 10% glucose should be administered intravenously.
- The baby should be reassessed every 30 seconds.
- If there was no heart rate at birth and there has been no response to resuscitation efforts after 10min, the baby is unlikely to survive and long term adverse neurological outcomes are highly likely. Senior advice should be obtained to aid decision making.

Further reading

Wyllie J et al. European Resuscitation Council Guidelines for Resuscitation 2015: Section 7. Resuscitation and support of transition of babies at birth. *Resuscitation* 2015; 95: 242–262.

Wyllie J et al. Resuscitation and support of transition at birth for babies. March 2015 https://www.resus.org.uk/resuscitation-guidelines/resuscitation-and-support-of-transition-of-babies-at-birth

A–Z of conditions in obstetric anaesthesia

David Leslie and Rachel Collis

Abdominal pregnancy

Characteristics

- Implantation of pregnancy outside the uterine cavity.
- Incidence of 10.9 per 100,000 births.
- Maternal mortality is up to 30%.
- Poor fetal outcome: 40–95% fetal mortality.
- Diagnosis can be difficult but MRI is useful and will help to identify other organ involvement.
- Associated with massive haemorrhage due to placental attachment to intra-abdominal organs.

Key points

Delivery

- Best managed in a tertiary unit, with advanced MDT planning and interventional radiology input.
- Placenta may not be completely excised and therefore at risk of sepsis after CS.
- GA ± invasive monitoring advised due to high risk of massive blood loss.
- Critical care facility for postoperative management.

Further reading

Huang K, Song L et al. Advanced abdominal pregnancy: an increasingly challenging clinical concern for obstetricians *International Journal of Clinical and Experimental Pathology* 2014; 7: 5461–5472.

Achondroplasia

Characteristics

- Spinal and craniofacial abnormalities include:
  - Large head, short limbs, saddle nose with normally proportioned trunk.
  - Kyphoscoliosis and lumbar lordosis.
  - Decreased neck movements.
  - Stenosis of foramen magnum and spinal canal.
  - Large tongue and mandible.
  - Atlantoaxial instability.
- May have restrictive lung disease with markedly decreased FRC.

Key points

Delivery

- Usually requires CS because of cephalo-pelvic disproportion.
- Associated with difficult intubation, therefore regional may be preferable.
- Difficult regional because of spinal deformities.
- Spinal canal stenosis can impair CSF flow, and dural puncture may be more difficult to recognize.

- CSE useful to control the block; however, increased risk of dural puncture with epidural needle.
- May have unpredictable spread of LA in epidural space.
- No neurological complications of regional techniques are documented.
- If GA needed:
  - Ensure facilities for awake fibreoptic intubation are available.
  - May require smaller endotracheal tube.
  - IV access may be difficult.
  - Avoid hyperextension of the neck.
- Aorto-caval compression may be severe.
- Invasive arterial monitoring and blood gases may be required in patients with cardiorespiratory compromise.

Further reading

Palomero MA et al. Spinal anaesthesia for emergency Caesarean section in an achondroplastic patient. *European Journal of Anaesthesiology* 2007; 24: 981–2.

Morrow MJ et al. Epidural anaesthesia for Caesarean section in an achondroplastic dwarf. *British Journal of Anaesthesia* 1998; 81: 619–621.

Acupuncture

Characteristics

- A technique of inserting and manipulating needles into acupuncture points on the body to restore health and well-being; has been used to treat pain.

Key points

Antenatal

- Has been used safely for the treatment of symphysis pubis dysfunction and lower back pain in pregnancy.

Delivery

- Acupuncture in labour can decrease pain and reduce the use of epidural analgesia.
- Some evidence for its use as an adjunct to conventional pain control.

Further reading

Dong C et al. Effects of electro-acupuncture on labor pain management. *Archives of Gynecology and Obstetrics* 2015; 291: 531–536.

Elden H et al. Effects of acupuncture and stabilising exercises as adjunct to standard treatment in pregnant women with pelvic girdle pain: randomised single blind controlled trial. *BMJ* 2005; 331: 249–250.

Addison's disease/crisis

Characteristics

- Adrenal insufficiency—either primary or secondary.
- Symptoms: weight loss, weakness, nausea, fatigue, abdominal pain, diarrhoea, postural hypotension.
- Can be life-threatening in pregnancy.
- Associated with fetal death *in utero* and postpartum adrenal crisis.
- Crisis more likely in labour, illness, and during delivery.
- Difficult to diagnose in pregnancy due to altered cortisol levels (1.5–3 times normal values).

Key points

Antenatal

- Continue with normal steroid replacement therapy in pregnancy.
- If nausea and vomiting, administer IV fluids and IV hydrocortisone.
- Monitor electrolytes in pregnancy.
- Stop mineralocortocoids if pre-eclampsia develops.
- Seek endocrine advice.

Delivery

- Consider extra dose of steroids during second stage.
- If CS—give 100mg hydrocortisone 6hly and IV saline for 24h. Decrease IV steroids over 3 days.
- Signs of crisis are hypotension, hypoglycaemia, and raised potassium.
- Treat crisis with IV fluids and IV steroids, and correct hypoglycaemia and reduce potassium levels with IV glucose and insulin infusion.

Further reading

Schneiderman M et al. Maternal and neonatal outcomes of pregnancy in women with Addison's disease: a population-based cohort study on 7.7 million births. *British Journal of Obstetrics and Gynaecology* 2017; 124: 1772–1779.

Amphetamine abuse

Characteristics

- Amphetamines (speed) are sympathomimetic amines acting as indirect CNS stimulants.
- Effects last for 3–6h.
- May be ingested orally, smoked, or injected IV.
- Symptoms of acute intoxication include: psychosis, paranoia, delirium, mania, decreased need for sleep, dilated pupils, raised HR and BP, nausea and vomiting, hyper-reflexia, respiratory depression, cardiac arrhythmias, seizures, coma, hyperpyrexia, proteinuria, and confusion.
- Chronic abuse causes dopamine depletion, memory impairment, and insomnia.
- High doses cause cardiovascular system collapse, myocardial infarction, cerebrovascular accident, seizures, renal failure, ischaemic colitis, and hepatotoxicity.
- There is an increased incidence of suicides and accidents.

Key points

- Universal precautions if thought to be an IV drug user.
- Difficult venous access if IV drug user.
- Send urine for toxicology.
- Associated with fetal anomalies, IUGR, fetal distress, and placental abruption.
- Regional block may cause severe hypotension.
- Response to vasopressors can be unpredictable. Direct-acting vasopressor may be more reliable.
- Need to rehydrate mother.
- If requires GA—acute ingestion increases MAC of volatile agents and chronic ingestion decreases it.

Further reading

Ladhani NN, Shah PS, Murphy KE; Knowledge Synthesis Group on Determinants of Preterm/LBW Births. Prenatal amphetamine exposure and birth outcomes: a systematic review and metanalysis. *American Journal of Obstetrics and Gynaecology* 2011; 20: 219.e1–e7.

Amyotrophic lateral sclerosis

Characteristics

- Progressive neurological disease of upper and lower motor neurones causing irreversible muscle weakness and spasticity.
- Often fatal within 3–5yrs and rare in the obstetric population.
- Maternal disease does not regress and may worsen due to increased respiratory and weight-bearing demands.
- Causes weakness, fasciculations, autonomic instability, and cardiac denervation.
- Uterine muscles are not involved in degeneration process and labour may be facilitated by pelvic floor weakness.

Key points

- Respiratory function should be regularly monitored in pregnancy and labour.
- Requires monitoring of oxygen saturation and blood gases in labour.
- Poor bulbar reflexes may increase risk of aspiration.
- Regional anaesthesia is possible. Spinal and GA have been used successfully for CS. CSE useful to control and avoid excessive height of block.
- Use suxamethonium with care and avoid if possible. Increased sensitivity to non-depolarizing muscle relaxants.
- Requires critical care facility for postoperative care.

Further reading

Xiao W et al. Total intravenous anaesthesia without muscle relaxant in a parturient with amyotrophic lateral sclerosis undergoing cesarean section: a case report. *Journal of Clinical Anesthesia* 2017; 36: 107–109

Lupo VR et al. Amyotrophic lateral sclerosis in pregnancy. *Obstetrics and Gynecology* 1993; 82: 682–685.

Ankylosing spondylitis

Characteristics

- Chronic inflammatory arthropathy with systemic involvement.
- Onset 15–25yrs olds. Males > females.
- Causes fibrosis, ossification, and ankylosis of joints, predominantly sacroiliac joints and the spine.
- 50% of patients have other joints involved.
- May be associated with psoriasis and inflammatory bowel disease.
- Can have restrictive lung defects and lung fibrosis.
- Decreased neck movements.
- Temporomandibular joint involvement.
- Can rarely affect cricoarytenoid joints.
- Can develop cardiovascular system disease—aortic and mitral regurgitation and conduction defects can occur.
- Severe ossification of the ligamentum flavum is very uncommon.

Key points

- Assess in pregnancy for lower spine mobility and difficult airway.
- Early respiratory function tests if there is evidence of respiratory involvement.
- May require oxygen saturation and blood gas monitoring in labour if lung disease present.
- ECG ± echocardiography is required during antenatal assessment.
- Regional anaesthesia is possible but may be difficult. The paramedian approach may be beneficial.
- May be difficult to remove epidural after labour—place in same position as insertion.
- If GA required, possible difficult intubation which may require awake fibreoptic intubation.
- Care with cervical spine positioning at all times.

Further reading

Giovannopoulou E et al. Ankylosing spondylitis and pregnancy: A literature review. *Currrent Rheumatology Reviews* 2017; 13: 162–169.

Antiphospholipid syndrome

Characteristics

- Syndrome of hypercoagulability, associated with autoimmune specific antibodies against phospholipids.
- Increased risk of thrombosis in pregnancy.
- Increased incidence of second trimester miscarriage.
- Can be primary or secondary to other systemic diseases, e.g. systemic sclerosis, SLE.
- Associated with venous and arterial thromboemboli.
- Causes prolonged APTT (not associated with bleeding risk) caused by lupus anticoagulant antibody interfering with assay.
- Adrenal insufficiency, pulmonary hypertension, and systemic hypertension are described. Antenatal investigations should be performed.
- May also be associated with Budd–Chiari syndrome.
- Increased risk of DVT postpartum—6-weeks prophylactic LMWH required.
- Predisposition to pre-eclampsia and placental abruption.

Key points

- A clear anticoagulation plan should be made in the antenatal period with haematology input.
- Usually on LMWH and aspirin, which is continued for 6 weeks postpartum. Regional anaesthesia is possible, but needs to be timed carefully with anticoagulation therapy. Continue with aspirin, as it is not a contraindication to regional anaesthesia.
- Regional anaesthesia can be performed if normal PT, no significant decrease in platelets, an isolated raised APTT (as increase is secondary to lupus anticoagulant) and an appropriate dosing interval post LMWH.
- May have occasional true clotting factor defects, which would contraindicate regional techniques.
- If emergency CS required and on heparin, GA should be used with protamine available (LMWH is incompletely reversed with protamine). Liaise with on-call haematologist.

Further reading

Fischer-Netz R et al. Pregnancy in systemic lupus erythematosus and antiphospholipid syndrome. *Best Practice & Research: Clinical Rheumatology* 2017; 31: 397–414.

Arthrogryposis multiplex congenita

Characteristics

- Non-progressive condition associated with multiple joint contractures, degeneration of anterior horn cells, skin and tissue abnormalities, micrognathia, and cervical spine and joint stiffness.
- Increased risk of spina bifida occulta.
- Scoliosis may occur with respiratory compromise.

- Associated with tracheal and laryngeal clefts and stenoses.
- May rarely have cardiac or pulmonary disease.

Key points
- Antenatal review essential with respiratory function tests. Skeletal review with radiological images that are available especially spine.
- Vascular access often limited and difficult, may require central venous access.
- Prone to bone fractures.
- Associated with difficult airway.
- Can have a hypermetabolic response to GA. This responds to active cooling.
- Regional anaesthesia may be technically difficult. Abnormal vertebral anatomy can complicate siting and spread of epidural and spinal blocks.
- Breech and transverse lies are more common, with increased need for CS.

Further reading
McGillivray K et al. Congenital arthrogryposis in pregnancy. *Journal of Obstetrics and Gynaecology* 2002; 22: 218–219.
Quance DR. Anaesthetic management of an obstetrical patient with arthrogryposis multiplex congenital. *Canadian Journal of Anaesthesia* 1988; 35: 612–614.

Budd–Chiari syndrome

Characteristics
- Hepatic venous outflow obstruction.
- May occur in the postpartum period.
- Either acute or chronic:
- The acute syndrome is due to a hypercoagulable state causing thrombosis of major hepatic veins resulting in liver cell necrosis.
- Caused by pregnancy, HELLP, SLE, severe pre-eclampsia, thrombotic thrombocythaemia purpura, malignancy, antiphospholipid syndrome, protein C deficiency, and factor V Leiden.
- The chronic syndrome is usually due to an IVC web and results in liver fibrosis.
- Treatment is aimed at preservation of liver function using stents and shunts. If untreated, leads to liver failure and death.

Key points
- Syndrome causes hepatomegaly, portal hypertension, ascites, and varices.
- There is poor platelet function and coagulopathy, therefore avoid regional techniques. Liaise with haematology.
- Avoid suxamethonium due to decreased pseudocholinesterase levels and therefore an unpredictable neuromuscular block.
- If acute presentation occurs in pregnancy and the fetus is adequately mature, a CS may be performed as a combined procedure with a liver transplant.

- If chronic with a shunt *in situ*, the patient will be on long-term warfarin, which may be converted to LMWH in pregnancy. Need LFTs and coagulation checked throughout pregnancy and regular monitoring of liver blood flow via ultrasound scanning. Severe cases should be managed in major hepatic units.

Further reading

Shukla A et al. Pregnancy outcomes in women with Budd Chiari syndrome before onset of symptoms and after treatment. *Liver International* 2018 ; 38:754–759.

Aggarwal N et al. Pregnancy outcome in Budd Chiari Syndrome—a tertiary care centre experience. *Archives in Gynecology and Obstetrics* 2013; 288: 949 952.

Cauda equina syndrome

Characteristics

- Damage to the cauda equina causing low back pain, unilateral or bilateral sciatica, saddle sensory disturbance, bowel and bladder dysfunction, and variable lower limb motor and sensory deficits.
- Caused by trauma, lumbar disc compression, abscess, spinal anaesthesia (more common in association with spinal catheters, but can occur with single-shot spinals), tumours, or idiopathic cause.

Key points

- Can occur during pregnancy and requires urgent decompression surgery.
- Surgery will require GA with gastric acid prophylaxis and rapid sequence induction.
- Prone position is not possible after 20 weeks gestation and position in left lateral position with abdomen supported is required.
- Aim to protect maternal safety, avoid fetal asphyxia, and prevent premature labour.
- Most anaesthetic agents are thought to be safe.
- After surgery and before consideration of regional techniques for delivery, a full review of neurology and radiological images are required in the antenatal period.
- Regional techniques can be difficult, with increased complications associated with previous surgery.
- Labour is not contraindicated.

Further reading

Jones CS et al. Presentation of caudal equine syndrome during labour. *BMJ Case Reports* 2015 18: 2015. pii: bcr2015212119. doi: 10.1136/bcr-2015-212119.

Tsen LC. Neurologic complications of labor analgesia and anesthesia (Review). *International Anesthesiology Clinics* 2002; 40: 67–88.

Cerebral tumours/craniotomy

Characteristics

- Cerebral tumours are rare in pregnancy, but symptoms such as headaches and vomiting may be mistaken for those of pregnancy itself.
- Needs multidisciplinary care. Management must be on an individual basis, with careful balance between maternal and fetal physiology.
- May remove tumour during the pregnancy or wait to deliver the fetus and perform a craniotomy at the same time.

Key points

- If craniotomy is required in pregnancy, use antacid prophylaxis, rapid sequence with cricoid pressure, maintain BP within 10% of normal during the procedure, obtund pressor response to laryngoscopy, and maintain left lateral tilt.
- Invasive BP monitoring is required and critical care postoperatively.
- If CS with tumour still *in situ*—GA.
- If any doubt about intracranial pressure (ICP)—need recent MRI/CT scan and neurological review.
- Epidural may increase ICP when boluses given.
- Dural tap may cause acute deterioration and coning.

Further reading

Wang LP et al. Neuroanaesthesia for the pregnant woman. *Anesthesia and Analgesia* 2008; 107: 193–200.

Cerebral venous sinus thrombosis

Characteristics

- Varied presentation. Features include headache, nausea and vomiting, decreased level of consciousness, seizures, focal neurological deficits, and cranial nerve palsies. Can be confused with other causes of epilepsy and eclampsia.
- Causes cerebral infarction secondary to tissue congestion and may be complicated by cerebral haemorrhage.
- Caused by infection, trauma, idiopathic and hypercoagulable states, e.g. pregnancy and the puerperium. An urgent MRI/CT with contrast studies is required.

Key points

- Avoid lumbar puncture.
- Local thrombolysis may be given.
- Anticoagulation is required.
- May require open thrombectomy.

Further reading

Swartz RH et al. The incidence of pregnancy-related stroke: a systematic review and meta-analysis. *International Journal of Stroke* 2017; 12: 687–697.

Edlow JA et al. Diagnosis of acute neurological emergencies in pregnant and post-partum women. *Lancet Neurology* 2013; 12: 175–185.

C1 esterase deficiency/angioneurotic oedema

Characteristics

- Autosomal dominant condition.
- Causes episodic local subcutaneous and submucosal oedema involving the upper respiratory tract and GIT.
- Episodes associated with stress, ovulation, menstruation, trauma, and infection.
- Does not respond to steroids or antihistamines.
- Disease is worse during pregnancy.

Key points

- A comprehensive plan is essential including the requirement and use of C1 inhibitor concentrate both for vaginal delivery or caesarean section. Should be delivered only in a centre with expertise in this disease.
- Epidural suitable for labour to decrease stress but patient must be turned regularly to prevent pressure-related oedema.
- Regional better than GA if possible.
- Avoid upper airway instrumentation; if necessary use a smaller endotracheal tube than usual.
- High risk of developing oedema postpartum; therefore, have a low threshold for a further dose of inhibitor at this time.
- Nurse in a high dependency area, as oedema can occur some hours after stress.

Further reading

Caballero T et al. International consensus and practical guidelines on the gynecologic and obstetric management of female patients with hereditary angioedema caused by C1 inhibitor deficiency. Journal of Allergy and Clinical Immunology 2012; 129: 308–320.

Chagas disease

Characteristics

- Tropical disease, endemic in Latin America, caused by infection with *Trypanosoma cruzi*.
- Transmission occurs through bites or through mucosal surfaces.
- 10–30% go on to develop chronic disease.
- Causes atrophy of cardiac and gastrointestinal tissues, cardiac dilation, thinning of ventricular walls, damage to the cardiac conduction system (causing RBBB and left anterior fascicular block progressing to complete AV block), and destruction of autonomic ganglia in the gut causing megacolon and megaoesophagus.
- Infection can transmit to the fetus.
- Severity of disease is varied and must be considered when making a plan for labour and delivery.

Key points

- ECG, Echo ± cardiology review antenatally.
- May require ECG monitoring in labour and invasive monitoring for CS depending on disease severity.
- Epidural suitable for labour but with slow incremental top-ups if severe cardiac disease.

Further reading

Gilson GJ et al. Chagas disease in pregnancy. *Obstetrics and Gynecology* 1995; 86: 646–647.

Charcot–Marie–Tooth disease

Characteristics

- Autosomal dominant condition causing chronic peripheral motor and sensory neuropathy.
- Characterized by muscle wasting, causing diaphragmatic weakness, and respiratory insufficiency.
- Disease often exacerbated in pregnancy.
- May require increased respiratory support as pregnancy progresses.
- Diaphragmatic splinting occurs in late pregnancy and exacerbates respiratory compromise.

Key points

- Careful antenatal assessment of the disease. Assessment of respiratory function essential, particularly in patients with upper limb involvement.
- May use non-invasive ventilation at home.
- Increased risk of operative delivery.
- Cautious use of suxamethonium due to risk of hyperkalaemia.
- Prolonged action of non-depolarizing muscle relaxants.
- No evidence of increased risk of malignant hyperpyrexia.
- Low dose CSE may be useful for CS.
- GA may be required dependent on severity of disease; admission to critical care may be required postoperatively ± ventilator support.

Further reading

Brock M et al. Anesthetic management of an obstetric patient with Charcot-Marie-Tooth disease: a case study. *Journal of the American Association of Nurse Anesthetists* 2009; 77: 335–337.

Chiari malformations

Characteristics

- Structural defects in the skull, dura, brain, spine, and spinal cord often associated with myelomeningocele. There is underdevelopment of cranial fossae and overcrowding of hindbrain structures.
- Type I is the most common where the lower part of the cerebellum, but not the brainstem, extends into the foramen magnum. It may be associated with syringomyelia, hydrocephalus, tethered cord, and scoliosis. It may present with headaches, neck pain, and mild

coordination problems, but often it is asymptomatic and discovered incidentally on cervical spine MRI scan.
- Type II Arnold-Chiari malformation both the cerebellum and the brain stem extend into the foramen magnum.
- Risk of descent of hindbrain structures through foramen magnum.
- CSF outflow obstruction through the 4th ventricle with raised ICP.
- Associated with obstructive sleep apnoea, inspiratory stridor, and scoliosis because of association with a syrinx in the spinal cord and syringomyelia.

Key points

- Successful decompression surgery with normal ICP can make regional techniques acceptable.
- A full antenatal neurological assessment with discussion from a neurosurgeon is required.
- No absolute recommendations with regards to regional vs general anaesthesia and vaginal vs CS delivery if ICP not raised.
- Safe use of regional anaesthesia is documented in type I.
- Avoid rises in ICP (i.e. hypercarbia, straining in labour).
- Avoid large boluses of solution into the epidural space (as this may increase ICP).
- Intubation can exacerbate upper limb neurological symptoms.

Further reading

Bolognese PA et al. Chiari I malformation and delivery. *Surgical Neurology International*. 2017; 8: 12.
Garvey GP et al. Anesthetic and obstetric management of syringomyelia during labour and delivery: a case series and systematic review. *Anesthesia and Analgesia* 2017; 125: 913–24.

Cocaine abuse

Characteristics

- Cocaine prolongs adrenergic stimulation by blocking presynaptic uptake of sympathomimetic neurotransmitters.
- Causes euphoria, hypertension, tachycardia, arrhythmias, seizures, hyper-reflexia, fever, dilated pupils, oedema, proteinuria, and emotional instability.
- Withdrawal causes fatigue, depression, and craving.
- Pregnancy causes increased cardiovascular sensitivity to cocaine.
- Increased risk of premature labour, fetal distress and IUGR, abruption, uterine rupture, hepatic rupture, cerebral ischaemia/infarction, and death.
- Patients may deny drug abuse.

Key points

- Perform a urine toxicology screen in high risk women.
- Regional anaesthesia is possible but must have recent platelet count and clotting study because of associated risks.

- May develop ephedrine-resistant hypotension—phenylephrine is a better option.
- May still have pain perception, despite adequate spinal or epidural sensory level.
- Prone to cardiovascular system instability. Esmolol infusion may help with cocaine-induced tachycardia, but may increase risk of cocaine-induced coronary vasospasm.
- Labetalol, GTN, and hydralazine may be useful to treat hypertension.
- Propofol and thiopental appear safe and effective. Volatile agents may increase risk of arrhythmia.

Further reading

Geary FH Jr et al. Management of the patient in labor who has abused substances. *Clinical Obstetrics and Gynecology* 2013; 56: 166–172.

Kuczkowski KM. Peripartum care of the cocaine-abusing parturient: are we ready? (Review). *Acta Obstetrica et Gynecologica Scandinavica* 2005; 84: 108–116.

CREST syndrome

Characteristics

- Systemic autoimmune condition—Calcinosis, Raynauds phenomenon, Oesophageal dysmotility, Sclerodactyly, and Telangectasia.
- May be complicated by aspiration and pulmonary disease, gastrointestinal bleeding, pulmonary hypertension, fibrosis of myocardium and arrhythmia, primary biliary sclerosis, renal disease, and entrapment neurological symptoms.
- May be taking NSAIDs and steroids outside pregnancy. An early pregnancy plan is required.
- Increased risk of premature labour.

Key points

- Pregnancy may worsen the disease; those with renal, cardiac, and pulmonary complications are most at risk. Assessment with sequential respiratory function tests and echocardiograms are required.
- May be difficult to differentiate between the disease itself and pre-eclampsia.
- A plan for difficult venous access and difficult airway must be made.
- Epidural and spinal possible after performing a coagulation screen. CSE may be useful, as a lower dose spinal may be required.

Further reading

Lidar M et al. Pregnancy issues in scleroderma. *Autoimmunity Reviews* 2012; 11: 515–519.

Cushing's syndrome

Characteristics

- Excess production of corticosteroids from the adrenal gland or by their exogenous administration.
- In general, most cases caused by an ACTH-secreting pituitary adenoma, but in pregnancy more are caused by adrenal adenomas.
- Increased maternal morbidity and mortality due to raised BP, hypokalaemia, diabetes, excessive weight gain, pre-eclampsia, cardiac failure, and poor wound healing.
- Treatment of the cause in pregnancy seems to improve outcome.

Key points

- Presentation in pregnancy can be difficult to diagnose due to normal weight gain, diabetes, and hypertension of pregnancy.
- Difficult control of blood sugar.
- Increased risk of difficult intubation.
- Muscle weakness may predispose to respiratory failure.
- May require steroid supplementation.
- May need surgical treatment in pregnancy. Laparoscopic adrenalectomy has been described.

Further reading

Andreescu CE et al. Adrenal Cushing's syndrome during pregnancy. *European Journal of Endocrinology* 2017; 177: K13–K20.

Lekarev O et al. Adrenal disease in pregnancy. *Best Practice & Research: Clinical Endocrinology & Metabolism* 2011; 25:959–973.

Demyelinating disease

Characteristics

- Multiple sclerosis is the most common and is caused by abnormalities of the myelin sheath.
- Causes limb weakness, visual disturbances, paraesthesia, incoordination, spasticity, hyper-reflexia, pain, mild dementia and dysarthria, respiratory muscle weakness, and bulbar weakness.
- Has an initial remitting and relapsing course, followed by secondary progressive disease.
- Exacerbations are related to stress, trauma, and infection.
- Exacerbations occur less frequently in pregnancy; however, may increase in the first 3 months postpartum.
- Exacerbations are not linked to choice of analgesia or mode of delivery.

Key points

- Antenatal assessment of condition with documentation of neurological deficit prior to regional technique and fully informed consent.
- Epidural and spinal not contraindicated.
- Neither mode of delivery or anaesthesia are related to relapse.
- Maximum safe dose of LA is lowered due to loss of blood–brain barrier.

- No evidence that volatile inhalation agents affect disease.
- Avoid suxamethonium as may cause hyperkalaemia associated with severe neurological deficit.
- Needs careful follow-up and early referral to a neurologist if problems develop.

Further reading

Amato MP et al. Management of pregnancy-related issues in multiple sclerosis patients: the need for an interdisciplinary approach. *Neurological Science* 2017; 38: 1849–1858.

Ghezzi A et al. Current recommendations for multiple sclerosis treatment in pregnancy and puerperium. *Expert Reviews of Clinical Immunology* 2013; 9: 683–692.

Whitaker JN. Effects of pregnancy and delivery on disease activity in multiple sclerosis. <u>New England Journal of Medicine</u> 1998; 339: 339–340.

Devic's syndrome

Characteristics

- Bilateral acute optic neuritis and transverse myelitis (causing functional transection of the spinal cord).
- Triggered by infection and autoimmune disease.
- Symptoms of back pain and progressive paraparesis.
- Increased risk of UTI, anaemia, and premature labour.

Key points

- Risk of autonomic hyper-reflexia causing hypertension, bradycardia, sweating, and cerebral haemorrhage.
- Epidural and spinal anaesthesia are effective at preventing autonomic hyper-reflexia.
- Epidural anaesthesia is easier to control with small incremental doses and regular assessment. May require smaller dose of LA than usual to provide adequate regional block. Avoid adrenaline in epidural.
- Avoid suxamethonium due to risk of hyperkalaemia. Use non-depolarizing muscle relaxants as normal.

Further reading

Sadana N et al. Anesthetic management of a parturient with neuromyelitis optica. *International Journal of Obstetric Anesthesia* 2012; 21: 371–375.

Gunaydin B et al. Epidural anaesthesia for Caesarean section in a patient with Devic's syndrome. *Anaesthesia* 2001; 56: 565–567.

Duchenne muscular dystrophy

Characteristics

- X-linked recessive disease of skeletal and cardiac muscle usually affecting males, causing progressive muscle weakness.
- Female carriers usually asymptomatic, but rarely can manifest signs and symptoms of the disease.
- A male fetus has a 50% chance of Duchenne muscular dystrophy.

Key points

- Perioperative complications include: cardiac arrhythmias and failure, cardiac arrest, malignant hyperpyrexia.
- Increased risk of cardiac arrhythmias.
- Regional anaesthesia advisable—CSE for surgery or early siting of labour epidural.
- Avoid suxamethonium and volatile anaesthetics. Suggested use of rocuronium and total IV anaesthesia if GA required.
- Prenatal administration of anaesthesia should not harm the male affected fetus.

Further reading

Molyneux MK. Anaesthetic management during labour of a manifesting carrier of Duchenne muscular dystrophy. *International Journal of Obstetric Anesthesia* 2005; 14: 58–61.

Dysfibrinogenaemia

Characteristics

- May be congenital or acquired.
- *Acquired* is secondary to abruption, intrauterine death, AFE, and massive haemorrhage.
- *Congenital* is rare and the woman will usually be under the care of a specialist haematologist.
- May be asymptomatic.
- Some patients have increased bleeding and some have a thrombotic tendency.

Key points

- Patients with congenital dysfibrogenaemia—liaise with haematologist preferably with an interest in haemostasis and thrombosis.
- Will need a comprehensive delivery plan with coagulation products.
- Increased risk of PPH and thrombosis.
- May need to treat with fibrinogen and/or heparin.
- Consider VHA for rapid assessment of coagulation.

Further reading

Mumford AD et al. Guideline for the diagnosis and management of the rare coagulation disorders: a United KingdomHaemophilia Centre Doctors' Organization guideline on behalf of the British Committee for Standards in Haematology. *British Journal of Haematology* 2014;167: 304–326.

Ebstein's anomaly

Characteristics

- Congenital anomaly in which the tricuspid valve is displaced apically and usually incompetent, so called atrialization of RV.
- If asymptomatic, usually well tolerated in pregnancy.
- Can be associated with an ASD or Wolf–Parkinson–White syndrome—in this situation arrhythmias and cyanosis may occur.
- In severe cases, a right to left shunt through an ASD may be present and cardiac failure may develop.

Key points
- ECG and echocardiogram as part of a comprehensive antenatal review with a cardiology opinion.
- Epidural safe in labour, but use with slow, incremental doses to avoid profound decrease in SVR.
- Maintain pre- and afterload.
- Avoid increases to PVR.

Further reading
Lima FV et al. Clinical characteristics and outcomes in pregannt women with Ebstein anomaly at the time of delivery in the USA: 2003–2012. *Archives of Cardiovascular Disease* 2016; 109: 390–398.
Zhao W et al. Pregnancy outcomes in women with Ebstein's anomaly. *Archives of Gynecology and Obstetrics* 2012; 286: 881–888.

Ehler's–Danlos syndrome

Characteristics
- Heterogenous group of hereditary connective tissue disorders.
- Classic types (type I, II, and III) cause joint hypermobility, skin hyper-elasticity, easily bruised, poor skin healing, excess bleeding, pneumothorax, and valvular prolapse.
- May have decreased response to LA agents. Pregnancy is likely to be uncomplicated in type I, II, and III.
- Type IV is due to abnormal type III collagen in the GIT, vascular tissue, and uterus ,and has a much poorer prognosis. Can have spontaneous rupture of bowel, major vessels, and uterus. Likely to have elective CS due to increased risk of uterine rupture. Sudden death in pregnancy reported.

Key points
- Reassurance is usually all that is required in types I–III.
- Type IV is a major concern—planned CS often advised.
- Careful assessment and discuss risks and benefits of GA vs regional techniques.
- GA usually preferable due to possible increased bleeding diathesis and risk of major bleed.
- Avoid sudden increases in BP.
- May have C-spine problems, therefore care with intubation necessary.
- Clotting usually normal but can be altered, and platelets may be low.
- Risk of coronary artery dissection or rupture of any vessel.

Further reading
Cereda AF et al. Spontaneous coronary artery dissection after pregnancy as first manifestation of a vascular Ehlers-Danlos syndrome. *Journal of Invasive Cardiology* 2017; 29: E67–E68.
Glynn JC, Yentis SM. Epidural analgesia in a parturient with classic type Ehlers–Danlos syndrome. *International Journal of Obstetric Anesthesia* 2005; 14: 78–79.
Kuczkowski KM. Ehlers–Danlos syndrome in the parturient: an uncommon disorder–common dilemma in the delivery room. *Archives of Gynecology and Obstetrics* 2005; 273: 60–62.

Epidermolysis bullosa

Characteristics

- Rare, inherited group of skin disorders.
- Causes blisters, pronounced scarring of skin and mucous membranes after minor trauma.
- Vaginal delivery is first choice, although in severe cases this may not be possible because of contractures.
- Varying degrees of severity.
- May have microstomia due to severe facial scaring.

Key points

- Assessment of airway and venous assess is required in antenatal period.
- Care with dressings; use paraffin gauze and light crepe bandages for IV cannulae. Never use adhesive dressings. Use minimal manual venous occlusion.
- Suxamethonium and non-depolarizing muscle relaxants are safe.
- Care with pressure points and eyes. Care with monitoring placement , e.g. saturation probe, BP cuff, and ECG electrodes. Invasive arterial BP monitoring may be useful.
- Tracheal intubation can be safe, with minimal examples in the literature of mucosal trauma. Lubricate laryngoscopes and oropharyngeal airways. May be a difficult intubation with very limited mouth opening.
- Spinal and epidurals are safe.

Further reading

Intong LRA et al. Retrospective evidence on outcomes and experiences or pregnancy and child-birth in epidermolysis bullosa in Australia and New Zealand. *International Journal of Womens Dermatology* 2017; 3(1 Suppl): S1–S5

Nandi R et al. Anesthesia and epidermolysis bullosa. *Clinics in Dermatology* 2010; 28: 319–324.

Epilepsy

Characteristics

- Many different types of seizures possible; grand mal seizures associated with increased risk to mother and fetus.
- Pseudoseizures characterized by resistance to open eyes, maintenance of papillary reflexes, response to pain, seizure lasting >90s without cyanosis, psychiatric history, or previous episodes.

Key points

- Women should be jointly managed with an epilepsy unit to optimize antenatal medication and prevent seizures.
- May have increased seizure frequency in pregnancy caused by changes in blood volume and poor compliance with medication.
- Fatigue, lack of sleep and starvation can increase risk of seizures in labour and regional techniques can help.

- If seizures in labour or delivery—protect and secure airway, support ventilation, and deliver fetus.
- Check blood sugar.

Further reading

Viale L et al. Epilepsy in pregnancy and reproductive outcomes: a systematic review and meta-analysis. *Lancet* 2015; 386: 1845–1852.

Familial Mediterranean fever

Characteristics

- A chronic inflammatory condition affecting serosal surfaces such as peritoneum, pleura, and joints.
- Associated with amyloidosis.
- Repeat bouts of fever associated with inflammation of serosal surfaces.
- Most common in patients of Mediterranean and Middle Eastern origin.
- Uncomplicated Familiar Mediterranean fever causes no additional problems for the anaesthetist.
- Renal failure most common cause of death. May have had renal transplant.
- In the presence of amyloid nephropathy, pregnancy has a deleterious effect on renal function.
- Cardiac disease causes LVF, conduction defects, and restrictive cardiomyopathy.
- High incidence of pre-eclampsia, thromboembolism, anaemia, and IUGR.

Key points

- Assessment in a multidisciplinary clinic assessing renal and cardiac function.
- Regional techniques good option but may need to be carefully titrated because of multisystem disease.
- If cardiac disease present—requires invasive monitoring.
- May require critical care support postpartum.

Further reading

Yasar O et al. Retrospective evaluation of pregnancy outcomes in women with familial Mediterranean fever. *Journal of Maternal-Fetal and Neonatal Medicine* 2014; 27: 733–736.

Friedreich's ataxia

Characteristics

- Autosomal recessive condition.
- Progressive degeneration of the spinocerebellar and corticospinal tracts.
- Mixed upper and lower motor neuron disease with cerebellar symptoms.
- Associated with scoliosis and hypertrophic cardiomyopathy.
- Prone to cardiac arrhythmias.

Key points

- Multidisciplinary antenatal assessment with cardiology review.
- Echocardiogram and 24h ECG is required.
- Assessment of scoliosis to plan for the possibility of regional analgesia. May have impaired respiratory function.
- Elective CS may decrease the cardiovascular stress associated with labour.
- Avoid suxamethonium due to risk of hyperkalaemia.
- No evidence of increased sensitivity to non-depolarizing muscle relaxants.
- CSE useful for CS ± invasive monitoring.

Further reading

Friedman LS et al. Pregnancy with Friedrich ataxia: a retrospective review of medical risks and psychosocial implications. *American Journal of Obstetrics and Gynecology* 2010; 203: 224.e1–5.

Gaucher's disease

Characteristics

- Autosomal recessive lysosomal storage disorder caused by enzyme deficiency managed with long-term enzyme replacement.
- Leads to accumulation of glycosphingolipids and multiple end-organ dysfunction.
- Type I–III—with type I and rarely type II surviving to reproductive age. Extremely heterogenous in onset and the organ involvement.

Key points

- Hepatosplenomegaly, thrombocytopenia, isolated clotting factor deficiency (factor IX and von Willebrand's disease), and anaemia.
- Risk of excessive bleeding; full haematological work-up required.
- Does not preclude regional technique after careful assessment.
- Skeletal involvement, i.e. osteopenia, pathological fractures, therefore care with positioning and transferring.
- Associated with lung parenchymal disease and pulmonary hypertension (rare), and neurological dysfunction, e.g. bulbar involvement, seizures, chronic aspiration.
- Difficult intubation associated with skeletal abnormalities and trismus.

Further reading

Ioscovich A et al. Anesthesia for obstetric patients with Gaucher disease: survey and review. *International Journal of Obstetric Anesthesia* 2004; 13: 244–250.

Gilbert's disease

Characteristics

- Autosomal dominant, benign condition with mildly elevated (up to 50mcmol/L) unconjugated serum bilirubin.
- Mild jaundice occurs with stress, infection, starvation, or surgery.
- Liver function otherwise normal.

Key points

- Not associated with HELLP syndrome.
- Stress of long labour/hyperemesis can precipitate attack.
- Post-delivery jaundice may occur.
- Avoiding long starvation times and use of IV glucose minimizes risk of jaundice.
- Not associated with abnormal clotting, therefore regional analgesia is useful.
- Use morphine and paracetamol more cautiously due to delayed metabolism.
- Nicotinic acid has been used to increase serum unconjugated bilirubin.

Further reading

Taylor S. Gilbert's syndrome as a cause of postoperative jaundice. *Anaesthesia* 1984; 39: 1222–1224.
Zusterzeel PL et al. Gilbert's syndrome is not associated with HELLP syndrome. *British Journal of Obstetrics and Gynaecology* 2001; 108: 1003–1004.

Glanzmann's thrombasthenia

Characteristics

- Rare, autosomal recessive platelet disorder caused by lack of glycoprotein IIb–IIIa.
- Diagnosed in childhood, usually presenting with marked mucocutaneous bleeding.
- Normal platelet numbers, but platelet function and aggregation are severely impaired.
- Women should be counselled about the high risk of severe peripartum bleeding before deciding whether to conceive.
- Late, severe PPH at 7–21 days is recognized, even after apparently adequate platelet transfusion at the time of delivery.
- Multiple platelet transfusions can lead to antiplatelet antibody production and a reduced effectiveness of further platelet transfusions.
- Neonatal allo-immune thrombocytopenia, due to fetal platelets inducing GpIIb–IIIa antibodies in the mother, may result in thrombocytopenia in the neonate.

Key points

- Must be managed jointly with a haemophilia centre.
- Regional anaesthesia absolutely contraindicated for labour and CS.
- Other treatments include immunoglobulins, plasmaphoresis, single donor platelet/HLA-matched platelet transfusion.

Further reading

Wijemanne A et al. Glanzmann thrombasthenia in pregnancy: optimising maternal and fetal outcomes. *Obstetric Medicine* 2016; 9: 169–170.

Huq FY, Kadir RA. Management of pregnancy, labour and delivery in women with inherited bleeding disorders. *Haemophilia* 2011; 17: 20–30.

Bolton-Maggs PH et al. A review of inherited platelet disorders with guidelines for their management on behalf of the UKHCDO. *British Journal of Haematology* 2006; 135: 603–633.

Guillain–Barré syndrome

Characteristics

- Acute or subacute ascending demyelinating polyradiculoneuritis, classically following viral infection, e.g. Epstein–Barr virus, leading to pain, paraesthesia, and paralysis extending proximally.
- Management involves symptomatic relief, thromboprophylaxis, nutrition, and physiotherapy, and regular monitoring of respiratory function (forced vital capacity).
- IV immunoglobulin and plasmapharesis for severe cases.

Key points

- Rarely presents in pregnancy but women who have recovered can have normal pregnancies.
- Full neurological assessment and respiratory function tests
- Guillain-Barre syndrome has no effect on uterine contraction or cervical dilatation, hence vaginal delivery preferred.
- May require assisted instrumental delivery.
- In cases with significant neurological deficit who require regional techniques for labour or CS, there is an increased sensitivity to LAs and autonomic instability. For this reason, care is necessary with spinal anaesthesia.
- Suxamethonium can cause hyperkalaemia.
- There is increased sensitivity to non-depolarizing neuromuscular blockers.

Further reading

Hukuimwe M et al. Guillain-Barré syndrome in pregnancy: a case report. *Women's Health (London)* 2017; 13(1): 10–13.

Karnad DR, Guntupalli KK. Neurologic disorders in pregnancy (Review). *Critical Care Medicine* 2005; 33 (10 Suppl): S362–S371.

Heart–lung transplant

Characteristics

- There are an increasing number of post-transplant patients of reproductive age who generally have a good outcome in pregnancy.
- Immunosuppressive therapy is responsible for increased risk of maternal and fetal complications including hypertension, pre-eclampsia, low birth weight, prematurity, and infection.
- Immunosuppressive therapy continues in pregnancy with the minimal dosage possible.
- Pregnancy does not increase the risk of graft rejection.
- Solid organ transplants have an increased association with PET.

Key points

- A denervated heart is devoid of functional autonomic innervation.
- The transplanted heart responds to haemodynamic changes seen in pregnancy by Frank–Starling mechanism.
- Upregulation of adrenoreceptors leads to increased sensitivity to circulating catecholamines.
- Women must be managed in a joint obstetric/cardiology clinic and have regular echocardiograms to assess cardiac function.
- Haemodynamic changes in labour are well tolerated if the transplant is functioning well.
- Mode of delivery is usually based on obstetric indications.
- Regional techniques are well tolerated.

Further reading

Wu DW, et al. Pregnancy after thoracic organ transplanttaion. *Seminars in Perinatology* 2007; 31: 354–362.
Padhan P. Pregnancy in recipients of solid-organ transplants. *New England Journal of Medicine* 2006; 354: 2726–2727.

Hereditary spherocytosis

Characteristics

- Autosomal dominant disorder causing early destruction of erythrocytes in the spleen.
- Patients suffer with haemolytic anaemia, marrow hyperplasia, splenomegaly, jaundice, and gallstones.
- Splenectomy is the treatment of choice in severe cases, improving Hb and platelet levels.
- Increased cholesterol levels may have detrimental effects on the patient, resulting in myocardial infarction or stroke.
- Pregnancy can be complicated by anaemia and haemolytic crises.

Key points

- Careful observation in pregnancy with folic acid supplementation and prevention of infection.
- Should be managed in joint haematology clinic.
- Post-splenectomy patients should have prophylaxis against infection.

Further reading

Pajor A et al. Pregnancy and hereditary spherocytosis. Report of 8 patients and a review. *Archives of Gynecology and Obstetrics* 1993; 253: 37–42.

Hereditary haemorrhagic telangiectasia (HHT)

Characteristics
- Hereditary haemorrhagic telangiectasia (HHT) is an autosomal dominant vascular dysplasia characterized by epistaxis, mucocutaneous telangiectasias, and arteriovenous malformations (AVM) in the brain, lung, liver, gastrointestinal tract, or spine.
- Arteriovenous malformations (AVMs) of pulmonary (30%), cerebral (20%), spinal (2%), and hepatic (30%) circulations can be asymptomatic.
- Pregnant women with HHT are known to have increased risks due to pulmonary and neurological AVMs.

Key points
- A careful antenatal review of symptoms and radiological imagining is important.
- As with other systemic AVMs, these can develop and increase in size during pregnancy.
- The presence of spinal AVMs is considered a relative contraindication to regional techniques and a conservative approach to regional techniques is appropriate.
- Epidural analgesia is relatively contraindicated if imaging is not available, but asymptomatic women can be offered a spinal anaesthetic because of the low risk of haemorrhagic complications.

Further reading

Lomax S, Edgcombe H. Anesthetic implications for the parturient with hereditary hemorrhagic telangiectasia. *Canadian Journal of Anaesthia* 2009; 56: 374–378.
de Gussem EM et al. Outcomes of pregnancy in women with hereditary hemorrhagic telangiectasia. *Obstetrics and Gynecology* 2014; 123: 514–520.

Herpes simplex infection

Characteristics
- Herpes simplex infection is common and can be in an active or inactive state.
- Patients may be immunocompromised due to co-existing disease and medication.

Key points
- CS delivery recommended in presence of active perineal infection.
- Regional anaesthesia is not contraindicated as long as active lesions are away from injection site.
- There are reports of epidural morphine being associated with reactivation of the infection and pruritus.

Further reading

Stankiewicz Karita HC et al. Invasive obstetric procedures and cesarean sections in women with known herpes simplex virus status during pregnancy. *Open Forum in Infectious Diseases* 2017; 4(4): ofx248.

Human immunodeficiency virus (HIV) infection

Characteristics

- Women of reproductive age are the fastest growing group of HIV sufferers.
- A multiorgan disease affecting cell-mediated immunity, which can be complicated by opportunistic infections, tumours, antiretroviral therapy, and substance abuse. The following manifestations have been reported:
  - Neurological (intracranial tumours, abscesses, neuropathies, myopathies).
  - Pulmonary (infections, tuberculosis, lymphomas).
  - Cardiac (myocarditis, pulmonary hypertension, cardiomyopathy, coronary artery disease).
  - Gastrointestinal (gastroparesis, hepatitis).
  - Haematological (hypercoagulable states, bone marrow failure).
- Monitoring of disease state with viral load and CD4 counts is important during pregnancy.
- Vertical transmission to the fetus *in utero* (4.5%), during childbirth (60%) and breastfeeding (35%) can occur. Transmission rates lower with antiretroviral therapy.

Key points

- With modern antiviral regimens, viral load can be undetectable with a low transmission rate to fetus.
- CS lessens the risk of transmission to the unborn baby. Antiretroviral therapy given prior to vaginal or caesarean delivery to reduce vertical transmission.
- HIV and drug therapy have minimal effect on complications associated with pregnancy and, in turn, pregnancy does not have a detrimental effect on the HIV disease process.
- Anaesthetic technique is governed by systemic effects of disease.
- Regional techniques and blood patch are safe in well controlled disease.

Further reading

Tricco AC et al. Safety and effectiveness of antiretroviral therapies for HIV-infected women and their infants and children: protocol for a systematic review and network meta-analysis. *Systematic Reviews* 2014; 3:51.

Horner's syndrome

Characteristics

- A triad of miosis, ptosis, and enophthalmus with facial flushing and anhydrosis.
- The patient complains of blurred vision, strange feeling over face, nasal stuffiness, and the sensation of respiratory difficulty, resulting from high epidural or spinal anaesthesia.
- Paralysis of sympathetic pathways from C6 to T1 leads to unopposed parasympathetic tone producing the clinical signs.

Key points

- Most common after regional techniques with excessive sympathetic block.
- Can cause confusion with other causes of acute neurological pathology in labour.
- Symptoms usually benign and resolve spontaneously. Patient reassurance is required.
- If prolonged, exclusion of other intracranial pathological causes of Horner's syndrome is important.

Further reading

Chambers DJ, Bhatia K. Horner's syndrome following obstetric neuraxial blockade—a systematic review of the literature. *International Journal of Obstetric Anesthesia* 2018; 35: 75–87.

Hypothyroidism/hyperthyroidism

Characteristics

Hypothyroidism

- Most common cause is autoimmune thyroiditis, which can affect 2.5% of pregnant women.
- Usually subclinical, with those affected being picked up by screening programmes.
- Evidence for impaired neuron intellectual development in the unborn child supports thyroid hormone replacement in these women.

Hyperthyroidism

- Autoimmune hyperthyroidism or Grave's disease is rare in pregnancy and treatment depends on the severity of the disease.
- Antithyroid drugs, i.e. propothiouracil is safe and can control the disease with good outcomes.
- Surgery may be indicated and is safe in the second trimester.
- Maternal complications include preterm labour, miscarriage, placental abruption, pre-eclampsia, cardiac failure, and thyroid storm.
- Thyroid antibodies can cross the placenta causing fetal abnormalities, IUGR, and neonatal hyperthyroidism.

Key points

- Early involvement of endocrinologist to control and monitor disease process.
- Pregnancy may ameliorate autoimmune thyroid disease.
- Surgery in the presence of uncontrolled hyperthyroidism is associated with a high mortality.

Further reading

Lazarus JH. Thyroid disorders associated with pregnancy: etiology, diagnosis, and management (Review). *Treatments in Endocrinology* 2005; 4: 31–41.

Hypoplastic anaemia

Characteristics

- Rare in pregnancy, with bone marrow failure and pancytopenia in peripheral blood posing a risk of infection and bleeding to the mother.
- Other complications include IUGR, fetal death, chorioamnionitis, and preterm delivery.
- Pregnancy may have a detrimental effect on the disease.
- Patients can present with bleeding gums and bruising.

Key points

- Appropriate replacement therapy of red cells, white cells and platelets is required under joint haematological guidance.
- Platelet antibody production can result in ineffective transfusions.
- Mode of delivery will depend on obstetric indication and severity of disease process.
- Regional anaesthesia may be contraindicated if severe thrombocytopenia, and there can be concern regarding the risk of infection with epidural placement.

Further reading

Bo L, et al Aplastic anemia associated with pregnancy: maternal and fetal complications. *Journal of Maternal-Fetal and Neonatal Medicine* 2016; 29: 1120–1124.

Implanted intrathecal pump

Characteristics

- Intrathecal opioid-delivering pumps are used for the treatment of severe refractory malignant and non-malignant pain.
- Implantation of an intrathecal catheter involves tunnelling the catheter and attaching it to an SC pump in the abdomen or thorax.
- Patients may be on multiple other medications.
- No reports of utilizing the pump alone for management of labour analgesia.
- Pumps can be dislodged in the pregnant abdomen.

Key points

- Seek expert advice on use of pump and position of catheter with appropriate imaging.
- Use of pump may be hazardous, and complications can include difficulty in finding the pump port, flushing of concentrated opioids through the catheter, and infection requiring antibiotic prophylaxis.
- Device does not preclude cautious use of regional techniques for labour/delivery. Epidural space may be scarred and spread of LA unpredictable. Attempts at epidural insertion should be made at a remote site to avoid shearing.

Further reading

Tarshis J et al. Labour pain management in a parturient with an implanted intrathecal pump. *Canadian Journal of Anaesthesia* 1997; 44: 1278–1281.

Intracranial mass-cyst

Characteristics

- Tumours and epidermoid cysts are rare in pregnancy, and growth may be increased by hormone excess.
- Patients present with symptoms of raised ICP—headache, seizures.
- Patients with stable neurology may progress to term with regular neurosurgical evaluation.

Key points

- Mode of delivery depends on tumour size and location, being largely led by a multidisciplinary approach to management.
- Epidural analgesia and spinal anaesthesia are potentially hazardous because of tentorial herniation and increases in ICP, but both have been safely reported.
- Meningitis after rupture of epidermoid cyst can occur.
- GA should include avoidance of fluctuation in ICP and maintenance of stable haemodynamics with remifentanil use, topical anaesthesia of larynx, and local infiltration of surgical site. Sufficient depth of anaesthesia and rapid recovery required, with multimodal analgesia and minimizing opioid use.

Further reading

Imarengiaye C et al. Goal oriented general anesthesia for Cesarean section in a parturient with a large intracranial epidermoid cyst. *Canadian Journal of Anaesthesia* 2001; 48: 884–889.

Jehovah's Witness

Characteristics
- Patients will not accept the transfusion of blood or blood products on religious grounds.
- There are differing views on accepting some concentrated products—fibrinogen concentrate etc. Patients can refuse stored whole blood, minor blood fractions (clotting factors, albumin), and non-stored autologous blood (cell salvage) to varying degrees.
- Ethical, moral, legal and practical issues make cases complicated, and each should be tackled with respect for the patient, with full informed consent and clear ideas about the patient's wishes.

Key points
- Detailed patient consent in presence of a witness including availability and acceptability of cell salvage techniques and individual clotting factors.
- Preoperative measures to optimize Hb levels: dietary, iron supplements (oral or IV), erythropoietin.
- Early warning of obstetric/anaesthetic staff on admission.
- Delivery in consultant-led unit—recommendation of Jehovah's Witness Association.
- IV and early use of oxytocins post delivery.
- Limit blood sampling and excessive blood loss with early recourse to surgical techniques, haemodilution, aprotinin, tranexamic acid, and desmopressin use.
- Epidural blood patch may also be refused.

Further reading
Mason CL, Tran CK. Caring for the Jehovah's Witness Parturient. *Anesthesia and Analgesia* 2015; 121: 1564–1569.
Zeybek B et al. Management of the Jehovah's Witness in obstetrics and gynecology: A comprehensive medical, ethical, and legal approach. *Obstetrical and Gynecological Survey* 2016; 71:488–500.

King–Denborough syndrome

Characteristics
- Rare disease of unknown inheritance.
- Presents with progressive myopathy, congenital skeletal and facial deformities.
- Marked kyphoscoliosis with respiratory failure which can be exaggerated in pregnancy.
- Increased physiological demands in labour can lead to significant cardiorespiratory compromise.

Key points
- Assessment of respiratory function and skeletal abnormalities.
- Regional technique desirable if anatomically possible.
- Craniofacial deformity can result in airway problems.
- Invasive monitoring may be useful, with serial arterial blood gas analysis.
- Avoid suxamethonium as susceptible to malignant hyperpyrexia.
- Ephedrine and oxytocin safe.

Further reading

Habib AS. Anesthetic management of a ventilator-dependent parturient with the King–Denborough syndrome. *Canadian Journal of Anaesthesia* 2003; 50: 589–592.

Klippel–Feil syndrome

Characteristics
- Inherited condition with skeletal, cardiac, and genitourinary abnormalities.
- Fusion of cervical vertebra can lead to progressive neurological damage and spinal cord anomalies. Scoliosis is common and other abnormalities of any vertebrae including spina bifida.
- Associated cardiac abnormalities include PDA, coarctation of aorta, and/or mitral valve prolapse.
- Maxillofacial abnormalities and deafness may occur.
- Obstructive sleep apnoea is reported.
- Short stature.

Key points
- Full assessment of airway, respiratory function, and vertebral abnormalities are required in the antenatal period.
- Women with a history of cardiac abnormalities should be seen in a joint obstetric/cardiology clinic.
- Difficult intubation, hypermobility, and neurological complications are common.
- Regional anaesthesia preferred.
- Awake fibreoptic reported for CS under GA.

Further reading

Hsu G et al. Anesthetic management of a parturient with type III Klippel-Feil syndrome. *International Journal of Obstetric Anesthesia* 2011; 20: 82–85.

Klippel–Trenaunay–Weber syndrome

Characteristics

- Rare, non-hereditary syndrome consisting of superficial and deep haemangiomata, hypertrophy of soft tissue and bone with extremity overgrowth and varicose veins.
- Can affect the trunk and epidural space.
- Cerebral and spinal cord arteriovenous fistulae predispose to haemorrhage and increased risk of DIC.

Key points

- Coagulation screen to eliminate chronic DIC.
- Regional techniques are not contraindicated if MRI evaluation of the epidural space is made.
- Mode of delivery depends on site of venous abnormalities.
- Multidisciplinary antenatal care with provision for cell salvage and alert to risk of haemorrhage/DIC.

Further reading

Horbach SE et al. Complications of pregnancy and labour in women with Klippel-Trénauny syndrome: a nationwide cross-sectional study. *British Journal of Obstetrics and Gynaecology* 2017; 124: 1780–1788.

Larsen syndrome

Characteristics

- Rare congenital condition inherited or caused by spontaneous mutation.
- Collagen malformation results in skeletal deformities; dislocated hips, knees and elbows, abnormal hands and feet, short stature, and cervical spine instability.
- Potential airway difficulties from: abnormal facies, tracheomalacia, laryngomalacia, subglottic stenosis.
- Cardiac defects: VSD, ASD, PDA, aortic dilatation, mitral valve prolapse.

Key points

- Assessment of airway, respiratory function, and spine.
- Kyphoscoliosis can result in restrictive lung disease.
- Epidural anaesthesia advisable if possible.

Further reading

Michel TC et al. Obstetric anesthetic management of a parturient with Larsen syndrome and short stature. *Anesthesia and Analgesia* 2001; 92: 1266–1267.

Laryngeal papillomatosis/ tracheal stenosis

Characteristics

- Recurrent laryngeal benign tumours caused by the human papillomavirus (HPV).
- Patients present with hoarseness, stridor, and airway obstruction.
- Pregnancy may lead to activation of HPV and worsening symptoms.
- Repeated surgical excision may be required in pregnancy.
- Vertical transmission to fetus can occur.

Key points

- Multidisciplinary approach (ENT, obstetrics, anaesthetics). Strictures can be monitored by respiratory function tests.
- Audible stridor requires urgent ENT referral for assessment.
- Preoperative nasal fibre-optic assessment of airway.
- May require resection in the third trimester of pregnancy with open airway technique. Severe cases should be managed in a specialist centre.
- Minimise risk of aspiration with antacid prophylaxis and head-up position.
- Regional techniques if possible.
- May need to use microlaryngeal tube for GA.

Further reading

Tripi PA et al. Anesthetic management for laser excision of recurrent respiratory papillomatosis in a third trimester parturient. *Journal of Clinical Anesthesia* 2005; 17: 610–613.

Lipomyelocele

Characteristics

- An intraspinal lipoma associated with disruption of the meninges, displacement of neural material, and spina bifida.

Key points

- Epidural space anatomy can be unpredictable, but well-planned regional anaesthesia for labour and CS has been reported.
- Radiological assessment of lesion required—MRI in second trimester ideal. Detailed patient consent.

Further reading

Thompson MD et al. Epidural blockade for labour and Caesarean section with associated L4–5 lipomyelocele. *Anesthesiology* 1999; 30: 1217–1218.

Lymphangioleiomyomatosis

Characteristics

- Rare idiopathic lung disease affecting women of reproductive age.
- Presents with cough, shortness of breath, bloody sputum, pleural effusions, and spontaneous pneumothoraces resulting in severe lung impairment.
- Diagnosis by lung biopsy.

Key points

- Detailed preoperative assessment with respiratory input.
- Regional anaesthesia technique of choice.

Further reading

McLoughlin L et al. Pregnancy and lymphangioleiomyomatosis: anaesthetic management. *International Journal of Obstetric Anesthesia* 2003; 12: 40–44.

Lymphocytic hypophysitis

Characteristics

- Autoimmune disorder associated with pregnancy where the pituitary is infiltrated with lymphocytes.
- Can present at any stage ante- or postpartum.
- Symptoms relate to mass effect—visual disturbance, headaches or hyperprolactinaemia or pituitary insufficiency.
- Can be self-resolving after delivery of the baby or a more chronic problem.
- Patients may require hormone replacement, steroid therapy, or surgery.

Key points

- Multidisciplinary approach with neurosurgeons and endocrinologists to confirm diagnosis.
- Regional anaesthesia if raised ICP has been excluded on CT/MRI.
- Increased risk of developing pituitary necrosis, i.e. Sheehan's syndrome from severe hypotension.
- PDPH may be difficult to diagnose.

Further reading

Buckland RH, Popham PA. Lymphocytic hypophysitis complicated by postpartum haemorrhage. *International Journal of Obstetric Anesthesia* 1998; 7: 263–266.

Malignant hyperthermia

Characteristics

- Rare pharmacogenetic condition of complex inheritance affecting muscle metabolism.
- Patients present with a personal history of MH or have been tested after a family history of MH.
- Presents with tachycardia, arrhythmias, rising temperature, and end-tidal CO_2 levels after exposure to certain triggers.
- Definitive diagnosis with muscle biopsy using caffeine–halothane contracture test.
- Aggressively treated with dantrolene sodium.

Key points

- Careful history and evaluation of susceptible patients or those with a strong family history.
- Plan for regional anaesthesia (with explanation to patient).
- Avoid suxamethonium and volatiles.
- Volatile-free anaesthetic machine must be available in case of emergency—flush with oxygen and change CO_2 absorber and rubber components prior to GA.
- Regional anaesthesia advised although a low risk labour can be managed in an alongside midwifery-led unit with an appropriate anaesthetic alert mechanism in place.
- Sodium citrate, ephedrine, thiopental, propofol, all non-depolarizing muscle relaxants, oxytocin, and local anaesthetics are safe in malignant hyperthermia.
- Total IV propofol anaesthesia for CS is well described.
- Dantrolene crosses placenta, so prophylaxis only for those with previous severe reaction and undergoing GA.
- Monitor temperature and end-tidal CO_2.
- Close temperature monitoring postoperatively.
- Fetus may have malignant hyperthermia.

Further reading

Lucy SJ. Anaesthesia for Caesarean delivery of a malignant hyperthermia susceptible parturient. *Canadian Journal of Anaesthesia* 1994; 41: 1220–1226.

Mediastinal masses

Characteristics

- Masses can be carcinoma, lymphoma, thyroid, or thymus in origin, or neurogenic.
- Patients can present with dyspnoea, haemoptysis, oedema, dilated neck veins, and cough.
- CT imaging of the thorax and rigid bronchoscopy are definitive investigations.

Key points

- Multidisciplinary approach to management in tertiary centre.
- Consider treatment options to reduce size of mediastinal mass if appropriate, e.g. radiotherapy or chemotherapy pre-delivery.
- Risk of cardiovascular collapse and complete airway obstruction on induction of GA due to loss of bronchial tone and lower lung volumes.
- Difficulty in lying flat can make regional anaesthesia a difficult but safe option.

Further reading

Kanellakos GW. Perioperative management of the pregnant patient with an anterior mediastinal mass. *Anesthesiology Clinics* 2012; 30: 749–758.

Dasan J et al. Mediastinal tumour in a pregnant patient presenting as acute cardiorespiratory compromise. *International Journal of Obstetric Anesthesia* 2002; 11: 52–56.

Motor neurone disease (amyotrophic lateral sclerosis)

Characteristics

- A progressive degenerative disease of the motor system of unknown aetiology.
- It involves upper and lower motor neurones and presents with weakness and fasciculations.

Key points

- Careful respiratory monitoring required.
- Increased physiological demands results in the disease presenting or deteriorating during pregnancy.
- CS and vaginal birth reported.
- Severe hyperkalaemia with suxamethonium. Increased sensitivity to non-depolarizing muscle relaxants.
- May require prolonged invasive or non-invasive postoperative ventilation.
- Regional techniques have been safely described.

Further reading

Maruotti GM et al. Anesthetic management of a parturient with spinal muscular atrophy type II. *Journal of Clinical Anesthia* 2012; 24(7): 573–577.

Moyamoya disease

Characteristics

- Stenosis of internal carotid arteries with hazy collateral circulation around base of brain. Most common in Japan.
- Risk of cerebral haemorrhage and ischaemia increased in pregnancy.
- Surgical (revascularization) and medical (antiplatelet, anticoagulant, vasodilator) treatment is often required.

Key points

- Most case reports describe CS delivery.
- Normotension and normocapnoea important to maintain cerebral flow.
- Vaginal delivery requires good analgesia and instrumental assistance.
- Epidural and low dose CSE techniques have been described.

Further reading

Kato R. et al. Anesthetic management for Caesarean section in moyamoya disease: a report of five consecutive cases and a mini-review. *International Journal of Obstetric Anesthesia* 2006; 15: 152–158.

Multiple endocrine neoplasia

Characteristics

- A group of inherited conditions (MEN1, 2A, 2B) with tumours in multiple endocrine glands (parathyroid, thyroid, pituitary, pancreas, adrenal medulla).
- Symptoms may be related to hyperparathyroidism, pituitary disease, and phaeochromocytoma.
- Most problems in pregnancy related to phaeochromocytoma—part of MEN 2A and 2B syndrome. Presents with hypertension at any time during pregnancy, headaches, sweating, and palpitations.
- Can be mistaken for pre-eclampsia; however, there is no proteinuria with phaeochromocytoma.

Key points

- Antenatal diagnosis improves outcome for mother and fetus.
- Avoidance of hypertensive crises, which can lead to cardiac failure and death.
- Elective CS delivery with perioperative A-blockade and B-blockade is recommended after 24 weeks gestation, followed by tumour resection after a recovery period.

Further reading

Ahn JT et al. Atypical presentation of pheochromocytoma as part of multiple endocrine neoplasia IIa in pregnancy. *Obstetrics and Gynecology* 2003; 102: 1202–1205.

Dugas G et al. Pheochromocytoma and pregnancy: a case review and report of anesthetic management. *Canadian Journal of Anaesthesia* 2004; 51: 134–138.

Myasthenia gravis

Characteristics

- Autoimmune disruption of postsynaptic acetylcholine receptors at the neuromuscular junction.
- Muscle fatigue in any muscle group; bulbar, pharyngeal, laryngeal, and respiratory muscles.
- Requires long-term anticholinesterase therapy which must be continue in labour; higher dose may need to be given IM.
- Pregnancy can alter course, with relapses most likely in first trimester and postpartum.

- 30% of infants are born with transient myasthenic syndrome.
- Myasthenic and cholinergic crises triggered by stress, exertion, or infection are differentiated by an edrophonium test.

Key points

- Thorough assessment of respiratory and bulbar function is required in the antenatal period.
- Vaginal delivery with assistance in second stage to reduce fatigue, with close monitoring of respiratory function intrapartum.
- Epidural or spinal anaesthesia encouraged.
- Cautious opioid use, only in a monitored environment.
- Very sensitive to non- depolarizing muscle relaxants—10% of standard dose recommended. Magnesium can significantly prolong their effect and precipitate weakness.
- Suxamethonium can be used safely in a bigger dose.
- Critical care support post delivery may be required.

Further reading

Almeida C et al. Myasthenia gravis and pregnancy: anaesthetic management—a series of cases. *European Journal of Anaesthesiology* 2010; 27: 985–990.
Chieza JT et al. Maternal myasthenia gravis complicated by fetal arthrogryposis multiplex congenita. *International Journal of Obstetric Anesthesia* 2011; 20: 79–82.

Myelodysplastic syndrome

Characteristics

- A group of haematological disorders with dysplastic haemopoiesis and blast cells present in peripheral blood and bone marrow.
- Present with anaemia and thrombocytopenia to varying degrees.
- Antiplatelet antibodies from multiple transfusions may be suppressed by immunoglobulins and steroids.
- Antenatal management must be jointly managed with a haematologist.

Key points

- Mode of delivery depends on obstetric indication and degree of thrombocytopenia.
- Maternal antibodies may cross placenta with unknown effect on fetus (risk of intracranial haemorrhage in fetus during vaginal delivery).
- Regional anaesthesia contraindicated in severe thrombocytopenia.
- Nitrous oxide implicated in bone marrow suppression.

Further reading

Hara K et al. Anaesthetic management of caesarean section in a patient with myelodysplastic syndrome. *Canadian Journal of Anaesthia* 1998; 45: 157–163.
Christiaens F et al. Anaesthetic management of Caesarean section in a parturient with acute myelodysplastic syndrome. *International Journal of Obstetric Anesthesia* 1997; 6: 270–273.

Myotonic dystrophy

Characteristics

- Autosomal dominant multisystem degenerative condition affecting skeletal, smooth, and cardiac muscle.
- Pregnancy is rare due to ovarian failure.
- Presents early in childhood with weakness and wasting of face, extremities, and respiratory muscles.
- Cardiac involvement commonly leads to destruction of the conducting system, heart block, and sudden death.
- Patients may be on oral anticoagulation.
- Cardiomyopathy and heart failure can also occur in pregnancy.
- Complications in pregnancy include polyhydramnios, premature labour, breech presentation, ineffective uterine contractions, retained placenta, and PPH.
- High risk of neonatal death.

Key points

- Thorough preoperative assessment to include cardiorespiratory investigation and airway assessment.
- Sensitive to premedication, opioids, non-depolarizing neuromuscular-blocking agents, and induction agents.
- Both regional and general anaesthesia can induce myotonia.
- Myotonia particularly associated with suxamethonium.
- Gastroparesis increases risk of aspiration.
- Higher incidence of difficult intubation.
- CSE is technique of choice for caesarean delivery.
- The theatre and IV fluids must be warmed to reduce myotonia.
- Respiratory failure is a frequent cause of postoperative morbidity.
- Higher risk of thromboembolism.

Further reading

Hopkins AN et al. Neurologic disease with pregnancy and considerations for the obstetric anesthesiologist. *Seminars in Perinatology* 2014; 38: 359–369.

Neurofibromatosis

Characteristics

- Autosomal dominant condition with variable expressivity: types I and II.
- A multisystem disorder with multiple neurofibromata and café au lait spots.
- Respiratory system: kyophoscoliosis, pulmonary fibrosis, pulmonary hypertension, and right heart failure.
- Cardiovascular system: hypertension, renovascular disease, phaeochromocytoma, coarctation of aorta, and mediastinal tumours.
- CNS: learning difficulties and epilepsy.
- Associated with carcinoid tumours.

Key points

- Full antenatal multidisciplinary assessment required.
- Pregnancy is associated with an increase in size and number of neurofibromata.
- Close monitoring of hypertension in pregnancy.
- Tumours in larynx and cervical cord can lead to airway management problems.
- Regional anaesthesia: CT/MRI of spinal cord and head late in pregnancy to evaluate presence of spinal tumours and raised ICP.
- No clear evidence of abnormal response to any neuromuscular-blocking drugs.

Further reading

Hirsch NP. Neurofibromatosis: clinical presentations and anaesthetic implications (Review). *British Journal of Anaesthesia* 2001; 86: 555–564.

Sakai T et al. A parturient with neurofibromatosis type 2: anesthetic and obstetric considerations for delivery. *International Journal of Obstetric Anesthesia* 2005; 14: 332–335.

Noonan's syndrome

Characteristics

- Non-chromosomal syndrome resembling Turner's syndrome affecting both males and females.
- Females have normal fertility.
- Features include short stature, joint contractures, webbed neck which may be fused, chest deformity, and typical facial appearances (flattened face, high arched palate, micrognathia, dental malocclusion).
- Congenital cardiac defects are classically right sided, pulmonary stenosis being most common. Others include ASDs, septal hypertrophy, PDA, aortic stenosis, and cardiomyopathy.
- Clotting derangement with hepatosplenomegaly can occur, but bleeding tendency is usually mild.
- Renal dysfunction, dermatological problems; hearing and visual abnormalities also reported.

Key points

- Early involvement of anaesthetic and obstetric team in pregnancy to formulate plan of care with cardiology and haematology involvement.
- Cardiac defects must be fully quantified and invasive monitoring considered.
- Regional technique desirable but can be difficult to site with unpredictable spread from kyphoscoliosis.
- If bleeding abnormality severe, regional may be contraindicated.
- Potentially difficult intubation.
- Chest deformity can be associated with kyphoscoliosis and respiratory compromise.

Further reading

McBain J et al. Epidural labour analgesia in a parturient with Noonan syndrome: a case report. *Canadian Journal of Anaesthesia* 2006; 53(3): 274–278.

McLure HA, Yentis SM. General anaesthesia for caesarean section in a parturient with Noonan's syndrome. *British Journal of Anaesthesia* 1996; 77: 665–668.

Opiate addiction

Characteristics

- Increased risk to mother and baby with high demand on obstetric anaesthetic services.
- High risk pregnancy with background of smoking and chronic poor health.
- Poor historians with varied ingestion of many different illicit substances either orally or IV.
- Often associated with poor venous access and viral blood-borne disease, i.e. hepatitis and HIV.
- Analgesia can be difficult with high pain scores, and unpredictable, with withdrawal and anxiety symptoms common.
- Women on methadone programmes should be closely monitored and methadone continued during antenatal and perinatal period.
- Partial agonist/antagonist opiates such as buprenorphine are sometimes used in drug cessation programs. They should be continued in the antenatal and perinatal period, however should not be given with high dose pure opiate agonists.

Key points

- Comprehensive anaesthetic review with the help of a substance misuse midwife is very useful to plan obstetric analgesia and venous access.
- Unpredictable response to drugs may highlight use of other substances.
- Opioid pain relief during labour, as part of regional analgesia and after CS is unreliable.

Further reading

Buckley DN, Ibrahim M. Brief review: obstetric care and perioperative analgesic management of the addicted patient. *Canadian Journal of Anaesthesia* 2014; 61: 154–163

Cassidy B, Cyna AM. Challenges that opioid-dependent women present to the obstetric anaesthetist. *Anaesthesia and Intensive Care* 2004; 32: 494–501.

Jones HE et al Buprenorphine treatment of opioid-dependent pregnant women: a comprehensive review. *Addiction*. 2012; 107 Suppl 1: 5–27.

Osteogenesis imperfecta

Characteristics

- Rare, inherited disorder of connective tissue with variable severity.
- Bone fragility (multiple fractures), short stature, blue sclera, and deafness.
- Types I: Is the mildest and women can usually have a normal pregnancy.
- Type III and IV are compatible with an almost normal life expectancy but are associated with multiple fractures, short stature, and severe skeletal deformity.

Key points

- Careful antenatal evaluation of respiratory function and skeletal abnormalities is essential.
- Platelet function should be checked.
- CS is often required.

- Care with positioning and transferring patient, including BP cuff placement to minimize risk of fractures. Laryngoscopy can cause damage to teeth, mandible fractures, or hyperextension of the neck.
- Reports of suxamethonium fasiculations causing fractures.
- Tendency to non-malignant hyperthermia—cooling blankets and fluids should be available.
- Regional anaesthesia can be technically difficult but remains technique of choice.

Further reading

Dinges E et al. Osteogenesis imperfecta: caesarean deliveries in identical twins. *International Journal of Obstetric Anaesthesia* 2015; 24: 64–68.

Yeo ST, Paech MS. Regional anaesthesia for multiple caesarean sections in a parturient with osteogenesis imperfecta. *International Journal of Obstetric Anesthesia* 1999; 8: 284–287.

Paroxysmal nocturnal haemoglobinuria

Characteristics

- Acquired defect of haemopoietic stem cells.
- Deficiency of cell surface proteins that regulate activation of complement.
- Haemolytic anaemia, severe thrombocytopenia, nocturnal haemolysis, haemoglobinuria, intra-abdominal and intracerebral thrombosis, infection, and haemorrhage can occur.
- Aim to maintain Hb >100g/L with folate and iron supplementation. Excess iron may precipitate haemolytic episode.

Key points

- Should be managed in a centre with expertise in the field.
- Issues are related to infection control, drug-induced complement activation, peripartum anticoagulation, and obstetric haemorrhage.
- Due to increased risk of thrombosis, frequently on LMWH.
- Attention to timing of epidural catheter insertion and removal, and the timing of subsequent re-dosing with heparin.
- Maintain normothermia, normovolaemia, and acid–base homeostasis as acidosis may precipitate haemolysis. Attention to asepsis, avoidance of stress responses and use of drugs and fluids that are unlikely to activate complement release.
- Irradiated, leukocyte-depleted RBCs are preferable for transfusion.
- GA may be required due to thrombocytopenia.

Further reading

Paech MJ, Pavy TJ. Management of a parturient with paroxysmal nocturnal haemoglobinuria. *International Journal of Obstetric Anesthesia* 2004; 13: 188–191.

Pemphigus vulgaris

Characteristics

- Immune-mediated bullous dermatosis.
- Autoantibodies against desmoglein 3, a desmosome transmembrane glycoprotein belonging to the cadherin family.
- Blisters due to loss of cell–cell adhesion in the basal and suprabasal layers of the deeper epidermis.

Key points

- Pregnancy may precipitate or aggravate disease.
- High dose prednisolone (60–360mg/day) for several weeks and gradual tapering to a maintenance dose.
- Some immunosuppressive drugs may need to be considered in pregnancy.
- Plasmapheresis has been proposed as a treatment option.
- The method of choice for delivery is vaginal, although local trauma may result in extension and worsening of local erosions.
- Delayed wound healing due to disease process and steroid therapy.
- Skin very fragile; airway instrumentation and adhesive skin dressings problematic.
- Regional anaesthesia has been described.

Further reading

Fainaru O et al. Pemphigus vulgaris in pregnancy: a case report and review of literature. *Human Reproduction* 2000; 15: 1195–1197.

Pneumomediastinum and pneumothorax (Hamman's syndrome)

Characteristics

- Hamman's syndrome consists of substernal pain, subcutaneous and retroperitoneal emphysema, obliteration of cardiac dullness, crunching sounds over the heart synchronous with the heart beat (Hamman's sign), increased mediastinal pressure, dyspnoea, cyanosis, engorged veins and circulatory failure, pneumothorax, and radiographic evidence of air in the mediastinum.
- Occurs during the second stage of labour during prolonged pushing.

Key points

- Surgical emphysema of the neck and face is pathognomonic and a chest X-ray will confirm the diagnosis.
- Conservative management with reassurance, oxygen supplementation, and analgesics.
- The use of nitrous oxide and oxygen mixture is contraindicated.
- Epidural anaesthesia avoids further exertion.
- High subarachnoid block may compromise respiratory function.

- If GA is indicated, facilities for insertion of a chest drain should be immediately available.
- Usually resolve spontaneously within 2 weeks, and the pneumothorax rarely needs to be drained.

Further reading

Miguil M, Chekairi A. Pneumomediastinum and pneumothorax associated with labour. *International Journal of Obstetric Anesthesia* 2004; 13: 117–119.

Polychondritis

Characteristics

- Relapsing polychondritis is characterized by episodic inflammation and degeneration of cartilage and connective tissue involving the upper airway.
- Diagnosis confirmed when 3 of the 6 features are present: bilateral auricular chondritis, non-erosive seronegative inflammatory arthritis, nasal chondritis, ocular inflammation, respiratory tract chondritis, and audiovestibular damage, and histological confirmation.

Key points

- The following can occur: Respiratory failure due to collapse of portions of the tracheobronchial tree; aortic or mitral valvular insufficiency, vasculitis, life-threatening aneurysms; spondyloarthropathy; connective tissue diseases; haematological diseases.
- Multidisciplinary management required—rheumatology, haematology, and obstetric anesthesia.
- Early epidural analgesia to decrease stress is preferable.
- A short second stage of labour with assisted delivery can be helpful.
- GA problems include propensity for gastro-oesophageal reflux; cricoid pressure may be relatively contraindicated if the woman has tracheal tenderness. A smaller tracheal tube may be required.

Further reading

Douglas MJ, Ensworth S. Anaesthetic management of the parturient with relapsing polychondritis. *Canadian Journal of Anaesthesia* 2005; 52: 967–970.

Polycythaemia rubra vera

Characteristics

- Overproduction of phenotypically normal myeloid cell lines independent of physiological stimulus.
- Characterized by: splenomegaly, generalized pruritus, increased blood viscosity, and thrombotic events of the liver, heart, brain, and lungs.
- Phlebotomy and cytotoxic chemotherapy (radioactive phosphorus, chlorambucil, hydroxycarbamide, and interferon alfa) are treatment options.

Key points

- Associated with pregnancy-induced hypertension, spontaneous abortion, maternal venous thromboembolism, and perinatal death.
- Pregnancy is associated with spontaneous control of the disease.
- No specific treatment is usually required except careful observation.
- Maintenance of the Hb level at 120g/L to avoid the thrombotic complications.
- Phlebotomy and low dose empirical acetylsalicylic acid treatment avoid teratogenic effects of cytotoxic agents.
- May be on LMWH, so a careful delivery plan should be in place.
- Regional anaesthesia is not contraindicated.

Further reading

Robinson S et al. The management and outcome of 18 pregnancies in women with polycythemia vera (Review). *Haematologica* 2005; 90: 1477–1483.

Porphyria

Characteristics

- Acute hepatic porphyrias are genetic diseases.
- Acute neurological symptoms, sometimes fatal, triggered by different factors including pregnancy and many anaesthetic drugs.

Key points

- Inhalational agents, opioids, depolarizing and non-depolarizing muscle relaxants, Las, and anticholinergic drugs are considered safe.
- Epidural analgesia has been used for labour analgesia.
- Avoid thiopental and diazepam, although midazolam considered safe.

Further reading

Harris C, Hartsilver E. Anaesthetic management of an obstetric patient with variegate porphyria. *International Journal of Obstetric Anesthesia* 2013; 22: 156–160.
Rigg JD, Petts V. Anaesthesia for the porphyric patient. *Anaesthesia* 1993; 48: 1009–1010.

Pseudoxanthoma elasticum

Characteristics

- Rare inherited disorder, either autosomal dominant and autosomal recessive, of connective tissue, involving skin, Bruch's membrane in eyes, and cardiovascular system.
- Elastic fibres are calcified and fragmented.
- Associated with visual loss from subretinal haemorrhage, gastrointestinal haemorrhage, angina, hypertension, and intermittent claudication.

Key points
- Regional techniques described. Theoretical risk of epidural haematoma but no case reports. Low dose CSE or epidural for caesarean delivery with gradual onset of sympathetic block and lower risk of hypotension.
- Shortening the second stage of labour may decrease retinal bleeding risk secondary to heavy straining.

Further reading
Douglas MJ et al. Anesthesia for the parturient with pseudoxanthoma elasticum. *International Journal of Obstetric Anesthesia* 2003; 12: 45–47.

Quadriplegia with autonomic hyper-reflexia

Characteristics
- Life-threatening complication associated with labour in parturient with spinal cord injury at or above T6, due to uncontrolled reflex sympathetic activity from a stimulus below the level of the lesion.
- Higher incidence of premature labour especially if lesion is above T5.
- Transection of the cord above the level of T10 may result in painless labour.
- The first indication of labour may be development of autonomic hyper-reflexia.
- Control of autonomic hyper-reflexia in labour without an epidural block has been unsatisfactory.

Key points
- Early establishment of regional anaesthesia to interrupt reflex arc and prevent triggering of autonomic hyper-reflexia is essential.
- During regional blockade, the block height cannot be measured easily. Height of block can assessed by eliciting muscle spasms in response to ethyl chloride spray or observing the level at which spastic paraparesis becomes flaccid.
- In high lesions the ability both to vasoconstrict the splanchnic bed (T5–L2) and to increase HR via the cardioaccelerator fibres (T1–4) is lost.
- Caution with vasopressors.
- Graded incremental boluses via epidural with arterial line has advantages.

Further reading
Sharpe EE et al. Anesthetic management of parturients with pre-existing paraplegia or tetraplegia: a case series. *International Journal of Obstetric Anesthesia* 2015; 24: 77–84.
Hambly PR, Martin B. Anaesthesia for chronic spinal cord lesions (Review). *Anaesthesia* 1998; 53: 273–289.

Rheumatoid arthritis

Characteristics

- Rheumatoid arthritis (Still's disease) is a chronic systemic disease with synovitis and extra-articular manifestations.
- Involvement of cervical spine with flexion deformities and atlantoaxial subluxation, temporomandibular and cricoarytenoid joints has implications for the management of the airway.
- New biological treatments have improved outcomes for women with severe disease and have been used successfully in pregnancy.

Key points

- Full assessment of airway and spine with appropriate X-rays if necessary.
- Systemic review for other manifestations of systemic disease.
- Plan for steroid cover for delivery with chronic steroid use.
- Caesarean delivery may be necessary if severe hip problems.
- Spinal or CSE techniques have been used.
- Stiff hips and scoliosis may complicate neuraxial anaesthetic technique and efficacy.
- Careful positioning of the patient is necessary.
- A difficult airway plan is required.

Further reading

Popat MT et al. Awake fibreoptic intubation following failed regional anaesthesia for Caesarean section in a parturient with Still's disease. *European Journal of Anaesthesiology* 2000; **17**: 211–214.

Sarcoidosis

Characteristics

- Systemic disease with non-caseating granulomata in tissues with fibrosis.
- Hilar lymphadenopathy, pleural and alveolar fibrosis, bronchial stenosis, atelectasis, RVF, conduction anomalies, cardiomyopathy, and hypercalcaemia can occur.
- Disease progression/relapse not clearly associated with pregnancy.

Key points

- Pulmonary and cardiac status should be evaluated in the antenatal period.
- Airway involvement may present with difficult intubation.
- May need increased steroid cover due to long-term use.
- Regional anaesthesia preferred if lung involvement is severe.
- Calcium should be maintained at normal level.
- Good postoperative analgesia after CS is essential to avoid pulmonary sequelae.

Further reading

Euliano TY et al. Sarcoidosis in a pregnant woman. *Journal of Clinical Anesthesia* 1997; 9: 78–86.
Freymond N et al. Infiltrative lung diseases in pregnancy. *Clinical Chest Medicine* 2011; 32: 133–146.

Scoliosis/corrected spinal surgery

Characteristics

- Untreated severe scoliosis can lead to death due to cardiorespiratory failure.
- Pregnancy and labour aggravate cardiorespiratory compromise.
- Surgical correction with instrumentation such as Harrington rods, or fusion with bone grafts, is usually performed as an adolescent.

Key points

- Serial assessment of respiratory function is important in severe cases.
- X-ray evaluation of previous surgery, if possible, looking at length of instrumentation and presence of bone grafts is very useful to guide management planning in the antenatal period.
- Neurological examination and documentation before regional technique is essential.
- Complicated epidural placement, with higher risk of failure, inadequate analgesia, and increased risk of dural puncture.
- Continuous spinal anaesthesia for labour and CS has been reported.
- Ultrasound-guided epidural placement has been successful.
- A one-shot spinal anaesthetic may be successful below instrumentation even if an epidural is not.

Further reading

Costello JF, Balki M. Cesarean delivery under ultrasound-guided spinal anesthesia [corrected] in a parturient with poliomyelitis and Harrington instrumentation. *Canadian Journal of Anaesthesia* 2008; 55: 606–11.

Yeo ST, French R. Combined spinal–epidural in the obstetric patient with Harrington rods assisted by ultrasonography. *British Journal of Anaesthesia* 1999; 83: 670–672.

Sickle cell disease

Characteristics

- Autosomal recessive disorder with sickling crises in infancy and chronic organ failure.
- Maternal mortality per pregnancy ranges between 1 and 2% and perinatal mortality remains as high as 5–6% in poorly managed cases.
- May cause preterm delivery, fetal growth retardation, anaemia, acute organ failure, UTIs, thrombosis, and sepsis.

Key points

- Systemic review of multisystem disease.
- Sickling crisis manifests as acute bone pain, chest syndrome, fever, leukocytosis, or abdominal pain.
- Treatment may include exchange transfusions in severe cases.
- Precipitating factors include pain, hypoxia, dehydration, cold, stress, and/or intercurrent infection.
- Intravaginal prostaglandins can precipitate a sickle crisis.
- Keep mother well warm, oxygenated, and hydrated in labour.

- Regional analgesia is preferable in labour for effective pain and stress management.
- Avoid aorto-caval compression to improve circulation.
- Avoid GA if possible.

Further reading

Management of Sickle Cell Disease in Pregnancy. Green–top Guideline No. 61 July 2011. Royal College of Obstetrics and Gynecology. https://www.rcog.org.uk/globalassets/documents/guidelines/gtg_61.pdf

Spina bifida

Characteristics

- Group of conditions that are categorized into spina bifida occulta and spina bifida cystica.
- Occulta is the most common (10–20%) and usually asymptomatic.
- Cystica is failed closure of the neural arch with herniation of the meninges (meningocele) or meninges and neural elements (myelomeningocele).
- Abnormal or tethered spinal cord may occur in spina bifida cystica, including the more unusual thoracic and cervical varieties of spinal dysraphism.

Key points

- Patients with all degrees of spina bifida should be assessed in the antenatal period, so that analgesia and anaesthesia can be planned.
- Radiological imaging of the vertebral level of the conus of the spinal cord helps decision making.
- Spinal bifida occulta involves failure of fusion of only one arch, no external lesion, and the spinal cord and nerves are normal. The patient does not have any neurological sequel. In these cases, spinal or epidural techniques are usually uncomplicated. An epidural should be performed above the level of the lesion and a spinal as low as possible.
- Patients with neurological abnormalities, cutaneous manifestations or involvement of more than one lamina may have a tethered cord and it is necessary to understand the extent of the defect before performing neuraxial anaesthesia. An MRI can be performed in pregnancy.

Further reading

Ali L, Stocks GM. Spina bifida, tethered cord and regional anaesthesia. *Anaesthesia* 2005; 60: 1149–1150.

Sturge–Weber syndrome

Characteristics

- Sturge–Weber syndrome (encephalotrigeminal angiomatosis) is a rare phakomatosis, with facial haemangioma encompassing at least part of cutaneous trigeminal nerve distribution and ipsilateral intracranial venous malformation.

Key points

- The leptomeningeal angiomatosis is predominantly venous. Arterial malformations are rare.
- The venous plexus may be extensive, causing the adjacent cortex to become atrophic.
- Intracranial haemorrhage and focal or generalized convulsions can occur.
- Difficult intubation has been described.
- The effects of pregnancy on this rare disorder remain undefined but of concern.

Further reading

Aziz AS et al. Successful pregnancy, epidural anaesthesia, labour, and delivery in a woman with Sturge-Weber syndrome and previous hemispherectomy. *Journal of Obstetrics and Gynaecology: Canada* 2013; 35: 917–919.

Tadrous R et al. Anaesthesia for Caesarian section in a patient with Sturge-Weber syndrome following acute neurological deterioration. *International Journal of Obstetrics and Anesthesia* 2011; 20: 259–262.

Subarachnoid haemorrhage

Characteristics

- Incidence of subarachnoid haemorrhage from aneurysms and AVMs in pregnancy is between 0.01 and 0.05%.
- Negative angiography does not exclude aneurysm with absolute certainty.

Key points

- History of clipped aneurysm does not preclude vaginal delivery, although a shortened second stage with epidural analgesia may be recommended.
- Assessment of neurological function should be carried out in the antenatal period with a neurological opinion.
- Spinal or epidural anaesthesia not contraindicated with a stable history.
- Following a recent bleed, epidural analgesia, because of fluid in lumbar extradural space, may increase ICP.
- Dural puncture and CSF leak may dislodge the clot and cause further bleeding.
- Invasive arterial pressure monitoring is recommended in recent unstable cases.

Further reading

Bateman BT et al. Peripartum subarachnoid hemorrhage: nationwide data and institutional experience. *Anesthesiology* 2012; 116: 324–333.

Subdural haematoma

Characteristics

- Cranial subdural haematomas may present acutely, subacutely or chronically, with headache, altered level of consciousness, seizures, or psychiatric symptoms.
- Subdural haematoma following dural puncture is rare and may be cranial or spinal. Persistent headache and deterioration of neurological status should elicit suspicion.

Key points

- Cause of subdural haematoma following dural puncture is low CSF pressure leading to traction and tearing of thin-walled meningeal blood vessels.
- An unusual or persistent presentation of PHPH should raise suspicion and requires neurological imaging.
- The management of subdural haematoma is either conservative, i.e. clinical observation with possible ICP monitoring, or surgery.
- Haematomas <5mm often resolve spontaneously.

Further reading

Cuypers V et al. Intracranial subdural haematoma following neuraxial anaesthesia in the obstetric population: a literature review with analysis of 56 reported cases. *International Journal of Obstetrics and Anesthesia* 2016; 25: 58–65.

Superior vena cava obstruction

Characteristics

- Rare and usually complicates tumours in the mediastinum.
- Affects venous drainage of the airway, leading to shortness of breath, stridor, and cough.

Key points

- Spinal anaesthesia with rapid sympathectomy and haemodynamic decompensation can be dangerous due to combined obstructed VR from the upper extremities, and obstruction from the lower extremities by the gravid uterus.
- Epidural anaesthesia is preferred with titration of vasopressors and IV fluids.
- The lateral position to reduce aortocaval compression is essential.
- GA with rapid sequence induction and femoral–femoral access to institute immediate cardiopulmonary bypass if intubation or ventilation were not possible has been described.
- IV drugs and fluids should be administered through an IV cannula in the lower limb.
- Intra-arterial monitoring is essential.
- CVP monitoring is unreliable.

Further reading

Buvanendran A et al. Perioperative management with epidural anesthesia for a parturient with superior vena caval obstruction. *Anesthesia and Analgesia* 2004; 98: 1160–1163.

Suxamethonium apnoea

Characteristics

- Prolonged neuromuscular blockade caused by altered enzymatic activity of plasma cholinesterase.
- May be inherited or acquired.
- Pregnancy itself is associated with reduced plasma cholinesterase activity, although not considered clinically relevant.

- Cholinesterase activity is investigated by measurement of the enzyme concentration and dibucaine number. However, this test may be unreliable in pregnancy due to its associated reduced cholinesterase level.

Key points

- A patient with a diagnosis of suxamethonium apnoea should be seen in the antenatal period, airway assessed and a clear plan made.
- Women who present after CS with suxamethonim apnoea should be followed up and fully investigated.
- Strategies used include giving suxamethonium and anticipating a prolonged period of postoperative ventilation, or administration of rocuronium 0.9mg/kg, which has been shown to have a similar onset time to suxamethonium. Sugammadex must be available for immediate reversal in the event of failed intubation.
- Intubation using alfentanil in varying doses and propofol without neuromuscular-blocking drugs has also been described.

Further reading

Davies P, Landy M. Suxamethonium and mivacurium sensitivity from pregnancy-induced plasma cholinesterase deficiency. *Anaesthesia* 1998; 53: 1109–1101.

Evans RT, Wroe JM. Plasma cholinesterase changes during pregnancy. Their interpretation as a cause of suxamethonium-induced apnoea. *Anaesthesia* 1980; 35: 651–654.

Alexander R, Fardell S. Use of remifentanil for tracheal intubation for Caesarean section in a patient with suxamethonium apnoea. *Anaesthesia* 2005; 60: 1036–1038.

Syringomyelia

Characteristics

- Progressive degenerative disease with cystic cavities within the spinal cord that cause severe neurological deficits.
- The clinical diagnosis is based on the triad: (1) loss of pain and temperature sensations with preservation of touch sensation over the neck, shoulders and arms; (2) amyotrophy; and (3) thoracic scoliosis.

Key points

- There is an overlap with Chiari malformations.
- Pre-anaesthetic assessment to document neurological deficit and assess respiratory function.
- Autonomic dysfunction if present necessitates invasive arterial monitoring and attention to normothermia.
- Caution with neuromuscular-blocking agents. Suxamethonium may cause hyperkalaemia.
- Syringobulbia, the extension of a syrinx into the brainstem, increases the risk of aspiration.
- Foramen magnum abnormalities may cause craniospinal pressure dissociation. A relatively higher CSF pressure in the head and lower

pressure in the spine contraindicates the use of subarachnoid anaesthesia.
• Epidural anaesthesia may be considered for patients with anticipated difficult intubation, but accidental dural puncture may be hazardous.

Further reading

Margarido C et al. Epidural anesthesia for Caesarian delivery in a patient with post-traumatic cervical syringomyelia. *Canadian Journal of Anaesthesia* 2011; 58: 764–768.
Garvey GP et al. Anesthetic and obstetric management of syringomyelia during labour and delivery: a case series and systematic review. *Anesthesia and Analgesia* 2017; 125: 913–924.

Systemic lupus erythematosus

Characteristics

• Multisystem inflammatory disorder characterised by autoantibody production and immune-mediated tissue injury.
• Clinical features depend on the severity of damage to organ systems such as musculoskeletal, renal, haematological, neurological, cardiac, and respiratory.

Key points

• Multidisiplinary approach with rheumatologist, haematologist, obstetrician, neonatologist, and anaesthetist is important.
• Increased incidence of fetal loss, hypertension, and pre-eclampsia.
• Associated with antiphospholipid syndrome and thrombosis, may need anticoagulation with LMWH. Lupus anticoagulant may cause isolated increase in APTT, not associated with increase bleeding risk.
• Management includes all types of anaesthesia, depending on severity of the organ involvement.
• Patients usually on aspirin and LMWH. An antenatal plan is required for timing of regional analgesia.
• The patients may be on long term steroids which may require supplementation in labour and CS.
• Ulcers on nasal and oral mucous membranes may increase trauma with tracheal intubation.
• Raynaud's phenomena complicates placement of arterial lines.
• Peripheral neuropathies or fixed neurological deficits should be documented before regional anaesthesia.
• Antibiotic prophylaxis for valvular lesions and prosthetic joints.

Further reading

Peart E, Clowse ME. Systemic lupus erythematosus and pregnancy outcomes: an update and review of the literature. *Current Opinion in Rheumatology* 2014; 26: 118–123.
Lateef A, Petri M. Managing lupus patients during pregnancy. *Best Practice and Research in Clinical Rheumatology* 2013; 27: 435–447.
Davies SR. Systemic lupus erythematosus and the obstetric patient—implications for the anaesthetist. *Canadian Journal of Anaesthesia* 1991; 38: 790–795.

Systemic sclerosis

Characteristics

- Multisystem disease of unknown aetiology, causing overproduction and growth of collagen, widespread vascular damage, microvascular obliteration, and Raynaud's phenomenon.

Key points

- Careful assessment of multisystemic condition.
- Review of cardiac function and exclusion of pulmonary hypertension, with assessment of airway and peripheral veins.
- Difficult venous access due to thickened skin, flexion contractures impair indirect BP measurement. Direct arterial cannulation may cause vasospasm and distal necrosis.
- Microsomia, nasal and oral telangiectasiae, oesophageal dysmotility and sphincter incompetence, pulmonary fibrosis, pulmonary hypertension, myocardial fibrosis, pericarditis, arrhythmia,s and conduction defects may occur.
- Gradual regional technique may reduce hypotension.
- May get prolonged sensory and motor blockade.
- Careful positioning—padding to avoid pressure necrosis, wrapping of limbs, warmth to avoid vasoconstriction.
- Avoid prolonged application of a pulse oximeter probe to one digit.

Further reading

Lidar M, Langevitz P. Pregnancy issues in scleroderma. *Autoimmunity Reviews* 2012; 11: A515–519.
Bailey AR et al. Spinal anaesthesia for Caesarean section in a patient with systemic sclerosis. *Anaesthesia* 1999; 54: 355–358.

Takayasu's disease

Characteristics

- Pulseless disease-occlusive thromboaortopathy is a rare inflammatory panendarteritis causing thrombosis and occlusion of systemic and pulmonary arteries.
- Cerebrovascular ischaemia occurs in one-third of patients, making maintenance of cerebral blood flow vital.
- Complications include hypertension, heart failure, and peripartum cerebral haemorrhage.

Key points

- Regional anaesthesia is a safe technique especially in cerebrovascular disease, which mandates monitoring for cerebral ischaemia.
- When regional anaesthesia is prohibited, short-acting opioid and relaxant drugs allow rapid awakening and easy assessment of cerebral function. The use of processed EEG monitoring, whilst not absolutely sensitive or specific, may be better than no monitor when the patient is asleep.

Further reading

Ioscovich A et al. Peripartum anesthetic management of patients with Takayasu's arteritis: case series and review. *International Journal of Obstetric Anesthesia* 2008; 17: 358–364.

Thalassaemia

Characteristics

- Inherited disorder of Hb synthesis, excess α chains precipitate in RBC precursors.
- Defective erythroid precursor maturation and shortened red cell survival.
- Hypertrophy of the bone marrow; skull and long bone changes and hepatosplenomegaly all result.
- Iron overload from transfusions damages myocardium, liver, and endocrine glands.
- Thalassaemia trait can cause resistant anaemia requiring blood transfusion in pregnancy.

Key points

- Hypertransfusion therapy corrects anaemia and suppresses hyperactive erthryopoiesis.
- Hb maintained above 80g/L during gestation or above this level if symptomatic.
- Leukocyte-depleted RBC concentrate prevents febrile non-haemolytic transfusion reactions, cytomegalovirus infections, and reduces immunomodulatory effect of transfusions.
- Regular folic acid supplementation.
- Intraoperative cell salvage is useful.
- Regional anaesthesia is contraindicated in patients with hypersplenic crises and thrombocytopenia.
- Severe maxillofacial deformities may present difficult airway problems.
- Osteoporosis, osteopenia, and scoliosis are common.

Further reading

Management of Beta Thalassaemia in Pregnancy. Green-top Guideline No. 66 March 2014. Royal College of Obstetrics and gynecology. https://www.rcog.org.uk/globalassets/documents/guidelines/gtg_66_thalassaemia.pdf

Leung TY, Lao TT. Thalassaemia in pregnancy. Best Practice & Research. Clinical Obstetrics & Gynaecology 2012; 26: 37–51.

Thrombotic thrombocytopenia purpura (TTP)

Characteristics

- TTP is a severe multisystem disorder affecting the microcirculatimn of many organ systems, with significant maternal and fetal morbidity.
- Comprises classic pentad of fever, severe thrombocytopenia, microangiopathic anaemia, neurological symptoms or signs, and renal failure.
- The presenting features have significant overlap with severe PET and HELLP syndrome and can be a diagnostic dilemma.
- ADAMTS13 inhibitor test <10% activity is diagnostic but is only available in specialist centres.
- A raised Troponin level is indicative of significant cardiac ischemia.
- Pregnancy can be an initiating event for acute TTP or produce a high risk of relapse if previously diagnosed.

Key points

- Close liaison with a specialist haemoatologist is essential.
- Treatment options include low dose aspirin, anticoagulation with LMWH, immunosuppression, and/or repeated plasma exchange.
- In severe cases plasma exchange within hours can be lifesaving and should be performed if ADAMTS13 test results are awaited.
- Analgesia/anaesthetic technique for delivery dictated by platelet count and anticoagulation therapy.
- High dependency care or ICU care is nearly always required.

Further reading

Kato R et al. ADAMTS13 deficiency, an important cause of thrombocytopenia during pregnancy. *International Journal of Obstetric Anesthesia* 2009; 18: 73–77.

Scully M et al. Thrombotic thrombocytopenic purpura and pregnancy: presentation, management, and subsequent pregnancy outcomes. *Blood* 2014; 124:211–219.

Urticaria pigmentosa

Characteristics

- Cutaneous manifestation of mastocytosis, proliferation, and accumulation of mast cells in various organs.
- Precipitants include trauma or mechanical irritation to the skin, psychological stress, extremes of temperature, spicy foods, alcohol, histamine-releasing drugs, and snake and bee venom.
- Symptoms include weakness, fatigue, urticaria, grand mal seizures, anaphylaxis, and/or cardiovascular collapse.

Key points

- Full assessment of drug-related problems with plan for labour analgesia.
- Premedication with H_1 and H_2 antihistamine agents and benzodiazepine to reduce anxiety.
- Close collaboration with obstetric team for the timely administration of prophylactic medications.
- Avoid histamine-releasing drugs.
- Effective analgesia to decrease anxiety—regional analgesia is recommended.
- Core temperature should be maintained.
- Repositioning should be kept to a minimum.
- If mast cell degranulation is suspected, corticosteroids, antihistamine drugs, and adrenaline should be used.
- Resuscitation equipment should be available for the duration of labour, delivery, and postpartum period to treat unanticipated hypotension and shock.

Further reading

Villeneuve V et al. Anesthetic management of a labouring parturient with urticaria pigmentosa. *Canadian Journal of Anaesthesia* 2006; 53: 380–384.

Varicella

Characteristics

- Varicella zoster virus causes a primary contagious and usually benign illness commonly known as varicella or chickenpox.
- Virus can lie dormant in the dorsal root ganglia and may be reactivated to cause localized cutaneous eruptions called 'herpes zoster' or 'shingles'.

Key points

- Pregnant women who are not immune to varicella can develop severe disease complicated by fetal abnormalities, pneumonia, and cerebral infection.
- Secondary bacterial superinfection, acute cerebellar ataxia, encephalitis, aseptic meningitis, and Guillain–Barré syndrome have been reported.
- Possibility of introducing the virus into the CNS during the placement of the regional block, resulting in meningitis or encephalitis, especially during the primary infection when viraemia is present.
- GA is the anaesthetic of choice if there are active or infected lesions on the skin at the site for placement of a spinal or epidural block.
- Consider use of IV aciclovir for severe infection.

Further reading

Janardhan AL et al. Anesthetic management of a parturient with varicella presenting for cesarean delivery. *International Journal of Obstetric Anesthesia* 2016; 28: 92–94.

Ventriculo-peritoneal shunts

Characteristics

- An artificial shunt to drain CSF into the peritoneum with various configurations, usually for the management of hydrocephalus.

Key points

- Headaches and other symptoms of shunt failure, i.e. vomiting, reduced level of consciousness, seizures, need MRI to evaluate ventricular dilatation and urgent neurological review.
- Mode of delivery is usually determined by obstetric reasons.
- A shortened second stage of labour may be desirable.
- Risk of intra-abdominal infection and adhesion formation around the distal end of the ventriculo-peritoneal shunt catheter after CS.
- Meticulous aseptic technique is essential for regional anaesthesia, and prophylactic antibiotics are generally recommended.
- There is a theoretical possibility of spinal anaesthetic leaking into the shunt with ineffective anaesthesia with a lumboperitoneal configuration.

Further reading

Schiza S et al. Management of pregnancy and delivery of a patient with malfunctioning ventriculoperitoneal shunt. *Journal of Obstetric Gynaecology* 2012; 32: 6–9.

Von Hippel–Lindau disease

Characteristics

- Rare autosomal dominant disease, causing diffuse haemangioblastomas of the CNS, mostly cerebellum, retina, and viscera.
- Associated with renal cell carcinoma, pancreatic cyst, and tumours, and phaeochromocytoma.

Key points

- Pregnancy can increase the size of haemangioblastomas with increased risk to mother and fetus.
- Review of medical notes and MRI scans essential with full antenatal MDT review.
- Epidural anaesthesia has been used successfully without neurological sequelae. The position of haemangioblastomas should be known.
- The choice of anaesthesia technique should be made after careful evaluation of the extent of the patient's disease.

Further reading

Hayden MG et al. Von Hippel-Lindau disease in pregnancy: a brief review. *Journal of Clinical Neuroscience* 2009; 16: 611–613.

Wegener's granulomatosis

Characteristics

- Wegner's granulomatosis is an uncommon systemic disease characterized by a necrotizing granulomatous vasculitis of the upper and lower respiratory tracts, with or without glomerulonephritis and disseminated small vessel vasculitis.

Key points

- Pulmonary haemorrhage is life threatening.
- Pre-eclampsia and prematurity associated with corticosteroids or prior renal diseases are the most serious complications.
- Head and neck manifestations of the disease may present a difficult airway problem.

Further reading

Auzary C et al. Pregnancy in patients with Wegener's granulomatosis: report of five cases in three women (Review). *Annals of the Rheumatic Diseases* 2000; 59: 800–804.

Wolff–Parkinson–White (WPW) syndrome

Characteristics

- Pre-excitation syndrome where activation of an accessory atrioventricular conduction pathway leads to early and rapid ventricular contractions.
- Short PR interval, anomalous QRS complexes, and a delta wave may be seen.
- Paroxysmal supraventricular tachycardias are common.

Key points

- Haemodynamic, hormonal, and emotional changes of pregnancy predispose to arrhythmias.
- The tachycardia in pregnancy along with an underlying WPW syndrome may induce unidirectional block in the re-entrant circuit, resulting in atrioventricular tachycardias.
- Tachyarrhythmias causing haemodynamic changes require immediate treatment.
- Vagal stimulation, sedation, propranolol, digoxin, calcium antagonists, and adenosine have been used.
- Adenosine is preferred due to its very short half-life.
- Electrical cardioversion during pregnancy has also been successful.

Further reading

Robinson JE et al. Familial hypokalemic periodic paralysis and Wolff–Parkinson–White syndrome in pregnancy. *Canadian Journal of Anaesthesia* 2000; 47: 160–164.

Index

Note: Tables, figures, and boxes are indicated by *t*, *f*, and *b* following the page number